T0309196

Handbook of Cardiac Electrophysiology

Handbook of Cardiac Electrophysiology

Second Edition

Edited by

Andrea Natale

Oussama M. Wazni

Kalyanam Shivkumar

Francis E. Marchlinski

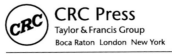

CRC Press
Taylor & Francis Group
Boca Raton London New York

CRC Press is an imprint of the
Taylor & Francis Group, an **informa** business

CRC Press
Taylor & Francis Group
6000 Broken Sound Parkway NW, Suite 300
Boca Raton, FL 33487-2742

© 2020 by Taylor & Francis Group, LLC
CRC Press is an imprint of Taylor & Francis Group, an Informa business

No claim to original U.S. Government works

International Standard Book Number-13: 978-1-4822-2439-9 (Hardback)

Visit the Taylor & Francis Web site at
http://www.taylorandfrancis.com

and the CRC Press Web site at
http://www.crcpress.com

CONTENTS

SECTION I
Basic EP Laboratory Setup and Equipment

SECTION II
Bradyarrhythmia

SECTION III
Supraventricular Tachyarrhythmia

SECTION IV
Ventricular Tachyarrhythmia

SECTION V
Syncope

SECTION VI
Device Procedures

SECTION VII
Performing Basic EP Studies

SECTION VIII
Catheter Ablation Techniques

PREFACE

This issue of the *Handbook of Electrophysiology* is a quick reference for EP fellows, allied health professionals, and electrophysiologists on the state-of-the-art management of rhythm disorders including discussions on how to set up an arrhythmia lab, different aspects of the catheter ablation procedure for atrial and ventricular arrhythmia, techniques of device implantation and lead extraction, and diagnostic testing and management of syncope. The current edition also addresses the different aspects of ECG-based origin of atrial flutter, indications for epicardial access, and ECG characteristics of normal heart PVCs. Lastly, the handbook details on the indications, techniques, and benefits of left atrial appendage closure.

It was our privilege to have a team of world-renowned experts contributing the latest information on the entire spectrum of EP knowledge in this handbook. We are confident that this handbook will not only be relevant to all clinicians and allied health professionals involved in the management of cardiac arrhythmia, but also will provide the readers an appreciation of the complexity of procedures that are performed every day in the electrophysiology labs.

ACKNOWLEDGMENTS

I wish to thank all the authors and staff that worked very hard to make this book possible. Additionally, I would like to thank my dearest wife Marina and daughters (Veronica and Eleanora) for supporting me in all my professional endeavors.

Dr. Andrea Natale

EDITORS

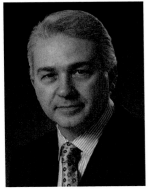

Dr. Andrea Natale is the Executive Medical Director of Texas Cardiac Arrhythmia Institute at St. David's Medical Center, Austin, Texas, and the EP National Medical Director for HCA Healthcare. A dedicated researcher and pioneer, Dr. Natale focuses on innovative advances in the treatment of atrial and ventricular arrhythmia. He perfected a circumferential ultrasound pulmonary vein-ablation system to correct atrial fibrillation and performed the procedure on the world's first five patients. He also developed some of the current catheter-based cures for atrial fibrillation, and was the first cardiac electrophysiologist in the nation to perform percutaneous epicardial radiofrequency ablation, which is a treatment for people who fail conventional ablation.

A very prolific author and speaker, he is the Editor-in-Chief of *JICE* and remains a leader of *JAFIB*, President of Venice Arrhythmia, and Director of several courses and summits. EP Live is one of the many pioneering accomplishments of Dr. Natale's passionate mission to train and educate: every two years, a 2-day intensive educational meeting is conducted under his direct guidance and supervision, where health care providers benefit from first-hand information on the recent advancements in arrhythmia treatment and research as well as get the opportunity to interact with authorities in electrophysiology. His EP Live concept was so well received by the electrophysiologists around the world that it is now extended to several countries outside USA, i.e., EPLATAM (Latin America), EP Live Europe, EP Live Dubai, and EP Live India.

Dr. Natale's greatest reward is restoring his patients to a life free of cardiac arrhythmia. In his own words, "I give all of myself to make sure my patient's heart does what it's supposed to do."

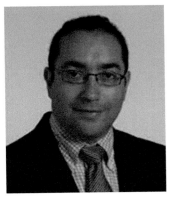

Dr. Oussama M. Wazni is currently the Section Head of Electrophysiology at the Cleveland Clinic. He specializes in electrophysiology with special interest in atrial fibrillation, ventricular tachycardia, and complex device management.

Dr. Wazni is principal investigator in several ongoing research studies related to device management, atrial fibrillation and ventricular tachycardia ablation, genetics of ventricular tachycardia, and long-term follow-up after AF ablation.

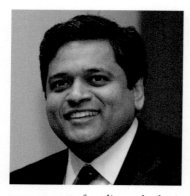

Dr. Kalyanam Shivkumar is a physician scientist who serves as the director of the UCLA Cardiac Arrhythmia Center & EP Programs (since its establishment in 2002). He is a graduate of the UCLA STAR Program (class of 2000) and his field of specialization is interventional cardiac electrophysiology. He leads a large group at UCLA (comprising a diverse group of fifteen faculty members, several trainees, and sixty staff + allied health professionals) involved in clinical care, teaching, research, and biomedical innovation. The team provides state of the art clinical care, has developed several innovative therapies (e.g., epicardial ablation, neuromodulation) for the non-pharmacological management of cardiac arrhythmias and other cardiac interventions. The team has a major focus on mechanistic research on the neural control of the mammalian heart. Dr. Shivkumar also serves as the director and chief of the UCLA Cardiovascular Interventional Programs. Dr. Shivkumar's research work relates to mechanisms of cardiac arrhythmias in humans especially the role of the autonomic nervous system and his research work transcends the perspective of a single organ and has implications for neurovisceral sciences in general. The UCLA Neurocardiology Research Program of Excellence was established by him as the specialized research arm of the Arrhythmia Center in 2014. Dr. Shivkumar and his colleagues are actively involved in human mechanistic studies and development of new intellectual property and medical technology for cardiovascular therapeutics. His IP has been incorporated into medical devices that are now FDA approved and in clinical use. He serves as an editor for several journals in cardiology and cardiac electrophysiology, and is a peer reviewer for several basic science and clinical journals. He also serves as a peer reviewer for the NIH in evaluating cardiac arrhythmia and neuroscience research. His research has been supported by grants from the American Heart Association, the Doris Duke Foundation, private donors, and from the NIH (continuously since 2006). Currently Dr. Shivkumar oversees a 15-university NIH consortium on neural control of the heart. Dr. Shivkumar has mentored several STAR awardees and has received several teaching awards. He has been appointed to serve on the board of examiners for Clinical Cardiac Electrophysiology Section of the ABIM (American Board of Internal Medicine). He has been elected to the membership of the American Society of Clinical Investigation (ASCI) and serves as the institutional representative of UCLA for the ASCI. He was elected as an honorary Fellow of the Royal College of Physicians (London) in 2016 and President of the ISAN (International Society of Autonomic Neuroscience) in 2019.

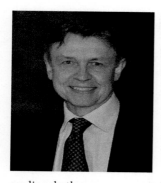

Dr. Francis E. Marchlinski is the Richard T and Angela Clark President's Distinguished Professor of Medicine at the Perelman School of Medicine at the University of Pennsylvania, the Director of Electrophysiology, University of Pennsylvania Health Care System, and the Director of the Electrophysiology Laboratory at the Hospital of the University of Pennsylvania. Dr. Marchlinski is a graduate of the University of Pennsylvania Medical School. He completed his postdoctoral internal medicine residency and cardiology/electrophysiology fellowship training at the Hospital of the University of Pennsylvania. For over thirty years Dr. Marchlinski has remained at the cutting edge of cardiac rhythm management. He has authored or co-authored over 450 original scientific articles and over 200 book chapters/reviews/editorials on a variety of topics in cardiac electrophysiology. His EP team at Penn has worked to successfully improve localizing and ablation techniques for the treatment of both atrial fibrillation and ventricular tachycardia and optimize device therapy for treating heart failure and preventing sudden cardiac death. Dr. Marchlinski has served on the International Heart Rhythm Society Committee to establish guidelines for the treatment of atrial fibrillation and ventricular tachycardia using catheter ablation techniques. He has been the recipient of the Luigi Mastroianni Clinical Innovator Award, the Venice Arrhythmia Distinguished Scientist Award and the ACTS Distinguished Investigator Award—Career Achievement—Translation from Early Clinical Use to Applicability for Widespread Clinical Practice. Dr. Marchlinski is on the editorial board of *Circulation, Arrhythmias and Electrophysiology, American Journal of Cardiology, Heart Rhythm Journal, Journal of Cardiovascular Electrophysiology, Journal of Interventional Cardiac Electrophysiology*, and *JACC-Electrophysiology* and is the Arrhythmia Section Editor for *Journal of the American College of Cardiology*. Dr. Marchlinski has organized and directed multiple fellowship training courses and regional and International EP symposia and has received numerous teaching awards at the University of Pennsylvania.

CONTRIBUTORS

Amin Al-Ahmad
Department of Electrophysiology
Texas Cardiac Arrhythmia Institute
Austin, Texas

Zaid Aziz
Center for Arrhythmia Care
Pritzker School of Medicine
The University of Chicago Medicine
Chicago, Illinois

Shiv Bagga
Department of Electrophysiology
St. Vincent's Medical Center
Indianapolis, Indiana

Rong Bai
Beijing Anzhen Hospital
Capital Medical University
Beijing, China

Mandeep Bhargava
Department of Electrophysiology
Cleveland Clinic
Cleveland, Ohio

Noel G. Boyle
Ronald Reagan UCLA Medical Center
Internal Medicine and Cardiology
UCLA Cardiac Arrhythmia Center
David Geffen School of Medicine at UCLA
Los Angeles, California

Jason S. Bradfield
UCLA Cardiac Arrhythmia Center
David Geffen School of Medicine at UCLA
Los Angeles, California

Michael P. Brunner
Department of Cardiology
Cardiovascular Medicine
Cleveland Clinic
Cleveland, Ohio

J. David Burkhardt
Department of Electrophysiology
Texas Cardiac Arrhythmia Institute
Austin, Texas

Daniel Cantillon
Cardiac Electrophysiology and Pacemaker
  Laboratories
Heart and Vascular Institute
Cleveland Clinic
Cleveland, Ohio

Mina K. Chung
Section of Cardiac Pacing and
  Electrophysiology
Department of Cardiovascular Medicine
Heart and Vascular Institute
and
Department of Cardiovascular and
  Metabolic Sciences
Lerner Research Institute
and
Cleveland Clinic Lerner College of
  Medicine
Case Western Reserve University
Cleveland, Ohio

Roy Chung
Section of Cardiac Electrophysiology and
  Pacing
Cleveland Clinic Heart and Vascular
  Institute
Cleveland, Ohio

Luigi Di Biase
Internal Medicine (Cardiology)
Albert Einstein College of Medicine
Montefiore Hospital
New York City, New York

Duc H. Do
Department of Cardiology
UCLA Cardiac Arrhythmia Center
David Geffen School of Medicine at UCLA
Los Angeles, California

Thomas Dresing
Cardiac Electrophysiology and Pacemaker
  Laboratories
Heart and Vascular Institute
Cleveland Clinic
Cleveland, Ohio

Andres Enriquez
Section of Cardiac Electrophysiology
Hospital of the University of Pennsylvania
Philadelphia, Pennsylvania

David S. Frankel
Electrophysiology Section
Cardiovascular Division
Perelman School of Medicine at the
    University of Pennsylvania
Philadelphia, Pennsylvania

Fermin Garcia
Section of Cardiac Electrophysiology
Hospital of the University of Pennsylvania
Philadelphia, Pennsylvania

Carola Gianni
Department of Electrophysiology
Texas Cardiac Arrhythmia Institute
Austin, Texas

Jonathan R. Hoffman
Department of Electrophysiology
Central Georgia Heart Center
Macon, Georgia

Rodney P. Horton
Department of Electrophysiology
Texas Cardiac Arrhythmia Institute
Austin, Texas

Ayman A. Hussein
Section of Cardiac Pacing and
    Electrophysiology
Heart and Vascular Institute
Cleveland Clinic
Cleveland, Ohio

Matthew C. Hyman
Department of Electrophysiology
University of Pennsylvania
Philadelphia, Pennsylvania

Amer Kadri
Department of Electrophysiology
Mercy Medical Center
Canton, Ohio

Ching Chi Keong
Department of Cardiology
National Heart Centre Singapore
Duke-NUS Graduate Medical School
Singapore

Houman Khakpour
UCLA Cardiac Arrhythmia Center
David Geffen School of Medicine at UCLA
Los Angeles, California

Decebal Gabriel Laţcu
Service de Cardiologie
Centre Hospitalier Princesse Grace
La Colle, Monaco

Jackson J. Liang
Department of Internal Medicine
    (Cardiology)
University of Michigan
Ann Arbor, Michigan

and

Hospital of the University of Pennsylvania
Philadelphia, Pennsylvania

John Lopez
Cardiac Electrophysiology and Pacemaker
    Laboratories
Heart and Vascular Institute
Cleveland Clinic
Cleveland, Ohio

Francis E. Marchlinski
Cardiology (Electrophysiology)
Perelman School of Medicine
University of Pennsylvania
Philadelphia, Pennsylvania

Kenneth Mayuga
Cardiac Electrophysiology and Pacemaker
    Laboratories
Heart and Vascular Institute
Cleveland Clinic
Cleveland, Ohio

Sanghamitra Mohanty
Department of Electrophysiology
Texas Cardiac Arrhythmia Institute
Austin, Texas

Daniele Muser
Electrophysiology Section
Cardiovascular Division
Hospital of the University of Pennsylvania
Philadelphia, Pennsylvania

Andrea Natale
Texas Cardiac Arrhythmia Institute
St. David's Medical Center
and
Department of Medicine
Dell Medical School
University of Texas at Austin
Austin, Texas

and

HCA National Medical Director
Cardiac Electrophysiology
and
Department of Medicine
Case Western Reserve University
Cleveland, Ohio

and

Interventional Electrophysiology
SCRIPPS Green Hospital
San Diego, California

Subramanya Prasad
Department of Electrophysiology
The Cleveland Clinic Foundation
Cleveland, Ohio

Kushwin Rajamani
Department of Electrophysiology
Cleveland Clinic
Cleveland, Ohio

Domenico G. Della Rocca
Department of Electrophysiology
Texas Cardiac Arrhythmia Institute
Austin, Texas

Jorge Romero
Department of Cardiology Arrhythmia
   Services
Montefiore Medical Center
New York City, New York

Walid Saliba
Department of Electrophysiology
Cleveland Clinic
Cleveland, Ohio

Mohamed Salim
Department of Electrophysiology
The Aga Khan Hospital Mombasa (AKHM)
Mombasa, Kenya

Javier E. Sanchez
Department of Electrophysiology
Texas Cardiac Arrhythmia Institute
Austin, Texas

Pasquale Santangeli
Electrophysiology Section
Cardiovascular Division
Hospital of the University of Pennsylvania
Philadelphia, Pennsylvania

Nadir Saoudi
Service de Cardiologie
Centre Hospitalier Princesse Grace
La Colle, Monaco

Robert D. Schaller
Department of Cardiac Electrophysiology
Hospital of the University of Pennsylvania
Philadelphia, Pennsylvania

Robert Schweikert
Department of Electrophysiology
Cleveland Clinic Akron General
Cleveland, Ohio

Kalyanam Shivkumar
Medicine (Cardiology), Radiology &
   Bioengineering
UCLA Cardiac Arrhythmia Center & EP
   Programs
UCLA Interventional CV Programs &
   Cardiac Catheterization Laboratories
David Geffen School of Medicine & UCLA
   Health System
Los Angeles, California

Gregory E. Supple
Department of Electrophysiology
University of Pennsylvania School of
   Medicine
Philadelphia, Pennsylvania

Patrick Tchou
Cardiac Electrophysiology and Pacemaker
   Laboratories
Heart and Vascular Institute
Cleveland Clinic
Cleveland, Ohio

Chintan Trivedi
Department of Electrophysiology
Texas Cardiac Arrhythmia Institute
Austin, Texas

Roderick Tung
Center for Arrhythmia Care
Pritzker School of Medicine
The University of Chicago Medicine
Chicago, Illinois

Marmar Vaseghi
UCLA Cardiac Arrhythmia Center
David Geffen School of Medicine at UCLA
Los Angeles, California

Oussama M. Wazni
Cardiac Electrophysiology and Pacemaker
    Laboratories
Heart and Vascular Institute
Cleveland Clinic
Cleveland, Ohio

Bruce L. Wilkoff
Department of Electrophysiology
Cleveland Clinic Lerner College of
    Medicine
Case Western Reserve University
Cleveland, Ohio

BASIC EP LABORATORY SETUP AND EQUIPMENT

DEVICE LAB SET-UP

John Lopez and Mina K. Chung

CONTENTS

The modern EP Laboratory caters to two general categories of diagnostic and interventional procedures. They can be classified as either ablation or device related. Ablation procedures are more involved and may require more equipment and time than device-related procedures. It is the purpose of Section II to encompass the whole spectrum when it comes to preparing the environment so as it is conducive to any of these general categories of procedures.

EP LAB

The EP Lab should be constructed following the Facility Guidelines Institute (FGI) (http://www.fgiguidelines.org/). The typical EP laboratory design has used the Cath Lab design settings for years but there needs to be a separate distinction due to the fact that the EP Laboratory houses more equipment and is sensitive to a different need that concentrates in the matter of interpreting clean electrical signals as opposed to pressures and hemodynamics.[1] The environment has also evolved to be able to accommodate emergent responses that may require cardiothoracic surgical interventions and general anesthesia services, which make it necessary for the environment to have adequate heat, ventilation, and air conditioning (HVAC) standards appropriate for operating room procedures.

It is ideal for the room to be considered as a wet location, which mandates the use of an isolated power system with line isolation monitoring.[2] This panel's purpose is to ensure that electrocution hazards are kept at a very minimum. A secondary benefit is that it also serves as a filter mechanism that can provide clean power to equipment, which helps reduce electrical noise due to the 60 Hz frequency of alternating current (AC). This shields the room from conducting noise from the main power source but consideration should be taken to troubleshoot equipment that may generate noise from within the room that can conduct to other equipment plugged in the same branch circuit.

DEVICE PROCEDURES

There have been many advances in cardiac implantable electrical devices (CIEDs), including pacemakers, implantable cardioverter-defibrillators, cardiac resynchronization devices, and implantable loop recorders. Newer models are capable of handling more sophisticated algorithms, they have more data storage capacity, and they are compact and now capable of interfacing wirelessly. This provides a new challenge and becomes an impetus for change in the ways that we traditionally pull paraphernalia needed in the procedure. Changes in interfaces can also create inadvertent issues that create problems between device communications. As technology advances, procedural considerations and need dynamically evolve and should be expected.

The equipment needed for CIED Implantation include:

- X-ray system
- EP recording system
- Defibrillator
- Device specific programmer
- Signal analyzer (usually a function provided by the device specific programmer)
- Electrocautery
- Temporary pacemaker
- Ultrasound (for emergent transthoracic scan and vascular access if needed)
- Suction apparatus (typically available as a wall source in procedural areas)
- Operating room instruments
- Open chest and emergency carts

X-RAY SYSTEM

The patient table should be radiolucent and freely movable to allow fluoroscopy from the patient's neck to groin. Ample space is necessary on the left and right side as well as the head of the bed, where personnel can monitor vital signs, oxygen saturation, patient status, and conscious sedation. Complex cases, such as device extractions or extractions with contralateral re-implants, may require space for bilateral pectoral, groin, or neck vascular access for a temporary pacer wire or arterial access for invasive blood pressure monitoring. It is helpful for a table to have options for Trendelenberg and reverse Trendelenberg positioning, although foam wedges may be placed under the legs to facilitate venous return during venous access or under the head for patients unable to lay flat.

Fluoroscopy remains essential to optimal lead placement. The fluoroscopy source can be either portable or fixed and should be maneuverable in oblique and lateral views. Maneuverability is important for obtaining access, venograms, and lead positioning. An option for magnification is used to visualize extension and retraction of the lead screw. The ability to record cine loops is helpful for guidance of vascular insertion and lead placement (e.g., coronary sinus venogram), as well as for teaching purposes. Cinefluoroscopy is the most commonly used recording mode, with some machines having the option to record loops from fluoroscopy.

Consideration should also be given to selectable default radiation dose exposure settings for procedures. While it is more a user preference, EP staff responsible for monitoring radiation exposure during procedures can opt to configure lower dose settings commensurate to preferred image quality with the equipment manufacturer engineers. This is preferably done during equipment installation but can be revisited upon request. Caution should be taken to include all members of the clinical team for approval to make it standard for their particular practice.

EP RECORDING SYSTEM, DEVICE SPECIFIC PROGRAMMER & SIGNAL ANALYZER

Once the pacing and/or defibrillation leads are positioned, lead impedance, capture threshold, and amplitude are tested. The electrodes are connected using alligator clips to a pacing system analyzer (PSA) and display. The signal can be displayed with standard bipolar intracardiac electrogram filtering (30 Hertz [Hz] high pass, 500 Hz low pass), as well as with a wider bandpass filter to facilitate assessment for an injury current on the intracardiac electrograms (0.5 Hz high pass filter and 500 Hz low pass filter). The injury current helps to confirm appropriate fixation to viable tissue. It is also helpful to have a secondary monitor to display the PSA or device programmer screens alongside the EP Recording system and X-Ray displays to the implanting physician.

EMERGENCY EQUIPMENT (DEFIBRILLATOR, TEMPORARY PACEMAKERS, OPEN CHEST, AND EMERGENCY CARTS)

Every lab should be equipped with emergency equipment. A combination defibrillator/external pacemaker is essential. The most frequent use of the defibrillator is for cardioversion and as a back-up to an internal cardiac defibrillator in defibrillation threshold testing. There should also be a cart stocked with emergency medications used for cardiopulmonary arrests (code cart), pericardiocentesis kit, and in centers performing high risk procedures, an open chest kit can be stocked. A pericardiocentesis kit should be available in the event of a lead perforation.

ELECTROCAUTERY

The use of electrocautery is essential for cutting through the dermal layers and also coagulating the vascularized tissue when creating a pocket for the device. While it has its advantages to scalpels to prevent nicks on lead insulation, strong electromagnetic interference (EMI) can be generated that has the potential to temporarily stun or damage device electronics.[3] This can be catastrophic in patients who are pacemaker dependent during device replacements. In some instances it may be advisable to insert a temporary pacing lead in patients who are pacemaker dependent, or to minimize cautery until leads can be secured for pacing. Temporary pacing should be available and ready for immediate activation, if needed.

OPERATING ROOM INSTRUMENTS & ROOM SUPPLIES

Many labs have instrument sets specially designed for device implantation. Basic sterile surgical instrument sets often include hemostats, forceps, fine forceps, suture scissors, Metzenbaum scissors, a needle holder, Weitlaner retractor, and manual retractors (Figure 1.1). Vascular ultrasound devices used to obtain vascular access may be helpful to avoid unnecessary arterial punctures when groin access is needed. Suction should be available in case of need.

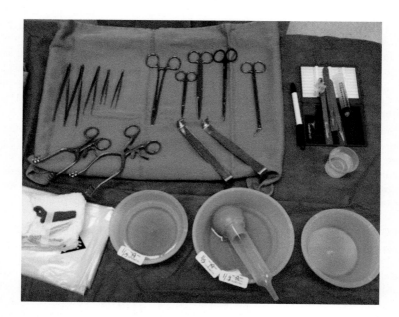

Figure 1.1 Example of a basic kit of instrument sets used and standardized on all implantable cardiac device procedures in an EP Lab setting.

In-room stocking or easy availability of single-use items adds to convenience during the procedure. Items that are used during device implantation include scalpels, absorbable and non-absorbable suture, splittable vascular sheaths, the implanted leads and device, stylets, sterile programming wand covers, drape clips, sterile fluoroscopy cover, and often steerable mapping catheters.

ADDITIONAL REFERENCE
There is also a recent document that was released by the Heart Rhythm Society that was created by a consensus of experts who aim to provide a standard framework for Cardiac Electrophysiology Labs in general. This document is entitled "2013 HRS Expert Consensus Statement on Electrophysiology (EP) Lab Standards: Process, Protocols, Equipment, Personnel and Safety" and is available for public download at http://www.hrsonline.org/ Practice-Guidance/Clinical-Guidelines-Documents/2013-Electrophysiology-EP-Lab-Standards-Process-Protocols-Equipment-Personnel-and-Safety#axzz3AklrR1h7.

REFERENCES

1. Haines, D., Beheiry, S., Akar, J., et al. (2014, May 8). *Heart Rhythm Society.* Retrieved May 26, 2015, from Heart Rhythm Society: http://www.hrsonline.org/Practice-Guidance/Clinical-Guidelines-Documents/2013-Electrophysiology-EP-Lab-Standards-Process-Protocols-Equipment-Personnel-and-Safety#axzz3AklrR1h7.

2. Earley, M.W., Sargent, J.S., Sheehan, J.V., & Buss, E.W. (Eds.) (2008). *NEC 2008 Handbook.* (pp. Article 517, Part VII). Quiny, MA: National Fire Protection Association.

3. Abdelmalak, B., Jagannathan, N., Arain, F., et al. (2011). Electromagnetic interference in a cardiac pacemaker during cauterization with the coagulating, not cutting mode. *J. Anaesthesiol. Clin. Pharmacol., 27*(4), 527–530.

ORGANIZATION OF THE ARRHYTHMIA LAB

Roy Chung and Oussama M. Wazni

CONTENTS

SETUP OF THE INTERVENTIONAL ELECTROPHYSIOLOGY LABORATORY MAPPING SYSTEMS

Setting up an electrophysiology laboratory for cardiac ablations requires specifics in the layout of laboratory, personnel, and equipment requirements. Conventional electrophysiology (EP) studies and ablation procedures should be performed with adequately trained personnel. One to two physicians are responsible for catheter manipulation and ablation. Two nurses are generally required, one to assist with tasks related to ablation and the other responsible for sedation of the patient. For most procedures, conscious sedation is preferred to allow for assessment of symptoms and minimization of risks associated with anesthesia, although general anesthesia is routinely employed now for pulmonary vein isolation.[1] To that effect, considerations are made to accommodate anesthesia cart and personnel. Support for complications related to EP studies and ablations should be readily available, including cardiac and vascular surgery and neurologic imaging modalities.

SETUP OF THE INTERVENTIONAL ELECTROPHYSIOLOGY LABORATORY

An electrophysiology laboratory capable of performing EP studies and ablations must be equipped with a radiographic system, the ability to separately monitor vital signs, and data acquisition capabilities.

- The *cinefluoroscopic equipment* includes the patient table and the C-arm, which allows for variable angulation of the X-ray beam. Biplane imaging provides simultaneous viewing of cardiac structures from different angles and can be useful in transseptal puncture. The video system should consist of 1–2 monitors and have the ability to store cine images. Above the patient table, one monitor displays fluoroscopic images and another displays tracings from the physiologic recorder and hangs from a mounted movable ceiling bracket, allowing the physician manipulating catheters to achieve the optimal viewing angle (Figure 2.1). Given the amount of fluoroscopy used in prolonged ablations or device implantation procedures, reduced fluoroscopy intensity is generally used in

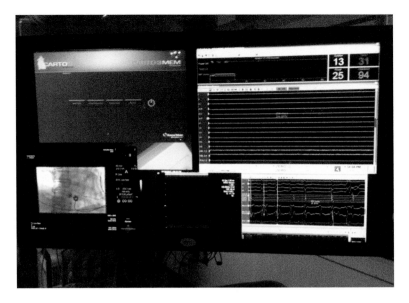

Figure 2.1 Mounted monitor with various displays, including fluoroscopy, electrophysiologic mapping system, real-time electrocardiograms.

the EP lab as compared to catheterization laboratories. These settings are typically done individually for each laboratories to physician's specification.

- *Vital signs monitoring* should be performed on independent equipment so that monitoring may continue if the data acquisition system fails. A cardioverter/defibrillator may be used for monitoring rhythm, and combined modality devices may be used to monitor vital signs. Through the defibrillation pads and ECG leads, several lead configurations can typically be viewed separately from the physiologic recorder. Additionally, non-invasive measurements of blood pressure and pulse oximetry can be followed. Capnography is of particular benefit in procedures with moderate sedation for a prolonged period of time. This also reduces over-dosing sedative and narcotic usage which may result in adverse events. Esophageal thermister probe allows monitoring of esophageal temperature for ablation performed along the posterior wall of the left atrium to avoid risk of atrial-esophageal fistula.
- The *data acquisition system* includes the physiologic recorder which displays and stores surface and intracardiac electrograms. The equipment console consists of this system as well as a slave monitor for radiographic images and an electrophysiologic stimulator. Input signals are displayed on computer screens and stored on archivable media, such as optical disks.

Electrical safety must be ensured in the setup of the electrophysiology laboratory to reduce the risk of current leakage to the patient which can precipitate ventricular arrhythmias. Leaking of current should remain less than 10 mA.

JUNCTION BOX

The junction boxes receive the intracardiac signals from the catheters and provide an interface into the physiologic recorder (Figure 2.2). Multiple switches within the junction box are

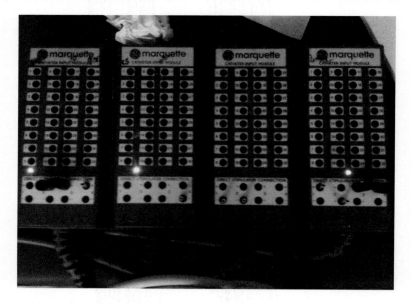

Figure 2.2 Junction boxes.

designated to a recording and stimulation channel which can be selected through the recording apparatus. The junction boxes are mounted at the foot of the patient table and connected to the physiologic recorder, which is kept as close as possible. This helps to minimize noise on the channels as well as reduce floor clutter.

RECORDING APPARATUS

The physiologic recorder records, displays, and stores intracardiac and surface recordings. It consists of filters, amplifiers, display screens, and recording software. From the junction box, the physiologic signals are introduced into the recorder. These signals are typically low in amplitude and require amplification prior to displaying and recording. The recording system amplifies and filters each input channel separately, with most current systems supporting up to 64 or more channels. The amplifiers have the ability to automatically or manually adjust gain control. The amplifiers should be mounted as close to the patient table as possible. This will reduce the cable length of the intracardiac connections and surface ECGs, which minimizes the signal noise. The amplifier is then connected to the main physiologic recorder through a floor channel, which, ideally, should run separately from electric power cables. Filters are used to eliminate unnecessary signals that distort electrograms (EGMs). High pass filters eliminate signals below a given frequency and low pass filters eliminate signals above a given frequency. Most intracardiac electrograms are clearly identified when the signal is filtered between a high pass of 40 Hz and a low pass of 500 Hz. Several pages can be simultaneously recorded and one of these typically includes a 12-lead ECG. The page displayed during studies typically shows several intracardiac electrograms with 3–4 surface ECG leads which allows for axis determination, activation timing, and P/QRS morphology (Figure 2.3). Pressure channels, if used, allow for simultaneous hemodynamic monitoring.

STIMULATOR

A programmable stimulator is necessary to obtain electrophysiologic data beyond measurements of conduction intervals. Stimulators are capable of various modes of pacing, including

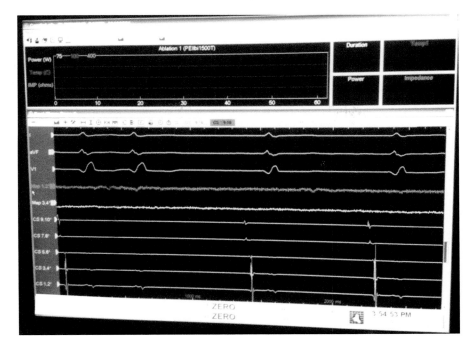

Figure 2.3 Intracardiac electrograms display with coronary sinus electrograms.

rapid pacing, delivery of single or multiple extra stimuli following a paced drive train, and delivery of timed extra stimuli following sensed beats. Stimulators should be capable of delivering variable currents, ranging from 0.1 to 20 mA. With satisfactory positioning of catheters, current thresholds under 2 mA (with 2 ms pulse width) can usually be achieved in both the atrium and ventricle. Higher outputs are seen with diseased myocardium, within the coronary sinus, and with the use of anti-arrhythmic medications. Output is usually set at twice the diastolic threshold. Most stimulators have the ability to pace through more than one channel; however, one channel generally suffices for all studies unless dual chamber pacing is required.

CARDIOVERTER/DEFIBRILLATOR

A primary and back-up cardioverter/defibrillator should be available throughout all EP studies (Figure 2.4). Current defibrillators deliver energy in a biphasic waveform which offers enhanced defibrillation success. Defibrillation pads are attached to the patient and electrically grounded. In our laboratory, the defibrillator and energy delivered by RFA share a common ground patch on the patient which connects through the *Booker box*. ECGs can be recorded through the defibrillation pads separate from the data acquisition system.[2,3]

RADIOFREQUENCY ABLATION

Radiofrequency ablation uses alternating current delivered between the catheter tip and grounding source to deliver energy to tissue, resulting in necrosis. Radiofrequency generators deliver current with a frequency between 300 and 750 kHz, with generation of heat occurring as a result of resistive and conductive heating. Monitoring of time, power, and

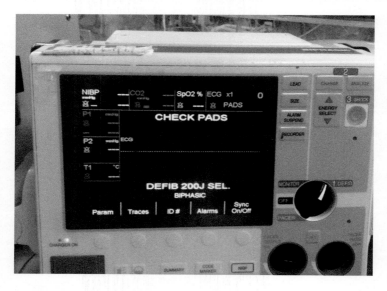

Figure 2.4 Cardioverter defibrillator.

impedance is necessary to ensure safe and effective ablation lesions. The new SmartAblate system comes with a generator, system pump, and remote control, is an integrated platform which streamlines the ablation procedure in an electrophysiology laboratory. Through the generator, limits on impedance and temperature are programmed and the desired power level is set (Figure 2.5).

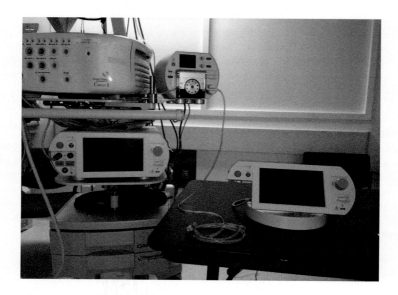

Figure 2.5 Biosense webster smart ablate generator.

Cardiac mapping is the process by which arrhythmias are characterized and localized. Conventional mapping involves acquiring electrogram data from fixed and moving catheters and creating mental activation maps with fluoroscopic two-dimensional (2D) images. More sophisticated mapping techniques provide three-dimensional (3D) anatomic localization of the catheter to assist in mapping and ablation. These technologies involve the acquisition of multiple electrogram locations to provide a high resolution activation, voltage, or propagation map. In addition to correlating local electrograms to 3D cardiac structures, these newer mapping techniques reduce the radiation exposure to the patient and physician. The most widely used is an electro-anatomic mapping system (e.g., the Biosense Webster CARTO system), which localizes the mapping and ablation catheter through a magnetic field. Three coils located beneath the patient generate ultra low magnetic fields that temporally and spatially code the area within the patient. With a magnetic field sensor in its tip that is referenced to an externally located patch on the patient, the catheter can be displayed and recorded in three dimensions with intracardiac electrograms (Figure 2.6). Another technology offers electro-anatomic mapping by creating electrical fields between opposing pairs of patch electrodes located on the patient's chest (e.g., St. Jude Endocardial Solutions, Incorporated, ESI). Six patches are placed on the body to create three orthogonal axes with the heart located centrally. A transthoracic electrical field is created through each pair of opposing patch electrodes and the mapping catheter delivers this signal for processing. Finally, Heart Rhythm Society has recently produced an expert consensus statement on electrophysiology laboratory standards, which serves as a great reference for physicians and hospital system to optimize patient care delivery.

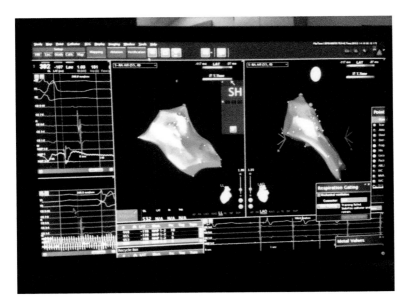

Figure 2.6 Three-dimensional display of the cardiac structure acquiring activation points for arrhythmia of interest.

1. Di Biase, L., Natale, A., et al. (2011). General anesthesia reduces the prevalence of pulmonary vein reconnection during repeat ablation when compared with conscious sedation: Results from a randomized study. *Heart Rhythm*, 8, 368–372.

2. Tracy, C.M., Akhtar, M., DiMarco, J.P., et al. (2006). Invasive electrophysiology studies, catheter ablation, and cardioversion: American college of cardiology/American heart association 2006 update of the clinical competence statement on. *J Am Coll Cardiol* 48, 1503–1517.

3. Haines, D.E., Beheiry, S., Akar, J.G., et al. (2014). Heart rhythm society expert consensus statement on electrophysiology laboratory standards: Process, protocols, equipment, personnel, and safety. *Heart Rhythm* 11(8), e9–e51.

HOLTER AND EVENT MONITOR LABORATORY SETUP

Roy Chung, Daniel Cantillon, and Mina K. Chung

CONTENTS

INTRODUCTION

- Cardiac arrhythmias are common, ranging from benign ectopic atrial or ventricular beats to atrial fibrillation or flutter, complete heart block, or ventricular tachycardia. Some of these are paroxysmal and not routinely identified through history or 12-lead electrocardiography (ECG). Some ventricular ectopies reflect triggered activity and can be intermittent or clustered. Therefore, daily event monitoring rather than an isolated ECG recording can provide higher yield.
- Ambulatory ECG (AECG) monitoring has become an essential tool in the diagnosis, characterization, quantification risk stratification and management, and prognostic stratification of cardiac arrhythmias, particularly among patients with structural and ischemic heart disease.[1] Contemporary light-weight monitoring technology and data processing capabilities now far eclipse the original 75 lb (34 kg) device introduced by Holter and Gengerelli.
- Various studies have demonstrated the increased sensitivity of ambulatory ECG monitoring for detecting spontaneous cardiac arrhythmias.[2,3]

- Though earlier monitors were designed to document tachycardia or bradycardia, due to improvements in solid-state digital technology and increased accuracy of software analysis systems, contemporary AECG monitors are used for:
  - Assessment and correlation of symptoms possibly related to arrhythmia.
  - Identification of high-risk post-MI patients with complex and frequent ventricular arrhythmias potentially benefitting from ICD implantation or other therapies.[4,5]
  - Assessment of etiologies of syncope.
  - Monitoring arrhythmia reduction after anti-arrhythmic drug or ablation treatment.[6]
  - Assessment of pacemaker and ICD function.

- Assessment of the burden of arrhythmias (e.g., atrial fibrillation or premature ventricular complexes [PVCs]).
  - Detection of changes in QRS complexes (e.g., bundle branch blocks), T-waves, or specific intervals (e.g., QT interval, T-wave changes).[7,8,9]
  - Documenting triggers of ventricular and supraventricular arrhythmias (PVCs, NSVT, PACs).

- A list of indications for Holter monitoring is given in Table 3.1.[10]

Table 3.1 Indications for Holter monitoring

Indication	Class I	Class IIa	Class IIb	Class III
Assess symptoms possibly related to rhythm disturbances	• Patients with unexplained syncope, near syncope, or episodic dizziness in whom the cause is not obvious • Patients with unexplained recurrent palpitation		• Patients with episodic shortness of breath, chest pain, or fatigue that is not otherwise explained • Patients with neurologic events when transient atrial fibrillation or flutter is suspected • Patients with symptoms such as syncope, near syncope, episodic dizziness, or palpitation in whom a probable cause other than an arrhythmia has been identified, but in whom symptoms persist despite treatment of this other cause	• Patients with symptoms such as syncope, near syncope, episodic dizziness, or palpitation in whom other causes have been identified by history, physical examination, or laboratory tests • Patients with cerebrovascular accidents, without other evidence of arrhythmia
Arrhythmia detection to assess risk for future cardiac events in patients without symptoms from arrhythmia	None		• Post-MI patients with LV dysfunction (ejection fraction ≤40%) • Patients with CHF • Patients with idiopathic hypertrophic cardiomyopathy	• Patients who have had sustained myocardial contusion • Systemic hypertensive patients with LV hypertrophy

(Continued)

Table 3.1 (*Continued*) Indications for Holter monitoring

Indication	Class I	Class IIa	Class IIb	Class III
				• Post-MI patients with normal LV function • Preoperative arrhythmia evaluation of patients for non-cardiac surgery • Patients with sleep apnea • Patients with valvular heart disease
Measurement of HRV to assess risk for future cardiac events in patients without symptoms from arrhythmia	None		• Post-MI patients with LV dysfunction • Patients with CHF • Patients with idiopathic hypertrophic cardiomyopathy	• Post-MI patients with normal LV function • Diabetic subjects to evaluate for diabetic neuropathy • Patients with rhythm disturbances that preclude HRV analysis (i.e., atrial fibrillation)
Assess anti-arrhythmic therapy	To assess anti-arrhythmic drug response in individuals in whom baseline frequency of arrhythmia has been characterized as reproducible and of sufficient frequency to permit analysis	• To detect pro-arrhythmic responses to anti-arrhythmic therapy in patients at high risk • To assess rate control during atrial fibrillation	• To document recurrent or asymptomatic non-sustained arrhythmias during therapy in the outpatient setting	None

(*Continued*)

Table 3.1 (*Continued*) Indications for Holter monitoring

Indication	Class I	Class IIa	Class IIb	Class III
Assess pacemaker and ICD function	• Evaluation of frequent symptoms of palpitation, syncope, or near syncope to assess device function to exclude myopotential inhibition and pacemaker-mediated tachycardia and to assist in the programming of enhanced features such as rate responsivity and automatic mode switching • Evaluation of suspected component failure or malfunction when device interrogation is not definitive in establishing a diagnosis • To assess the response to adjunctive pharmacologic therapy in patients receiving frequent ICD therapy		• Evaluation of immediate postoperative pacemaker function after pacemaker or ICD implantation as an alternative or adjunct to continuous telemetric monitoring • Evaluation of the rate of supraventricular arrhythmias in patients with implanted defibrillators	• Assessment of ICD/pacemaker malfunction when device interrogation, ECG, or other available data (chest radiograph and so forth) are sufficient to establish an underlying cause/diagnosis • Routine follow-up in asymptomatic patients
Ischemia monitoring	None	• Patients with suspected variant angina	• Evaluation of patients with chest pain who cannot exercise • Preoperative evaluation for vascular surgery of patients who cannot exercise • Patients with known CAD and atypical chest pain syndrome	• Initial evaluation of patients with chest pain who are able to exercise • Routine screening of asymptomatic subjects

(*Continued*)

Table 3.1 (*Continued*) Indications for Holter monitoring

Indication	Class I	Class IIa	Class IIb	Class III
Monitoring in pediatric patients	• Syncope, near syncope, or dizziness in patients with recognized cardiac disease, previously documented arrhythmia, or pacemaker dependency • Syncope or near syncope associated with exertion when the cause is not established by other methods • Evaluation of patients with hypertrophic or dilated cardiomyopathies • Evaluation of possible or documented long QT syndromes • Palpitation in the patient with prior surgery for congenital heart disease and significant residual hemodynamic abnormalities • Evaluation of anti-arrhythmic drug efficacy during rapid somatic growth • Asymptomatic congenital complete AV block, non-paced	• Syncope, near syncope, or sustained palpitation in the absence of a reasonable explanation and where there is no overt clinical evidence of heart disease • Evaluation of cardiac rhythm after initiation of an anti-arrhythmic therapy, particularly when associated with a significant pro-arrhythmic potential • Evaluation of cardiac rhythm after transient AV block associated with heart surgery or catheter ablation • Evaluation of rate-responsive or physiologic pacing function in symptomatic patients	• Evaluation of asymptomatic patients with prior surgery for congenital heart disease, particularly when there are either significant or residual hemodynamic abnormalities, or a significant incidence of late postoperative arrhythmias • Evaluation of the young patient (<3 years old) with a prior tachyarrhythmia to determine if unrecognized episodes of the arrhythmia recur • Evaluation of the patient with a suspected incessant atrial tachycardia • Complex ventricular ectopy on ECG or exercise test	• Syncope, near syncope, or dizziness when a non-cardiac cause is present • Chest pain without clinical evidence of heart disease • Routine evaluation of asymptomatic individuals for athletic clearance • Brief palpitation in the absence of heart disease • Asymptomatic Wolff–Parkinson–White syndrome

COMPONENTS OF AN AMBULATORY ECG MONITORING LABORATORY

- The three main components of a long-term ambulatory ECG monitoring laboratory setup are (Figure 3.1):
  - Recording devices
  - Storage of recorded or transmitted data
  - Playback and analysis systems.

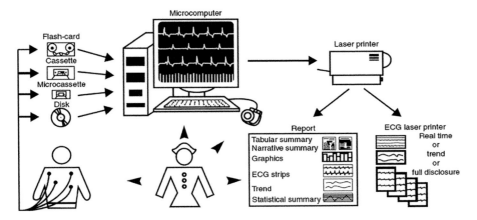

Figure 3.1 Multiple components of a long-term ambulatory ECG monitoring set up.

RECORDING DEVICES AND STORAGE OF TRANSMITTED DATA

- AECG monitoring can be continuous or intermittent.
- Continuous AECG is usually performed for 24–48 h (e.g., Holter monitors), but there are patch-type devices approved for longer (e.g., 2 weeks) continuous recording. Some mobile cardiac outpatient telemetry (MCOT) units provide real-time 24 h/day telemetry for up to 30 days. This can provide a wireless ECG transmission with automatic arrhythmia detection.
- Intermittent ambulatory recordings (obtained for longer periods) can be achieved by using transtelephonic transmitters that transmit real-time recordings over the phone, or by using memory loop recorders that are worn continuously but activated by an event button, which triggers storage of ECG from a programmable period prior to activation of the event button to a programmable period of time after activation of the button. Implantable loop recorders (ILRs) can provide even longer term intermittent monitoring, currently up to 2–3 years.
- Improvements in digital technology have allowed superior transtelephonic recordings increasing the potential uses of long-term ambulatory recording devices.
- Table 3.2 lists the various types of recording devices and their features.

Table 3.2 Recording, scanning, and transmitting features of the two types of recorders

Type	Recording	Scanning	Transmitting	Comments, advantages, and disadvantages
Holter				
Analog	• Battery powered device; records at extremely slow speeds at frequencies (0.05–100 Hz) similar to the standard ECG • All ECG complexes "full disclosure"	• Technicians digitize data with computer assistance, templating, area determination, and superimposition.	None	• Discrepancies in the range of recording frequency among devices can cause inaccuracies in measuring dynamic ST segment changes. • Irregularities in the tape drive can create artifacts that simulate bradycardia/tachycardia.
Digital—continuous recording	• Recording on digital or compact disk or flash card. ECG from multiple channels is stored in solid-state memory. • Unlike older systems, newer systems record each beat within a 24 h period. This creates full disclosure similar to tape systems. • All ECG complexes "full disclosure."	• Technician with computer assistance, templating, area determination, and super-imposition. • Algorithms for arrhythmia recognition measuring HRV and tabulation of ectopics enable real-time analysis by microprocessor with retrospective technician editing.	Transtelephonic	• Patient-activated markers or time-encoded markers enable symptom arrhythmia correlation. The playback instrument system which is operator-interaction-dependent has an arrhythmia analyzer, ST segment detector, RR interval analyzer, and a signal-averaging computer with software capable of generating ECG recordings, trends, or statistical summaries.

(Continued)

Table 3.2 (*Continued*) Recording, scanning, and transmitting features of the two types of recorders

Type	Recording	Scanning	Transmitting	Comments, advantages, and disadvantages
Digital—real-time analysis	• Computer analysis of ECG and selected ECG	• With microprocessor and electronic memory real-time analysis of digitized recordings online[12]	None	• Though usually done for 24 h, can be extended up to 5 days with battery change.[11] • Though reports can be generated upon completion of the test, absence of continuous storage of ECG data makes subsequent analysis and verification difficult.
In-hospital telemetry	• Recent improvements permit ECG recording from 2 channels with arrhythmia and ST segment change analysis.[13]	• Solid-state storage of ECG recordings online permits full disclosure with capability for re-examining at a later date.		• The continuously looping stored telemetry signal is presented as hourly full disclosures for review of all continuous events during the previous 12–24 h.[14]
Event recorder				
Post-event non-looping, without memory Hand-held (including credit card size) wristwatch type	• ECG selected by patient activation	• Direct visualization	Transtelephonic	• When compared to continuous recorders, they can provide recordings during events thus increasing the likelihood of symptom event correlation.

(*Continued*)

Table 3.2 (Continued) Recording, scanning, and transmitting features of the two types of recorders

Type	Recording	Scanning	Transmitting	Comments, advantages, and disadvantages
Automatic electronic sensor, in DDD pacemaker	• ECG when activated automatically by sensor	• Direct visualization of analysis or ECG	Direct telemetry	
Pre-event looping, with memory	• Various electrodes are placed and the device is worn continuously for 3–4 weeks.	• After activation, permanently stored ECG recordings are obtained, 1–4 min before and 30–60 s after device activation.[15]	While the older versions required immediate telephone access for transmitting, newer devices have limited (2–5 min) of solid-state memory which can be transmitted telephonically at the patient's convenience.	• Though these devices are invaluable in documenting the onset and offset of a paroxysmal cardiac arrhythmic event, patient error, and device malfunction are potential limitations.[16]
Wristwatch type monitor worn with attached electrodes	• ECG, selected by patient activation, with memory of pre-event. • The circuitry is completed by index finger and thumb or hand contact.	• Direct visualization	Solid-state storage of ECG data on the device is transmitted transtelephonically at the patient's convenience.	• Solid-state technology allows 1–5 min of ECG recording up to 3–5 times during events.

(Continued)

Table 3.2 (Continued) Recording, scanning, and transmitting features of the two types of recorders

Type	Recording	Scanning	Transmitting	Comments, advantages, and disadvantages
ILR (implantable loop recorder) subcutaneous, implanted digital recorder	• ECG selected by patient activation with memory of pre-event. After event, patient places a pager-like device over the loop recorder. By pressing a button, the ECG data are recorded to the hand-held device, which is available for later analysis by the physician.	• Direct visualization	Direct telemetry	• Though it involves an invasive procedure, the ability to record pre- and post-event, independent of patient activation, which is available for microprocessor-based analysis is a significant advantage. The ILR permits ECG recordings during water immersion, unlike other event recorders.
Automatic electronic sensor, in ICD or pacemaker	• ECG, when activated by firing of ICD or recognized by sensor in pacemaker, with memory	• Direct visualization of analysis of ECG	Direct telemetry	
Real-time				
Real-time transtelephonic monitoring	• ECG at central monitoring station—no recording at device	• Direct visualization	Transtelephonic	

CONTINUOUS AMBULATORY ECG MONITORING

- Mainstream continuous recording systems are mostly digital at present.

INTERMITTENT AND MEMORY LOOP AECG MONITORING (TABLE 3.2)

- Intermittent recorders are light-weight patient-activated devices that may have limited capacity for storage, but which can be useful in patients with infrequent symptoms.
- Though the memory loop recorders have to be worn continuously, they provide ECG data prior to the onset of the event, which could aid in the diagnosis of the mode of onset of arrhythmia. This is particularly useful in patients with significant symptoms that occur infrequently or very brief symptoms.
- A study of transtelephonic transmissions in 5052 patients after pacemaker implantation showed that 95% of events with suspected transient cardiac arrhythmias occurred within 5 weeks of using the device, with serious arrhythmia in 52% of these.[15] When this device was used in patients with recurrent syncope, a diagnosis was made in 25% of them.[16] Despite adequate patient education, improper device activation was seen in 20% of patients.
- Recent use of implantable memory loop recorders allows continuous ECG recordings for extended periods of up to 3 years.[17] The device can be patient-activated or programmed to record automatically based on preset heart rate limits.
- A study using ILR in 85 patients with recurrent syncope (negative HUT, AECG, and EPS), showed recurrent syncope in 68% at a mean of 10.5 months post-implantation, 30% of which were secondary to bradycardia.[17]

ARTIFACTS AND ERRORS

- Due to technical problems during recording and analysis, a large amount of invalid data during AECG recording is possible.
- For accurate analysis and interpretation of AECG recordings it is important to recognize artifacts that can simulate arrhythmia.
- With earlier tape-based recorders, tape slippage, excessive damping, inappropriate calibration, or saturation of the amplifier could cause artifacts.[18] Tape distortion can falsely prolong intervals that simulate sinus pauses.
- Changes in body position (supine vs erect) and breathing patterns can change P-wave, QRS, and T-wave morphology.
- A major cause of inaccurate arrhythmia and ST segment recognition and analysis is noise interference from multiple sources.
- Electrical artifacts can simulate pacemaker malfunction.
- Most current devices use digital recordings, rendering the problems associated with tape recordings obsolete. However, it is important to recognize event markers that may appear to simulate depolarizations.

SCANNING AND ANALYSIS TECHNIQUES

- Current scanning systems incorporate computer-assisted analysis with algorithm-based software systems capable of generating ECG recordings, arrhythmia analysis, ST segment detection, RR interval analysis, and providing trends or statistical summaries.
- It has been shown that when operator analysis is done without computer assistance, up to a third of supraventricular or ventricular arrhythmias are missed.[19] Computer-assisted analytic systems significantly improve the sensitivity and specificity of ECG monitoring.[20,21]

PERSONNEL, TRAINING REQUIREMENTS, AND QUALITY CONTROL

- In addition to a technician/nurse trained in the technical aspects of the device recorder who places the electrodes and hooks up the device, the base station must be equipped with a cardiovascular technician or nurse on a 24-h basis, or with a microcomputer capable of receiving and storing data for later analysis.
- Guidelines established by the American College of Cardiology/American Heart Association (ACC/AHA) have outlined the minimum knowledge and training necessary for acquiring and maintaining competence in AECG interpretation.
- Table 3.3 lists the ECG diagnoses that can be made with AECG.

Table 3.3 Technical and clinical differences of ambulatory ECG and transtelephonic loop recorder

	Ambulatory ECG	Transtelephonic loop
Technical		
ECG data	24–48 h of 2- or 3-channel ECG Continuous ECG data	4–5 min of 1-channel ECG intermittent and patient-activated ECG data
Resources needed	Holter recorder Holter playback analysis system Operator interaction	Transtelephonic loop recorder Telephone communication with audio modem Base station printout recorder (24 h availability) Operator interaction
Cost	24 h $150–300	30-day surveillance $200–300
Patient participation	Minimal (diary for symptoms)	Moderate/substantial (sending and recording ECG data)
Clinical		
Indications	To diagnose cardiac arrhythmias with qualitative/quantitative assessment	To diagnose infrequent or rare cardiac arrhythmias qualitatively only
As first-line diagnostic test	Often	Never
As arrhythmic follow-up	Often	Rarely or special situation (e.g., sudden death cohorts or effects on QT interval)
As pacemaker follow-up	Often	Often

Source: Knoebel, S.B. et al., *Am. J. Cardiol.*, 38, 440–447, 1976.

- Due to various technical differences among devices, physicians who interpret AECG need to
    - Acquire cognitive skills which in addition to basic electrocardiography include assessment of heart rate variability (HRV), cardiac pacemakers, and ICDs (Table 3.4).
    - Understand the equipment and computer algorithms including problems during editing.
    - Have knowledge of artifactual and transient physiologic changes and the false-positive and false-negative findings during arrhythmia detection and classification (Table 3.5).
- A minimum of 150 supervised AECG interpretations is recommended to expose the trainee to most of the technical and physiologic phenomena known to confound AECG interpretation.[22]
- Hands-on experience with operation of the Holter instrumentation enables the trainee to appreciate artifacts and errors encountered during recording and analysis.
- A minimum of 25 interpretations per year is recommended to maintain competence in AECG interpretation.[22]
- Quality assurance in AECG interpretation by physicians can be achieved by conducting periodic reviews of random samples of their prior AECG interpretations by an acknowledged expert.

Table 3.4 List of AECG diagnoses

Type of AECG disorder	List of diagnoses
Sinus node rhythms and arrhythmias	Sinus rhythm Sinus tachycardia (>100 beats per minute) Sinus bradycardia (<50 beats per minute) Sinus arrhythmia Sinus arrest or pause Sino-atrial exit block
Other supraventricular rhythms	Atrial premature complexes Atrial premature complexes, non-conducted Ectopic atrial rhythm Ectopic atrial tachycardia, unifocal Ectopic atrial tachycardia, multi-focal Atrial fibrillation Atrial flutter Junctional premature complexes Junctional escape complexes or rhythm Accelerated junctional rhythm Junctional tachycardia, automatic Supraventricular tachycardia, paroxysmal
Ventricular arrhythmias	Ventricular premature complexes Ventricular escape complexes or rhythm Accelerated idioventricular rhythm Ventricular tachycardia Ventricular tachycardia, polymorphous (including torsade de pointes) Ventricular fibrillation

(*Continued*)

Table 3.4 (*Continued*)   List of AECG diagnoses

Type of AECG disorder	List of diagnoses
Atrial ventricular conduction	First-degree AV block Mobitz type 1 second-degree AV block (Wenckebach) Mobitz type 2 second-degree AV block AV block or conduction ratio, 2:1 AV block, varying conduction ratio AV block, advanced (high-grade) AV block, complete (third-degree) AV dissociation
Intraventricular conduction	Left bundle branch block (fixed or intermittent) Right bundle branch block (fixed or intermittent, complete or incomplete) Intraventricular conduction disturbance, non-specific Aberrant conduction of supraventricular beats Left posterior fascicular block Ventricular pre-excitation (Wolff–Parkinson–White pattern)
QRS axis and voltage	Right axis deviation (−90 to −180 degrees) Left axis deviation (−30 to −90 degrees) Low voltage (less than 0.5 mV total QRS amplitude in each extremity lead and less than 1.0 mV in each precordial lead)
Chamber hypertrophy or enlargement	Left atrial enlargement, abnormality, or conduction defect Right atrial abnormality Left ventricular hypertrophy with secondary ST-T abnormality Right ventricular hypertrophy with or without secondary ST-T abnormality
Repolarization (ST-T, U) abnormalities	Early repolarization (normal variant) Juvenile T-waves (normal variant) Non-specific abnormality, ST segment, and/or T-wave ST and/or T-wave suggests ischemia ST suggests injury ST suggests ventricular aneurysm Q-T interval prolonged Prominent U waves
Pacemaker	Ventricular-paced rhythm Atrial-sensed ventricular-paced rhythm AV dual-paced rhythm Failure of appropriate capture, atrial Failure of appropriate capture, ventricular Failure of appropriate inhibition, atrial Failure of appropriate inhibition, ventricular Failure of appropriate pacemaker firing Retrograde atrial activation Pacemaker mediated tachycardia

Source: Kadish, A.H. et al., *Circulation*, 104, 3169–3178, 2001.

Table 3.5   Skill sets required for competency in AECG interpretation

Cognitive skills needed to interpret AECGs competently (from ACC/AHA guidelines 2001)[22]	
1.	Knowledge of the appropriate indications for ambulatory electrocardiography
2.	Knowledge of cardiac arrhythmias, their diagnosis, and significance in normal subjects and in patients with heart disease
3.	Appreciation of the wide range of variability in arrhythmia occurrence in the ambulatory patient throughout a diurnal cycle, and the influence of the autonomic nervous system on the rhythm of the heart
4.	Knowledge of changes in the ECG that may result from exercise, hyperventilation, conduction disorders, electrolyte shifts, drugs, meals, temperature, Valsalva maneuvers, ischemia, and transient repolarization phenomena related to a variety of cardiac diseases
5.	Knowledge of cardiac drugs and how they may affect conduction and repolarization on the ECG, particularly for suspected pro-arrhythmic phenomena
6.	Knowledge of the sensitivity, specificity, and diagnostic accuracy of ambulatory electrocardiography in various age groups and populations, particularly with respect to ST segment changes and the application of Bayes' theorem
7.	Knowledge of the most widely accepted criteria for ischemic ST segment changes
8.	Knowledge of ambulatory electrocardiographic evidence of failure to capture, failure to sense, or failure to pace for cardiac pacemakers and ICDs
9.	Knowledge of ambulatory electrocardiographic evidence of appropriate and inappropriate anti-tachycardia pacing or defibrillation in the ICD patient
10.	A basic understanding of the advantages and disadvantages of the instrumentation used in continuous and intermittent ambulatory electrocardiography from a recorder, and the possible causes for false-positive or false-negative test results that are due to inherent instrumentation or signal processing limitations
11.	Knowledge of the particular characteristics of the AECG instrumentation used to process the recordings for which the electrocardiographer is responsible
12.	Appreciation of the skills required by the technologist to interact with the AECG instrumentation in editing the computer output, and the need to be assured of the competence of the technologist

Source: Kadish, A.H. et al., *Circulation*, 104, 3169–3178, 2001.

HOLTER MONITORING

RECORDER MAINTENANCE AND PREPARATION

- Optimal and reliable performance of Holter monitors requires routine maintenance depending on the frequency of use. Continuous recording Holters need weekly maintenance.

PREPARATION

- Before device application to the patient, a blank magnetic tape should be inserted into the recorder.
- Adequately charged or new batteries should be available. If rechargeable batteries are used they must be charged for 4–16 h prior to use depending on the manufacturer's recommendation.
- Calibration standards of 1 mv are available in most Holter recorders. Brief ECG recordings with these standards should be obtained on each tape, to serve as a baseline for subsequent analysis.

SELECTION OF LEAD SYSTEM

- Ambulatory Holter monitors are available in 1, 2, 3, 6, and full 12-channel systems. Using fewer leads improves the recording reliability, minimizes noise artifact, and improves patient mobility and satisfaction with the monitoring system at the expense of diagnostic information gained from multiple leads, including the ability to discern artifact from true signal. In contrast, full 12 lead Holters are utilized for ambulatory ST segment monitoring, morphology evaluation for ventricular arrhythmias, and emerging parameters such as T-wave-alternans where a multi-lead evaluation is essential.
- Despite a lack of studies establishing the superiority of using one lead vs the other, the expert consensus is that a modified V1 lead system (P-wave and QRS morphology) and V3 to V5 lead system (ST segment depression or elevation) are best for identifying ectopic beat patterns and myocardial ischemia, respectively[23] (Figure 3.2).

ELECTRODE PLACEMENT (FIGURE 3.3)

- The ground electrode is placed in the lateral one-third of the right infraclavicular fossa immediately medial to the shoulder.
- For V1, the positive exploring electrode is placed in the fourth intercostal space (ICS) on the anterior chest 1 inch from the right sternal border; the negative electrode is placed in the lateral one-third of the left infraclavicular fossa medial to the shoulder.
- For V3, the positive electrode is placed in the left lower fourth ICS midway between the left sternal border and the left midclavicular line (MCL); the placement of the negative electrode is similar to V1.
- For V5, the positive electrode is placed on the anterior chest in the fifth ICS space midway between the left MCL and the left midaxillary line; the negative electrode is located 1 inch below the inferior angle of the right scapula on the posterior chest.

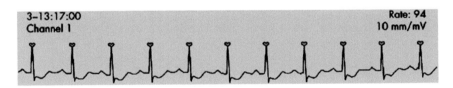

Figure 3.2   Modified V1 system for P wave and QRS morphology.

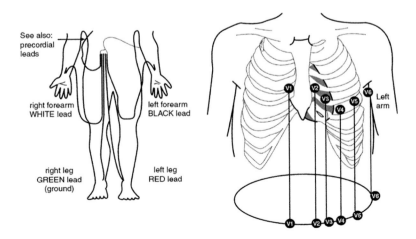

Figure 3.3   Electrode placement for limb leads and precordial leads.

- For AVF, the positive electrode is placed in the ninth to tenth ICS at the left anterior axillary line; the negative electrode is placed in the lateral third of the left infraclavicular fossa medial to the shoulder.[24]

PREPARATION OF ELECTRODE SITE

- The patient removes clothing from the waist up and the positions of the five electrodes as described earlier are prepared.
- Body hair in and around the site of the electrode placement should be removed by light shaving.
- Skin surface oil and dirt are rubbed off with alcohol-soaked gauze. Adequate skin preparation is crucial for optimum ECG signal. Alcohol prep pads lack the abrasive quality of gauze, and therefore should not be used.
- The central area of the electrode where the skin will make contact with the electrode pad should be gently abraded by wiping 3–4 times with extra fine grade sandpaper. Removal of this extra layer of dead superficial skin will enhance contact and improve the quality of the electrode signal.
- The adhesive disk should be securely attached to the skin. A longer period (72 h) of contact is achieved with some ambulatory monitoring electrodes. Applying a thin layer of tincture of benzoin serves as a useful adjunct, particularly on hot humid days, to negate the effect of excessive sweating. In patients with hypersensitivity to electrode gel or adhesive material, a non- or hypoallergenic electrode type or tape should be used to avoid serious local skin reactions.
- After the electrodes are placed, the electrical impedance between the poles of each bipolar lead should be checked to ensure optimal ECG signal. Using a standard impedance meter with a 10 Hz signal the impedance should always be 5000 ohms, preferably 3500 ohms.[25]
- An electrode lead wire is snapped on to each of the electrode pads. The five lead wires are connected to a single patient cable. Accidental pull-out of the lead wires is avoided by using a lead wire brace retainer around the area of the patient's cable interface to serve as a stabilizing support. Additional protection with adhesive tape wrapping around the lead wire retainer is desirable.

PATIENT INSTRUCTION, PRE-EXAMINATION PROCEDURES

- A log book containing patient identifiers, contact information, diagnosis, date, the serial number of the recorder used, and battery identification, if it is rechargeable, should be kept in the Holter recording examination area.
- In the patient's diary, in addition to demographic information and dates of examination, the patient records the time of activities (including major changes), symptoms with time of occurrence, and medications that are ingested during AECG examination. This facilitates correlation of activities and symptoms with detected electrocardiographic phenomena.
- It should be emphasized that the patient should engage in his routine activities.
- The recording starts either with the connection of the patient cable to the Holter recorder or by activation of the recorder. The start time per the patient's watch is noted in the patient's diary and also entered into the clock of the Holter recorder.
- Once recording begins, the clarity of the electrical signal has to be verified before the patient is sent home. The clarity of ECG signal should be tested while manually tapping the various electrodes and vigorously moving the corresponding lead wires for both bipolar leads. If a wandering baseline or muscular or electrical artifacts are seen, the electrode/lead wire responsible for the artifact is identified using an impedance meter and replaced.
- Due to assumption of different positions by the ambulatory patient, ECG rhythm strips should be recorded in at least 5 positions (standing, sitting, supine, left lateral supine, and right lateral supine). This provides accurate baseline comparisons for the changes that normally occur during a 24-h AECG.

- Finally, the lead wire retainer and the patient cable should be taped to the anterior chest wall. The Holter recorder can be worn on the hip (with a belt) or carried over the shoulder (with a strap).

REMOVAL OF THE HOLTER RECORDER

- Following completion of the time period (usually 24 h), the Holter recorder is removed as follows:
    - The patient cable is disengaged from the Holter recorder.
    - The diary and recorder are removed from the patient.
    - Lead wires are removed from the electrodes.
    - Micropore tape holding the patient cable to the chest wall is removed.
    - Electrode pads can be removed by the patient or the technician.
    - Excessive electrode gel is wiped off with alcohol pads; any skin irritation or reaction is treated by application of 1% hydrocortisone gel.
    - The patient's diary is always kept with the corresponding patient's tape.

DEVICE SELECTION AND DURATION OF RECORDING FOR AECG MONITORING

- Selection of continuous vs intermittent ECG recording is individualized based on the frequency and duration of symptoms.
- Table 3.6 shows the type of device to be selected depending on the symptoms and the diagnostic yield.[26]

Table 3.6   Technical pitfalls responsible for false-positive/negative findings

Causes of technical false-positive/false-negative findings in arrhythmia detection and classification	Causes of false-positive/false-negative findings in detection and interpretation of cardiac ischemia
1. Inadequate computer QRS detection and classification algorithms 2. Noise interference or lead-electrode baseline drift or artifact 3. Low-voltage recording 4. Recorder malfunction with variable tape drive or inaccurate storage 5. Physiologic variations in QRS form and voltage 6. Incomplete degaussing or erasure of data from previously used tapes or memory storage 7. Inadequate or incorrect technician interpretation during analysis 8. Incorrect time stamping of AECG tracings	1. Positional changes on the ST segment 2. Hyperventilation 3. Sudden excessive exercise-induced ST segment changes 4. Vasoregulatory or Valsalva-induced ST segment changes 5. Intraventricular conduction disorders 6. Undiagnosed or unappreciated left ventricular hypertrophy 7. ST segment changes secondary to tachyarrhythmias 8. False ST segment changes from atrial fibrillation or atrial flutter 9. ST segment changes secondary to electrolyte disturbance or drugs 10. Inadequate lead system employed 11. Incorrect or lack of lead calibration 12. Inadequate recording fidelity 13. Recording signal processing that compresses or filters the data, altering the ST segment characteristics

Source: Kadish, A.H. et al., *Circulation*, 104, 3169–3178, 2001.

- The presence of symptom–arrhythmia correlation is diagnostic.
- While most patients are monitored for 24–48 h, it is possible to monitor for longer periods (e.g., days up to 4 weeks).
- While the presence of arrhythmia without associated symptoms does not contribute towards diagnosis, lack of arrhythmia during symptoms excludes arrhythmia as a possibility.
- A randomized cross-over trial of 43 patients with palpitations randomized to event monitoring and 48-h monitoring showed that event monitors were more than twice as likely to detect a clinically important arrhythmia.[27]

CONCLUSIONS

- AECG monitoring is an important tool for evaluating patients with suspected arrhythmias that are not easily detected through routine electrocardiography.
- Rapidly emerging technologic advances have not only changed the size and ease of carrying recording devices but have added a wide spectrum of possibilities ranging from recognition of ectopic beats and recognizing ST segment changes to complex QT interval analysis, diagnosing unexplained syncope by ILR implantation, and HRV assessment.

REFERENCES

1. Buxton, A.E., Lee, K.L., Fisher, J.D. et al. (2000). A randomized study of the prevention of sudden death in patients with coronary artery disease. Multicenter Unsustained Tachycardia Trial Investigators. *N Engl J Med* 1999; 341(25): 1882–90. Erratum in *N Engl J Med* 342(17), 1300.

2. Boudoulas, H., Schaal, S.F., Lewis, R.P., & Robinson, J.L. (1979). Superiority of 24-hour outpatient monitoring over multi-stage exercise testing for the evaluation of syncope. *J Electrocardiol* 12(1), 103–8.

3. Poblete, P.F., Kennedy, H.A.L, & Caralis, D.G. (1978). Detection of ventricular ectopy in patients with coronary heart disease and normal subjects by exercise testing and ambulatory electrocardiography. *Chest* 74(4), 402–407.

4. Cairns, J.A., Connolly, S.J., Roberts, R., & Gent, M. (1997). Randomised trial of outcome after myocardial infarction in patients with frequent or repetitive ventricular premature depolarisations: CAMIAT. Canadian Amiodarone Myocardial Infarction Arrhythmia Trial Investigators. *Lancet* 1997; 349(9053): 675–82. Erratum in *Lancet* 349(9067), 1776.

5. Julian, D.G., Camm, A.J., Frangin, G., et al. (1997). Randomised trial of effect of amiodarone on mortality in patients with left-ventricular dysfunction after recent myocardial infarction: EMIAT. European Myocardial Infarct Amiodarone Trial Investigators. *Lancet* 1997; 349(9053): 667–74. Erratum in *Lancet* 1997; 349(9059): 1180, *Lancet* 349(9067), 1776.

6. Kennedy, H.L. (1992). Ambulatory (Holter) electrocardiography technology. *Cardiol Clin* 10(3), 341–59.

7. Yan, G.X., Antzelevitch, C. (1999). Cellular basis for the Brugada syndrome and other mechanisms of arrhythmogenesis associated with ST-segment elevation. *Circulation* 100(15), 1660–1666.

8. Brugada, R., Brugada, J., Antzelevitch, C., et al. (2000). Sodium channel blockers identify risk for sudden death in patients with ST-segment elevation and right bundle branch block but structurally normal hearts. *Circulation* 101(5), 510–515.

9. Kennedy, H.L., Bavishi, N.S., & Buckingham, T.A. (1992). Ambulatory (Holter) electrocardiography signal-averaging: A current perspective. *Am Heart J* 124(5), 1339–1346.

10. Crawford, M.H., Bernstein, S.J., Deedwania, P.C. et al. (1999). ACC/AHA Guidelines for Ambulatory Electrocardiography. A report of the American College of Cardiology/ American Heart Association Task Force on Practice Guidelines (Committee to Revise the Guidelines for Ambulatory Electrocardiography). Developed in collaboration with the North American Society for Pacing and Electrophysiology. *J Am Coll Cardiol* 34(3), 912–948.

11. Kennedy H.L. and Podrig P.J., Role of Holter monitoring and exercise testing for arrhythmia assessment and management. In: Podrig PJ, Kowey PR, eds. *Cardiac Arrythmia*, 2nd edn. Lippincott, Williams & Wilkins. Philadelphia, PA. 2001, 168.

12. Kennedy, H.L., & Wiens, R.D. (1987). Ambulatory (Holter) electrocardiography using real-time analysis. *Am J Cardiol* 59(12), 1190–1195.

13. Hasin, Y., Freiman, I., & Gotsman, M.S. (1984). Two-channel ECG monitoring in the coronary care unit. *Clin Cardiol* 7(2), 102–108.

14. Aly, A.F., Afchine, D., Esser, P., et al. (2000). Telemetry as a new concept in long term monitoring of SIDS-risk infant. *Eur J Med Res* 5(1), 19–22.

15. Reiffel, J.A., Schulhof, E., Joseph, B., et al. (1991). Optimum duration of transtelephonic ECG monitoring when used for transient symptomatic event detection. *J Electrocardiol* 24(2), 165–168.

16. Linzer, M., Pritchett, E.L., Pontinen, M., et al. (1990). Incremental diagnostic yield of loop electrocardiographic recorders in unexplained syncope. *Am J Cardiol* 66(2), 214–219.

17. https://www.medtronic.com/patients/fainting/device/our-insertable-cardiac-monitors/reveal-linq-icm/

18. Krasnow, A.Z., & Bloomfield, D.K. (1976). Artifacts in portable electrocardiographic monitoring. *Am Heart J* 91(3), 349–357.

19. Report of Committee on Electrocardiography, American Heart Association. (1967) Recommendations for standardization of leads and of specifications for instruments in electrocardiography and vectorcardiography. *Circulation* 35(3), 583–602.

20. Stein, I.M., Plunkett, J., & Troy, M. (1980). Comparison of techniques for examining long-term ECG recordings. *Med Instrum* 14(1), 69–72.

21. Knoebel, S.B., Lovelace, D.E., Rasmussen, S., & Wash, S.E. (1976). Computer detection of premature ventricular complexes: A modified approach. *Am J Cardiol* 38(4), 440–447.

22. Kadish, A.H., Buxton, A.E., Kennedy, H.L., et al. (2001). American College of Cardiology/ American Heart Association/American College of Physicians–American Society of Internal Medicine Task Force; International Society for Holter and Noninvasive Electrocardiology. ACC/AHA clinical competence statement on electrocardiography and ambulatory electrocardiography: A report of the ACC/AHA/ACP–ASIM task force on clinical competence (ACC/AHA Committee to develop a clinical competence statement on electrocardiography and ambulatory electro-cardiography) endorsed by the International Society for Holter and noninvasive electro-cardiology. *Circulation* 104(25), 3169–3178.

23. Kennedy, H.L., & Underhill, S.J. (1975). Electrocardiographic recognition of ventricular ectopic beats in lead V1—a preliminary report. *Heart Lung* 4(6), 921–926.

24. Cristal, N., Gueron, M., & Hoffman, R. (1972). Vi-like and VF-like leads for continuous electrocardiographic monitoring. *Br Heart J* 34(7), 696–698.

25. Hinkle, L.E. Jr. (1985). The role of long-term ambulatory electrocardiography and computer-assisted techniques in the identification of cardiac arrhythmias. *Cardiovasc Clin* 16(1), 139–49.

26. Enseleit, F., & Duru, F. (2006). Long-term continuous external electrocardiographic recording: A review. *Europace* 8(4), 255–266.

27. Kinlay, S., Leitch, J.W., Neil, A., et al. (1996). Cardiac event recorders yield more diagnoses and are more cost-effective than 48-hour Holter monitoring in patients with palpitations. A controlled clinical trial. *Ann Intern Med* 124(1 Pt 1), 16–20.

BRADYARRHYTHMIA

BRADYCARDIA

Shiv Bagga and Mandeep Bhargava

CONTENTS

BRADYCARDIA—PATHOPHYSIOLOGY

Bradyarrhythmias and conduction blocks are common electrocardiographic findings. These arrhythmias can result from a wide variety of disorders of the cardiac conduction system. Bradycardias are generally divided into disorders involving either the sinus node or atrioventricular conduction or as neurally mediated arrhythmias. Bradyarrhythmias may be discovered as incidental electrocardiographic abnormalities or may be found after investigation for symptoms suggestive of their presence. A wide variety of symptoms may be caused by the different etiologies of bradycardia, often times adding diagnostic difficulty to patients with coexisting medical problems.

DISORDERS OF THE SINUS NODE

Sinus node dysfunction (SND) includes a spectrum of heart rhythm disturbances related to abnormal sinus impulse formation and/or propagation with a wide array of electrocardiographic presentations such as inappropriate sinus bradycardia, sinus arrest, sinoatrial exit block, and tachycardia–bradycardia syndrome.[1-3] In other words, SND manifests primarily as inappropriate heart rate responses for a given level of exertion; known as chronotropic incompetence (CI).[4,5] The clinical presentation may include fatigue, dyspnea, poor effort intolerance, dizziness, or frank syncope while palpitations may be the primary complaint in patients with tachycardia–bradycardia syndrome. The most common etiology of sinus node dysfunction includes idiopathic degenerative disease with the incidence increasing with age. Other intrinsic factors include coronary disease, hypertension, and infiltrative disorders. Extrinsic factors include drug effects, autonomic influences, and electrolyte imbalances.

Sinus bradycardia exists in an adult when the sinus node discharges less than 60 beats per minute (bpm). This occurs normally in young adults from vagal tone or in older individuals from medications or underlying sinus node dysfunction. During sleep, the normal heart rate can decrease to 35–40 bpm with marked sinus arrhythmia and asymptomatic pauses. In contrast bradycardia due to SND is typically observed even during the day, with minimal or no variation during physical activities. Slowing of sinus rate allows for the emergence of low-frequency atrial ectopic rhythms with similar or slightly higher rate. This phenomenon of wandering pacemaker may even be seen in normal subjects during vagal hypertonia.

Sinus arrest, or sinus pause, is a disorder of automaticity in which no impulses are generated within the sinus node and may last from seconds to several minutes. The length of the pause is not an exact multiple of the P–P interval, suggesting that the mechanism is loss of automaticity of sinus node and not conduction block. On the contrary, a third-degree sinoatrial (SA) block is a disorder of sinus impulse conduction and electrocardiographically manifests as a sudden pause with the pause being an exact multiple of the basic P–P interval. However it must be emphasized that, this condition can be diagnosed only when the sinus rate is relatively regular before and after the pause. SA exit block can be divided into type I (SA Wenkebach), type II (SA Mobitz II), and high-degree SA block (Figure 4.1). Type I SA block can be recognized electrocardiographically as a group beating of P waves with shortening of the P–P intervals and pauses that amount to less than twice the shortest P–P cycle. In contrast, type II SA block demonstrates intermittent failure of conduction of the sinus impulse to the atrium as manifested by fixed PP intervals with pauses that equal twice the P–P interval. Type II SA exit block with a 2:1 periodicity, manifests as an alternant sequence of shorter and longer P–P cycles, with the longer measuring the double of the shorter cycles.

SND may contribute or coexist with atrial tachyarrhythmias, mainly atrial fibrillation, what is commonly referred to as the tachycardia–bradycardia syndrome.[3] Pauses are often observed after cessation of tachycardia, posing difficulty in pharmacologically managing the tachyarrhythmia. Atrial fibrillation is likely associated with SND due to the increased dispersion of refractoriness or early after depolarizations (EADs) occurring in the setting of bradycardia. Atrioventricular (AV) conduction disturbances occur in approximately half of patients with SND. Marked first-degree AV block at long sinus cycle lengths or slow ventricular rates in absence of AV nodal blocking medications in patients with atrial flutter or fibrillation should alert one to the presence of diffuse conduction system disease.

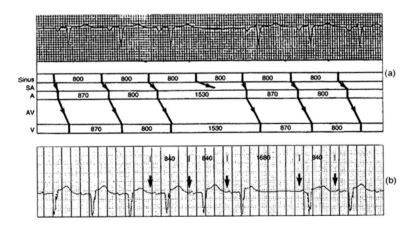

Figure 4.1 (a) SA Wenkebach with 4:3 conduction to the atrium. The PP interval is greatest in the initial cycle with subsequent decrease in PP interval until block in the atrium. (b) Mobitz II block—no change in the PP interval is seen prior to a dropped P-wave. (Reprinted from *The ECG in Emergency Decision Making*, 2nd edition, Wellens, H.J.J., Saunders Elsevier, Copyright 2006, with permission from Elsevier.)

The most common etiologies of AV conduction disturbances include fibrosis, degeneration of the conduction system, ischemia, and drugs. In the young, the most common etiology is congenital AV block or AV block from surgery for congenital heart disease. Among the elderly, idiopathic fibrosis and calcification of the conduction system is a frequent cause. Ischemic heart disease accounts for approximately one-third of cases of AV block, either the result of chronic coronary disease or myocardial ischemia. AV nodal conduction disturbances are seen frequently in acute coronary syndromes (described below). Lev's disease refers to the sclerotic process that is seen in older individuals involving the fibrous ring. Associated echocardiographic findings include calcification of the mitral and aortic valves. Though advanced AV conduction abnormalities are uncommon in young or middle-aged adults, coronary artery disease, autoimmune disorders such as systemic lupus erythematosus or rheumatoid arthritis, acute or chronic infectious or hypersensitivity myocarditis, infiltrative processes, hypothyroidism, congenital cardiomyopathies such as left ventricular noncompaction or Ebstein anomaly, Lamin AC mutations, and pathologic hypervagotony and idiopathic degenerative scleroatrophy of the AV junctional specialized tissue (Lenegre's disease) are among the most frequent etiologies in this age group of patients and warrant a thorough evaluation for the etiology of AV conduction disease in this age group before proceeding with pacemaker implantation.[6] A comprehensive list of causes of AV conduction disorders is given in Table 4.1.

Table 4.1   Etiologies of atrioventricular conduction disorders

Drug effects
Diagoxin
Beta-blockers
Non-dihydropyridine calcium-channel blockers
Membrane-active anti-arrythmic drugs
Ischemic heart disease
Acute myocardial infarction
Chronic coronary artery disease
Idiopathic fibrosis of the conduction system
Lenègre's disease
Lev's disease
Congenital heart disease
Congenital complete heart block
Ostium primum atrial septal defect
Transposition of the great vessels
Maternal systemic lupus erythematosus
Calcific valvular disease
Cardiomyopathy
Infiltrative disease
Amyloidosis
Sarcoidosis
Hemochromatosis
Infectious and inflammatory diseases
Endocarditis
Myocarditis (Chagas diseases, Lyme disease, rheumatic fever, tuberculosis, measles, mumps)
Collagen vascular diseases (Scleroderma, rheumatoid arthritis, Reiter's syndrome, systemic lupus erythematosus, ankylosing spondylitis, polymyositis)
Metabolic
Hyperkalemia
Hypermagnesemia
Endocrine: Addison's disease

(Continued)

Table 4.1 (*Continued*) Etiologies of atrioventricular conduction disorders

Trauma
Cardiac surgery
Radiation
Catheter trauma
Catheter ablation
Tumors
Mesothelioma
Hodgkin's disease
Malignant melanoma
Rhabdomyosarcoma
Neurally mediated
Carotid sinus syndrome
Vasovagal syncope
Neuromyopathic disorders
Myotonic muscular dystrophy
Slowly progressive X-linked muscular dystrophy

Source: Reprinted from *Textbook of Cardiovascular Medicine*, 1st edition, Topol, E.T., Lippincott-Raven, Philadelphia, PA, Copyright 1998, with permission from Elsevier.

AV conduction disturbances are classified as first-, second-, or third-degree (complete) block and these can occur at various levels in the AV conduction system. First-degree AV block is a misnomer in that every P-wave is conducted to the ventricles, however with an abnormal prolongation of the PR interval (greater than 0.20 s). Though a prolonged PR conduction may be the result of conduction delay within the atrium, AV node, His bundle, or bundle branches, it is usually secondary to delay at the level of AV node.

Second-degree AV block is characterized by a failure of one or more atrial impulses to reach the ventricles and is further sub-classified as type I and type II which define the electrocardiographic pattern rather than the anatomical site of block. Type I second-degree AV block or Wenkebach pattern is defined as the occurrence of a single non-conducted sinus P wave associated with inconstant PR intervals before and after the blocked impulse provided there are at least two consecutive conducted P waves (i.e., 3:2 AV block) to determine behavior of the PR interval.[7] The term inconstant PR interval is important because the majority of type I sequences are atypical and do not conform to the traditional teaching about the mathematical behavior of the PR intervals.[7] The PR intervals may shorten or stabilize and show no discernible or measurable change anywhere in a type I sequence. The description of "progressive" prolongation of the PR interval is misleading because PR intervals may shorten or stabilize and show no discernible or measurable change anywhere in a type I sequence. Indeed, atypical type I patterns in their terminal portion can exhibit a number of consecutive PR intervals showing no discernible change before the single blocked beat. However, even in such cases the post-block PR interval is always shorter. Slowing or an increase of the sinus rate does not interfere with the diagnosis of type I block.

It must be emphasized that a type I second-degree AV electrocardiographic pattern does not necessarily localizes the site of conduction disturbance to the AV node. Type I second-degree AV block with narrow QRS is practically AV nodal. An intra-Hisian site of block should be suspected in the presence of a narrow QRS if the block shows a paradoxical improvement in conduction with carotid pressure or fails to improve with isoproterenol or atropine. Although uncommon, type I second-degree AV block with bundle branch block (BBB) is due to conduction delay in the His Purkinje system (HPS) in 60%–70% of cases.[8]

The definition of type II second-degree AV block continues to be problematic in clinical practice.[7] It is defined as the occurrence of a single non-conducted sinus P wave associated with constant PR intervals before and after the blocked impulse, provided the sinus rate or the P–P interval is constant and there are at least two consecutive conducted P waves (i.e., 3:2 AV block) to determine behavior of the PR interval. The pause encompassing the blocked P wave should equal two (P–P) cycles. The diagnosis of type II block is incomplete unless there is a statement about the unchanged PR interval of the first conducted beat after the blocked impulse.[7] Stability of the sinus rate is an important criterion because a vagal surge can cause simultaneous sinus slowing and AV nodal block, generally a benign condition that can superficially resemble Type II second-degree AV block.

Regardless of QRS duration, type II second-degree AV block is always infra-nodal (intra or infra-Hisian) and often is associated with a bundle branch block pattern.[7,9] When confronted with a pattern that appears to be type II with a narrow QRS complex (especially in Holter recordings), one must consider the possibility of type I block without discernible or measurable increments in the PR intervals.[7] In addition, sinus slowing with AV block rules out type II block and indicates a vagally-induced AV block as it is unlikely that a disease process will suddenly involve two levels of the conduction system simultaneousl.[7] Type II second-degree AV block often progresses to complete AV block and can manifest as syncope. When development of this type of block with new bundle branch block is seen in association with anterior myocardial infarction, it implies a proximal left anterior descending artery occlusion.

When AV conduction occurs in a 2:1 pattern, the block cannot be classified unequivocally as type I or type II, as it is essential to have two consecutive conducted P waves to characterize second-degree AV block in terms of type I or type II block. The site of the lesion in 2:1 AV block can often be determined by seeking the company that the 2:1 AV block keeps. An association with either type I or type II second-degree AV block helps localization of the lesion. Outside of an acute myocardial infarction, sustained 2:1 AV block with a wide QRS complex occurs in the HPS in 80% of cases and emphasizes the fact that 2:1 AV block with bundle branch block may not always be infra-nodal.[10] In general, a 2:1 AV block with a normal width QRS and/or a P–R interval greater than 300 ms localizes the conduction delay to the level of AV node but nearly a third of 2:1 AV blocks with narrow QRS complex are due to intra-Hisian delay.[8] The response to a change in vagal tone is a less reliable but occasionally helpful indicator of location of the site of block, since vagal tone affects AV nodal tissue far greater than the HPS. Maneuvers such as Valsalva and carotid sinus massage, which enhance vagal tone thereby decreasing AV nodal conduction, are expected to worsen AV nodal block but improve infra-nodal block because a slowed AV nodal conduction allow the refractory His Purkinje tissue more time to recover, thereby improving the transmission of supraventricular impulses (Figure 4.2). The reflex use of atropine in 2:1 AV block is strongly discouraged.[10] In HPS disease, atropine increases the sinus rate without a concomitant improvement in infra-nodal conduction and may thus aggravate the degree of AV block. In general, an asymptomatic patient with sustained 2:1 AV block and equivocal response to the above said maneuvers may merit an EP study to elucidate the site of conduction delay and hence the need for pacemaker therapy.

Not all atrial impulses that fail to conduct to the ventricles are necessarily second-degree AV block. If an atrial impulse reaches the AV junction early enough in the cycle while the node is refractory, the impulse is not conducted. This is a common scenario seen with early premature atrial complexes (PACs). Block, which infers pathology of conduction, is an incorrect description of this phenomenon. Likewise, 2:1 conduction, rather than block, is a more apt description of atrial flutter that conducts to the ventricles in this pattern.

Advanced second-degree AV block refers to the blocking of two or more consecutive P waves with some conducted beats indicating some preservation of AV conduction but nevertheless carries an ominous prognosis. On the other hand, third-degree AV block (complete heart block) signifies absence of AV conduction. Block can occur in either the AV node or HPS. The site of block can be somewhat inferred by the nature of the escape rhythm, with narrow QRS escape complexes and rates greater than 40 bpm suggestive of block in the AV node or proximal His. Conversely, block within the distal His or the branching structures will manifest as wide QRS escape complexes with slower rates. Third-degree heart block may be acquired or congenital. Congenital third-degree AV block occurs in approximately 1 in

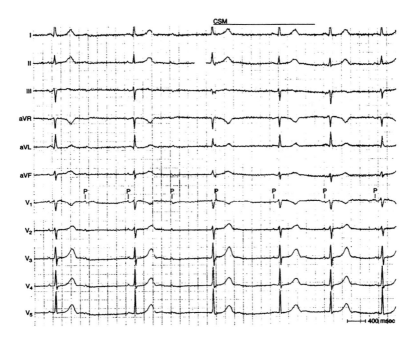

Figure 4.2 Improvement in AV conduction with carotid sinus pressure. Two-to-one AV block improves to one-to-one AV block with prolongation of the cycle length, indicating His Purkinje disease. (Reprinted from *The ECG in Emergency Decision Making*, 2nd edition, Wellens, H.J.J., Saunders Elsevier, Copyright 2006, with permission from Elsevier.)

20,000 children. In over half, AV block is discovered as a result of bradycardia in utero or neonatally and is secondary to maternal lupus in over 90% of cases. Mortality in AV block from neonatal lupus tends to be high. When AV block is diagnosed later in childhood, maternal lupus is rarely responsible and etiologies include structural heart defects and myocarditis. Initially, AV block may be transient but most often progresses to permanent AV block with junctional escape.

INTRAVENTRICULAR CONDUCTION DISTURBANCES

Intraventricular conduction disturbances (IVCDs) occur below the AV node and do not in themselves result in bradyarrhythmias. Conduction delay can occur anywhere along the HPS and etiologies are similar to those causing AV block. The most common etiologies include idiopathic fibrosis and ischemia. IVCDs are more commonly seen in structurally abnormal hearts. These are generally classified by the number of fascicles affected. The HPS is a trifascicular system, with bifascicular block referring to conduction delay within either both the right bundle and left anterior or posterior fascicle or the left bundle branch in itself. Chronic bifascicular block in asymptomatic patients has a low risk of progression to AV block; however, in the setting of an anterior infarction and new bifascicular block, the risk is substantial. Once a diagnosis of bifascicular block is made, maintenance of AV conduction hinges on the continuing integrity of the remaining third fascicle.

The term, trifascicular block is a confusing description often applied loosely to describe the electrocardiographic (ECG) pattern of prolonged PR interval in association with bifascicular block. In true sense, trifascicular block is present when bifascicular block is associated with a prolonged His-Ventricular (HV) interval. A prolonged PR interval does not identify patients who have prolonged HV intervals in such cases. In fact, nearly half of patients with bifascicular block and prolonged PR intervals have prolongation of the Atrial-His (AH) interval (i.e., AV nodal conduction time). A strict definition of trifascicular block is block documented in all three fascicles, whether simultaneously or at different times. Thus the term, trifascicular block should be applied only to the ECG patterns of alternating RBBB and LBBB or RBBB with intermittent LAFB and LPFB. These patients are at high risk for progression to sudden development of complete AV block and have a class I indications for permanent pacing, even in asymptomatic individuals.

PAROXYSMAL AV BLOCK

Paroxysmal AV block, an unusual but formidable form of conduction block, occurs when one-to-one conduction abruptly changes to complete AV block. Thus it is the onset of a paroxysm of high-grade AV block associated with a period of ventricular asystole before conduction returns or a subsidiary pacemaker escapes. In recent times three different types of paroxysmal AV blocks have been recognized. Intrinsic paroxysmal AV block due to a sudden pause-dependent phase 4 AV block occurring in diseased conduction tissue, extrinsic vagal paroxysmal AV block occurring in association with vagal reactions and idiopathic paroxysmal AV block with its distinct clinical presentation characterized by a long history of recurrent syncope without prodromes, absence of cardiac and ECG abnormalities, absence of progression to persistent forms of AV block, and efficacy of cardiac pacing therapy.[11–13]

Intrinsic paroxysmal AV block is regarded as a manifestation of an intrinsic disease of the AV conduction system (Stokes–Adams attack) and is usually initiated by atrial, His, or ventricular premature extrasystole.[11] This may manifest either as tachycardia-dependent AV block in the HPS (also called phase 3 or voltage-dependent block) during or after exertion or as an abrupt onset of bradycardia or AV block after a pause (phase 4 block).[14] Paroxysmal AV block in these patients is a marker for His Purkinje disease with an unpredictable escape mechanism. The outcome is characterized by a rapid progression toward permanent AV block.[11]

CONDUCTION ABNORMALITIES AFTER MYOCARDIAL INFARCTION

Both bradyarrhythmias and conduction disturbances can be seen with myocardial infarctions and are generally related to ischemia or autonomic disturbance. The clinical features and management of bradyarrhythmias and conduction block depend on the location of the infarction. The right coronary artery supplies the SA node in 60% of people and the left circumflex the remaining. In over 90% of people, the RCA feeds the AV node and proximal His. The terminal portion of the His bundle and the main left bundle and the right bundle branch are supplied by septal perforators of the LAD.[15] Sinus bradycardia, prolonged PR conduction with Wenkebach, and complete heart block are common in inferior myocardial infarctions (IMIs). Complete AV block occurs in approximately 10% of patients with IMI. This rarely occurs suddenly, being most often seen with prolonged PR conduction gradually progressing to complete AV block. AV block occurs within the node in over 90% of cases and typically results in a transient block. The escape complex is usually narrow and infrequently requires pacing. Bradyarrhythmias occurring in the setting of inferior infarctions are generally responsive to atropine. With anterior infarctions, conduction disturbances are not as benign and are related to the size of the infarction. The development of fascicular or bundle branch block is correlated to the size of infarct.[16] Complete AV block in anterior MI can occur abruptly in the first 24 h, developing without warning. AV block may also be preceded by the development of an intraventricular conduction disturbance or by type II second-degree block. Complete heart block occurs secondary to necrosis of the distal His and bundle branches within the septum. Escape complexes are unstable and have a wide QRS, thereby necessitating permanent pacing When AV block occurs with anterior infarctions, mortality is greatly increased.

In patients with AV block in the setting of an acute anterior wall MI, the major determinant of the need for permanent pacing beyond symptomatic bradycardia is the presence of intraventricular conduction defects. Patients who demonstrate bundle branch block have an unfavorable prognosis and a higher risk of sudden death. Although these patients may be at risk for serious bradyarrhythmias in the post-hospitalization period, their adverse prognosis is not necessarily related to the development of high-grade AV block. These patients are at high risk for other post-MI complications, including pump failure and ventricular tachyarrhythmias. In the contemporary practice, most patients with acute anterior wall MI with AV block and BBB have LV dysfunction and thus are eligible for implantation of an implantable cardioverter-defibrillator for primary prevention of sudden death. Often, they may even be candidates for a cardiac resynchronization device.

NEURALLY MEDIATED BRADYCARDIA

Autonomic stimulation can lead to sinus node slowing or AV nodal blockade in the absence of sinus or AV node dysfunction. Neurocardiogenic syncope and carotid sinus hypersensitivity are the most common etiologies of autonomically mediated bradycardia.[17] Both occur in the setting of excess vagal tone and have similar clinical manifestations which include a cardioinhibitory response. This results from an increase in parasympathetic tone which can lead to sinus bradycardia, prolonged PR conduction, and second- and third-degree AV block. The pathophysiology involving the cardioinhibitory response in neurocardiogenic syncope is felt to result from an exaggerated response to a physiologic reflex. The syndrome begins with relative hypovolemia that triggers a sympathetic reflex with an increase in heart rate, myocardial contractility, and peripheral vasoconstriction. Increased contractility results in ventricular cavity obliteration which, in turn, generates pressure sensed by mechanoreceptors (c-fibers).[18,19] In predisposed individuals, this results in vasodepression and cardioinhibition manifested as hypotension and slowing of the sinus rate or AV nodal block, respectively.

POST-SURGICAL BRADYARRHYTHMIAS

Bradyarrhythmias following open heart surgery are common. Most commonly, AV block is seen following aortic and mitral valve surgery. Due to the lower position of the aortic valve, surgeries following this site result in an AV nodal block involving more often the infranodal portion of the AV junction and may often not resolve and need a permanent pacemaker. The mitral valve sits higher and surgeries at this site result in nodal blocks which are more likely to resolve spontaneously as the post-operative edema settles and are less likely to need a pacemaker. Multi-valvular surgeries have a higher risk of causing AV block than uni-valvular surgeries.

Septal myectomy invariably leads to resection of the left bundle and can often require permanent pacing secondary to subsequent AV block. Permanent pacing is required in 2%–3% of surgeries involving valve replacement and in approximately 10% of cardiac transplant recipients.[20] Sinus node dysfunction occurs in 50% of patients postoperatively resulting from prolonged donor ischemia or injury to the SA nodal artery. Injury to the SA node or artery can be avoided by performing bicaval, rather than atrial anastomosis. AV block is infrequently seen postoperatively in cardiac transplants.[20] The most frequent intraventricular conduction disturbance is right bundle branch block, likely secondary to repeated biopsies required in these patients.

POST TRANSCATHETER AORTIC VALVE REPLACEMENT BRADYARRHYTHMIAS

In recent years, transcatheter aortic valve replacement (TAVR) has become a well-accepted option for treating patients with aortic stenosis at intermediate to high surgical risk.[21-23] However, conduction disturbances, mainly new-onset LBBB and advanced AV block requiring permanent pacemaker implantation, remain the most common complication of this procedure. New-onset LBBB has been reported in about one-fourth of TAVR procedures using first generation valves with an increased incidence reported with implantation of self-expandable valves.[24,25] As compared to surgical aortic valve replacement, the incidence of complete heart block and pacemaker implantation has been higher than expected, with rates of implantation up to 25% being reported.[26-28] A recent study reported a high burden of arrhythmic events at 1-year follow-up in nearly one-half of patients with new onset LBBB, leading to a treatment change in more than one-third. Significant bradyarrhythmias were detected in 20% of the patients, with a permanent pacemaker required in nearly one-half of them.[29]

Conduction disturbances in the setting of TAVR, result primarily from a direct mechanical insult to the conduction system as well as association between aortic stenosis and conduction disturbances due to calcium deposition on the conduction system because of its proximity to the aortic valve complex.[30-32] In addition, inter-individual variability of the antero-posterior relationship of the AV node with respect to the apex of the triangle of Koch, as well as the length of the non-penetrating portion of the His bundle predisposes patients to a higher risk of TAVR-induced conduction disturbances.[33,34]

BRADYARRHYTHMIAS SECONDARY TO MEDICATIONS

Multiple cardiac medications are known to cause bradycardia. Beta-blockers, calcium-channel blockers, digoxin, and anti-arrhythmic medications include the most common agents. The mechanisms involve blockade of beta receptors or calcium channels resulting in slowing of sinus depolarization and AV conduction or alteration of autonomics. In patients presenting with drug-induced AV block, drug therapy can be stopped entirely, reduced in dosage, or continued if there is no acceptable alternative (permanent pacemaker is indicated in these circumstances). More recent data suggests that in the majority of patients presenting with presumed drug-induced AV block, discontinuation of the offending medications does not obviate the need for pacemaker implantation with nearly one-third of the patients having recurrence of AV block in those with initial resolution after discontinuation of the offending drug.[34,35] This indicates that the drugs may in fact be unmasking an already underlying AV conduction abnormality.

DIAGNOSTIC TESTING

Diagnostic testing for suspected bradyarrhythmias is generally limited to noninvasive methods. The initial work-up includes a 12-lead ECG followed by 24–48 h Holter monitoring. For patients with infrequent symptoms, an event monitor may be used to monitor the cardiac rhythm for up to 4 weeks. Implantable loop recorders are also available for prolonged continuous diagnostic monitoring. In instances where inappropriate sinus bradycardia is suspected, stress testing can be performed to assess chronotropic competence. Assessment of autonomic tone includes carotid sinus massage and tilt table testing. Carotid sinus pressure with concomitant ECG monitoring can be helpful in identifying patients with carotid sinus hypersensitivity. Pauses exceeding 3 s in response to carotid pressure are abnormal. Carotid sinus pressure should not precipitate sinus pauses, although slowing in the sinus rate or AV block can be normal responses. Tilt table testing can be helpful in differentiating bradycardia from sinus node disease and autonomic dysfunction. Bradycardic responses to tilt testing are the result of autonomic dysfunction.

Pharmacologic testing can also be useful in differentiating sinus node dysfunction from autonomic dysfunction. Autonomic blockade with atropine (0.4 mg/kg) and propranolol (0.2 mg/kg) can be used to determine the intrinsic heart rate (IHR), which represents the sinus node rate without autonomic influences. IHR can be calculated from the formula: $118 - (0.57^*age)$. Intrinsic sinus rates lower than the calculated value suggest sinus node dysfunction while sinus rates over this value represent autonomic dysfunction.

Electrophysiologic evaluation of bradyarrhythmias includes assessment of sinus node function and AV conduction. Sinus node function cannot be measured directly. The two most common tests for sinus node function measure SA function indirectly. Sinus node recovery time (SNRT) is the time taken for sinus rhythm to resume after 30 s of overdrive atrial pacing. This interval is measured in the high right atrium from the last paced beat to the first spontaneous sinus beat. A delay of longer than 1500 ms is abnormal. The corrected value (CSNRT) can be determined by subtracting the intrinsic sinus cycle length from the SNRT value. Values of CSNRT longer than 550 ms suggest sinus node dysfunction. The second indirect measurement of sinus node function is the sino-atrial conduction time (SACT). This technique is used for detecting delayed conduction between the sinus node and surrounding atrial tissue. This involves resetting the sinus node with atrial extra stimuli delivered in the high right atrium. After measurement of the intrinsic sinus rate, atrial extra stimuli are delivered during sinus rhythm over a range of coupling intervals (A1A2). Earlier coupled atrial extra stimuli invade and reset the sinus node. The interval of the returning sinus impulse following the atrial extra stimulus is measured and SACT is calculated as: (A2A3 – A1A1)/2. SACT values greater than 115 ms are considered abnormal.

BIBLIOGRAPHY

1. Ferrer, M.I. (1968). The sick sinus syndrome in atrial disease. *JAMA* 206, 645–646.

2. Ferrer MI. The sick sinus syndrome. *Circulation* 1973;47:635–641.

3. Short DS. The syndrome of alternating bradycardia and tachycardia. *Br Heart J* 1954;16:208–214.

4. Melzer C, & Dreger H. Chronotropic incompetence: A never-ending story. *Europace* 2010;12:464–465.

5. Brubaker PH, & Kitzman DW. Chronotropic incompetence causes, consequences, and management. *Circulation* 2011;123:1010–1020.

6. Barra SN, Providencia R, Pavia L, et al. A review on advanced atrioventricular block in young or middle-aged adults. *Pacing Clin Electrophysiol* 2012;35:1395–1405.

7. Barold SS, & Hayes DL. Second-degree atrioventricular block: A reappraisal. *Mayo Clin Proc* 2001;76:44–57.

8. Barold SS. Lingering misconceptions about type I second-degree atrioventricular block. *Am J Cardiol* 2001;88:1018–1020.

9. Barold SS, Herweg B, & Gallardo I. Acquired atrioventricular block: The 2002 ACC/AHA/NASPE guidelines for pacemaker implantation should be revised. *Pacing Clin Electrophysiol* 2003;26:531–533.

10. Barold SS. 2:1 Atrioventricular block: Order from chaos. *Am J Emerg Med.* 2001;19:214–217.

11. Lee S, Wellens HJJ, Josephson ME. Paroxysmal atrioventricular block. *Heart Rhythm* 2009;6:1229–1234.

12. Zysko D, Gajek J, Kozluk E, et al. Electrocardiographic characteristics of atrioventricular block induced by tilt testing. *Europace* 2009;11:225–230.

13. Brignole M, Deharo JC, Roy LD, et al. Syncope due to idiopathic paroxysmal AV block. Long term follow-up of a distinct form of atrioventricular block. *J Am Coll Cardiol* 2011;58:168–173.

14. El-Sherif N, Jalife J. Paroxysmal atrioventricular block: Are phase 3 and phase 4 block mechanisms or misnomers? *Heart Rhythm* 2009;6:1514–1521.

15. Lei KI, Wellens HJ, Schuilenburg RM. Bundle branch block and acute myocardial infarction. In: Wellens HJ, Lie KI, Janse MJ, editors. *The Conduction System of the Heart: Structure, Function and Clinical Applications*. Philadelphia, PA: Lea and Febiger, 1976:666.

16. De Guzman M, Rahimtoola SH. What is the role of pacemakers in patients with coronary artery disease and conduction abnormalities? In: Rahimtoola SH, editor. *Controversies in Coronary Artery Disease*. Philadelphia, PA: Davis, 1983:191–207.

17. Colman N, Nahm K, Ganzeboom KS, et al. Epidemiology of reflex syncope. *Clin Auton Res* 2004;14(Suppl 1):9–17.

18. Kosinski D, Grubb BP, Temesy-Armos P. Pathophysiological aspects of neurocardiogenic syncope: Current concepts and new perspectives. *Pacing Clin Electrophysiol* 1995;18:716–724.

19. Mosqueda-Garcia R, Furlan R, Tank J, et al. The elusive pathophysiology of neutrally mediated syncope. *Circulation* 2000;102:2898–2906.

20. Chung MK. Cardiac surgery: Postoperative arrhythmias. *Crit Care Med* 2000;28 (suppl.):N136–N144.

21. Leon MB, Smith CR, Mack M, et al. PARTNER Trial Investigators. Transcatheter aortic-valve implantation for aortic stenosis in patients who cannot undergo surgery. *N Engl J Med* 2010;363:1597–1607.

22. Smith CR, Leon MB, Mack MJ, et al. PARTNER trial investigators. transcatheter versus surgical aortic-valve replacement in high-risk patients. *N Engl J Med* 2011;364:2187–2198.

23. Nishimura RA, Otto CM, Bonow RO, et al. American College of Cardiology/American Heart Association Task Force on Practice Guidelines. 2014 AHA/ACC guideline for the management of patients with valvular heart disease: Executive summary: A report of the American College of Cardiology/American Heart Association Task Force on Practice Guidelines. *J Am Coll Cardiol* 2014;63:2438–2488.

24. Vahanian A, Urena M, Walther T, et al. Thirty-day outcomes in patients at intermediate risk for surgery from the SAPIEN 3 European approval trial. *Euro Intervention* 2016;12:e235–e243.

25. Manoharan G, Linke A, Moellmann H, et al. Multicentre clinical study evaluating a novel resheathable annular functioning self-expanding transcatheter aortic valve system: Safety and performance results at 30 days with the Portico system. *Euro Intervention* 2016;12:768–774.

26. Guetta V, Goldenberg G, Segev A, et al. Predictors and course of high-degree atrioventricular block after transcatheter aortic valve implantation using the core valve revalving system. *Am J Cardiol* 2011;108:1600–1605.

27. Toggweiler S, Stortecky S, Holy E, et al. The electrocardiogram after transcatheter aortic valve replacement determines the risk for post-procedural high-degree AV block and the need for telemetry monitoring. *JACC Cardiovasc Interv* 2016;9:1269–1276.

28. Fadahunsi OO, Olowoyeye A, Ukaigwe A, et al. Incidence, predictors, and outcomes of permanent pacemaker implantation following transcatheter aortic valve replacement: Analysis from the US Society of Thoracic Surgeons/American College of Cardiology TVT Registry. *JACC Cardiovasc Interv* 2016;9:2189–2199.

29. Rodes-Cabau J, Urena M, Nombela-Franco L, et al. Arrhythmic burden in patients with new-onset LBBB post-TAVR. *JACC Cardiovasc Interv* 2018;11:1495–1505.

30. Moreno R, Dobarro D, López de Sá E, et al. Cause of complete atrioventricular block after percutaneous aortic valve implantation: Insights from a necropsy study. *Circulation* 2009;120:e29–e30.

31. MacMillan RM, Demorizi NM, Gessman LJ, Maranhao V. Correlates of prolonged HV conduction in aortic stenosis. *Am Heart J* 1985;110:56–60.

32. Urena M, Hayek S, Cheema AN, et al. Arrhythmia burden in elderly patients with severe aortic stenosis as determined by continuous electrocardiographic recording: Toward a better understanding of arrhythmic events after transcatheter aortic valve replacement. *Circulation* 2015;131:469–477.

33. Kawashima T, Sato F. Visualizing anatomical evidences on atrioventricular conduction system for TAVI. *Int J Cardiol* 2014;174:1–6.

34. Hamdan A, Guetta V, Klempfner R, et al. Inverse relationship between membranous septal length and the risk of atrioventricular block in patients undergoing transcatheter aortic valve implantation. *JACC Cardiovasc Interv* 2015;8:1218–1228.

35. Zeltser D, Justo D, Halkin A, et al. Drug-induced atrioventricular block: Prognosis after discontinuation of the culprit drug. *J Am Coll Cardiol* 2004;44:105–108.

36. Osmonov D, Erdinler I, Ozcan KS, et al. Management of patients with drug-induced atrioventricular block. *Pacing Clin Electrophysiol* 2012;35:804–810.

37. Wellens HJJ. *The ECG in Emergency Decision Making*, 2nd ed., St. Louis, MO: Saunders Elsevier, 2006.

38. Topol ET. *Textbook of Cardiovascular Medicine*, 1st ed. Philadelphia, PA: Lippincott-Raven, 1998.

INDICATIONS FOR PERMANENT PACING AND CARDIAC RESYNCHRONIZATION THERAPY

Shiv Bagga, J. David Burkhardt, and Mandeep Bhargava

CONTENTS

INTRODUCTION

Since the initial publication of the American College of Cardiology (ACC) and the American Heart Association (AHA) guidelines for device based therapy in 1984, the indications for pacemaker therapy have increased over recent years and now include both the treatment of bradyarrhythmias and heart failure. These guidelines were most recently revised in 2008 in conjunction with the Heart Rhythm Society (HRS) with a focused update published in 2012.[1] The guidelines are based on the concept of evidence based medicine and strive to guide patient care on the basis of the best available clinical trial data. The guidelines rank the strength of evidence in a standard ACC/AHA format by class complimented by a grading system based on the relative benefit versus risk as a statement of certainty of treatment effect. These guidelines discuss indications for pacing in patients with bradycardia due to sinus node and acquired atrioventricular (AV) dysfunction, chronic bifascicular and trifascicular block, hypersensitive carotid sinus, and neurally mediated syndromes as well as pacing for hemodynamic indications including cardiac resynchronization therapy for heart failure. This chapter will also introduce the concept of His bundle pacing and pacing in post TAVR patients.

SINUS NODE DYSFUNCTION

Sinus node dysfunction (SND) includes a spectrum of heart rhythm disturbances related to abnormal sinus impulse formation and/or propagation with a wide array of electrocardiographic presentations such as inappropriate sinus bradycardia, sinus arrest, sino-atrial exit block, and tachycardia–bradycardia syndrome. Another manifestation of sinus node dysfunction frequently encountered is chronotropic incompetence (CI), which is broadly defined as an inadequate sinus rate response to stress or exercise. These patients may not exhibit evidence of SND at rest; however, symptoms of fatigue and dyspnea occur reproducibly with exertion.

The non-specificity of symptoms, especially in elderly as well as intermittency of symptoms and electrocardiographic features of SND make it difficult to establish a cause–effect relationship in many cases. In addition, there is a great deal of disagreement about the absolute heart rate or length of pause required before pacing is indicated. The guidelines emphasize the importance of documenting the presence of "symptomatic" bradycardia in patients with SND. Correlation of episodic bradycardia with symptoms compatible with cerebral hypoperfusion is imperative when deciding whether a permanent pacemaker is indicated or not. Work-up should start with a 12-lead electrocardiogram (ECG), followed by a 24- to 48-h ambulatory monitoring or an event monitor in case extended monitoring is required. Implantable loop recorders increase the diagnostic yield for patients with infrequent events and in fact, this approach has been shown in selected patients to be more cost-effective than a strategy of serial non-invasive studies followed by invasive studies.

Finally if non-invasive tests fail to make a diagnosis, invasive electrophysiological (EP) study to evaluate sinus node function may be rarely be considered. However, these studies are limited by low sensitivity and specificity and the variable significance of the abnormalities revealed. The severity of chronotropic incompetence can be diagnosed and documented with the use of an exercise stress test. Most clinicians would define CI as an inability to achieve 80% of the maximal age predicted heart rate, generally calculated using the Astrand's formula, i.e., 220 minus age.

The natural history of untreated SND may be highly variable. The majority of patients with history of syncope because of SND will have recurrent syncope, while in others, symptomatic SND may be separated by long periods of normal sinus node function. The mean annual incidence of complete AV block based on data from patients implanted with single-chamber atrial pacemakers for SND is 0.6% (range 0%–4.5%) with an overall prevalence of 2.1% (range 0%–11.9%).[2] The incidence of sudden death is low and SND very rarely affects survival regardless of whether or not it is treated with a pacemaker. Hence, the main rationale for permanent pacing in the setting of SND is symptomatic bradycardia with its attendant risk of injuries, especially in elderly.

Symptomatic bradycardia is defined by the ACC/AHA/HRS document as a documented bradyarrhythmia that is directly responsible for development of the clinical manifestations of syncope or near syncope, transient dizziness or light headedness, or confusional states resulting from cerebral hypoperfusion attributable to slow heart rate. Fatigue, exercise intolerance, and congestive heart failure may also result from bradycardia. These symptoms may occur at rest or with exertion. As alluded to above, direct correlation of the symptoms to the bradycardia must be established. The indications for implantation of a PM for SND based on the evidence based guidelines are listed below.

- Class I
  - (1) Sinus node dysfunction with documented symptomatic bradycardia, including frequent sinus pauses that produce symptoms *(Level of Evidence: C)*
  - (2) Symptomatic chronotropic incompetence *(Level of Evidence: C)*
  - (3) Symptomatic sinus bradycardia that results from required drug therapy for medical conditions *(Level of Evidence: C)*
- Class IIa
  - (1) Reasonable for sinus node dysfunction with heart rate less than 40 bpm when a clear association between significant symptoms consistent with bradycardia and the actual presence of bradycardia has not been documented *(Level of Evidence: C)*
  - (2) Reasonable for syncope of unexplained origin when clinically significant abnormalities of sinus node function are discovered or provoked in electrophysiological studies *(Level of Evidence: C)*

- Class IIb
  (1) May be considered in minimally symptomatic patients with chronic heart rate less than 40 bpm while awake *(Level of Evidence: C)*
- Class III
  (1) Sinus node dysfunction in asymptomatic patients *(Level of Evidence: C)*
  (2) Sinus node dysfunction in patients whom the symptoms suggestive of bradycardia have been clearly documented to occur in the absence of bradycardia *(Level of Evidence: C)*
  (3) Sinus node dysfunction with symptomatic bradycardia due to non-essential drug therapy *(Level of Evidence: C)*

ATRIOVENTRICULAR BLOCK

AV block is classified as first-, second-, or third-degree (complete) block; anatomically, it can occur at various levels in the AV conduction system; above the His bundle (supra-His), within the His bundle (intra-His), and below the bundle of His (infra-His). The site of AV block largely determines the adequacy and reliability of the underlying escape rhythm and hence the need for a permanent pacemaker. First-degree AV block is defined as abnormal prolongation of the PR interval (greater than 0.20 s) and is usually secondary to delay at the level of AV node. Pacing for patients with first-degree AV block is rarely an indication unless the patient has symptoms suggestive of pacemaker syndrome. This has been found in patients with marked (PR greater than 300 ms) first-degree AV block (Class IIb indication).[3]

Second-degree AV block is sub-classified as type I and type II which define the electrocardiographic pattern rather than the anatomical site of block. It must be emphasized that type I second-degree AV block should not be automatically labeled as AV nodal without mention of QRS duration. Type I second-degree AV block with narrow QRS is practically AV nodal. This can be physiological, especially during sleep in normal individuals with high vagal tone and these people need no treatment. Asymptomatic type I second-degree AV block with narrow QRS is generally considered benign (Class III indication). His bundle recordings are unnecessary in an asymptomatic patient with type I second-degree AV block and a narrow QRS. However, an intra-Hisian site of block should be suspected in the presence of a narrow QRS if the block shows a paradoxical improvement in conduction with carotid pressure or fails to improve with isoproterenol or atropine. Although uncommon, type I second-degree AV block with BBB requires special consideration because the site of conduction delay could be in the His Purkinje system (HPS) in 60%–70% of cases.[4] A His bundle recording is thus required to confirm the site of block. Type II second-degree AV block, based on the strict electrocardiographic definition is always infranodal and an indication for pacing regardless of QRS duration, symptoms, or whether it is paroxysmal or chronic. When confronted with a pattern that appears to be type II with a narrow QRS complex (especially in Holter recordings), one must consider the possibility of type I block without discernible or measurable increments in the PR intervals. In addition, simultaneous sinus slowing with AV block (P–P prolongation along with PR prolongation) rules out type II block and indicates a vagally-induced AV block.[5]

When AV conduction occurs in a 2:1 pattern, the block cannot be classified unequivocally as type I or type II, as it is essential to have two consecutive conducted P waves to characterize second-degree AV block in terms of type I or type II block. The site of the lesion in 2:1 AV block can often be determined by seeking the company that the 2:1 AV block keeps. An association with either type I or type II second-degree AV block helps localization of the lesion.

Outside of an acute myocardial infarction, sustained 2:1 AV block with a wide QRS complex occurs in the HPS in 80% of cases and 20% in the AV node.[4,6] This data emphasizes the fact that 2:1 AV block with bundle branch block may not always be infranodal and hence not necessarily an indication for a pacemaker in an asymptomatic patient. In general, a 2:1 AV block with a normal QRS and/or a P–R interval greater than 300 ms is usually associated with delay at the level of AV node, nearly a third of 2:1 AV block with narrow QRS complex are due to intra-HIS delay. The response to a change in vagal tone is a less reliable but occasionally helpful indicator of the location of the AV block, since vagal tone affects AV nodal tissue far greater than the HPS. Maneuvers such as Valsalva and carotid sinus massage, which enhance vagal tone thereby decreasing AV nodal conduction, are expected to worsen AV nodal block but improve infra-nodal block because a slowed AV nodal conduction allow the refractory His Purkinje tissue more time to recover, thereby improving the transmission of supraventricular impulses. In general, an asymptomatic patient with sustained 2:1 AV block and equivocal response to the above said maneuvers may merit an EP study to elucidate the site of conduction delay and hence the need for pacemaker therapy. The reflex use of atropine in 2:1 AV blocks is discouraged, as it increases the sinus rate and accelerates AV node conduction without giving an opportunity for the diseased HPS to recover from refractoriness, thereby worsening the AV conduction.

Advanced second-degree AV block refers to the lack of conduction of two or more consecutive P waves with some conducted beats, which indicates some preservation of AV conduction and not a complete heart block. In the setting of atrial fibrillation, a prolonged pause (e.g., greater than 5 s) should be considered a manifestation of advanced second-degree AV block (Class I indication). On the other hand third-degree AV block (complete heart block) is defined as complete absence of AV conduction. Third-degree AV block or complete heart block often presents with a wide QRS escape rhythm and symptomatically may manifest with fatigue, dyspnea, pre-syncope, or frank unheralded syncope. Rarely, ventricular fibrillation and torsades de pointes can result from marked bradycardia and prolonged pauses.

Similar to patients with SND, indications for pacing in patients with acquired AV block are also influenced by the presence or absence of symptoms. However, in patients with second-degree AV block, an intra or infra-Hisian site of conduction delay as discussed earlier, mandates pacing (class IIa indication) even if the patient is asymptomatic as these patients have a high risk of progression to third-degree AV block. Similarly, in patients with third-degree AV block, irrespective of the symptomatic status, it is the site of origin of the escape rhythm rather than an arbitrary escape rate cut-off which determines the stability of the rhythm and hence most of them need implantation of a permanent pacemaker. This is reflected in the guidelines by the fact that permanent cardiac pacing is strongly considered in patients with asymptomatic advanced or third-degree AV block. Last but not the least, potential reversible causes must be ruled out and corrected before deciding to implant a permanent pacemaker in a patient with AV block. One exception is drug-related AV block that has been shown to have a high recurrence rate even after discontinuation of the drug (Class IIb indication).[7,8]

Certain neuromuscular diseases (NMD) are associated with a high risk of unpredictable progression of AV conduction disease. Waiting for the development of complete AV block in these patients may expose them to significant risk of sudden death or syncope related to AV block. Permanent pacing should be considered early in the course of neuromuscular disease and should be offered to the asymptomatic patient once any conduction abnormality is noted (Class IIb indication). However a few of these NMDs are also associated with a higher risk of ventricular arrhythmias and sudden death so that an implantable cardioverter-defibrillator placement rather than a pacemaker may be a more reasonable option.[9] Another disease associated with a high risk of progressive conduction disturbances is cardiac sarcoidosis and a permanent pacemaker is generally warranted even if a patient has had transient AV block. Similar to NMDs, patients with cardiac sarcoid are at high risk for ventricular tachyarrhythmias and sudden death and an ICD implantation may be more appropriate based on recent expert consensus recommendations.[10]

Exercise induced AV block though relatively rare, usually indicates a diseased HPS (phase 3 or tachycardia-dependent AV block), is associated with poor prognosis and is a class I indication for permanent pacing even if transient and not associated with any symptoms. Similarly phase 4 block induced by a premature beat (intrinsic paroxysmal AV block) is also most often associated with significant HPS disease and merits implantation of a permanent pacemaker.

Indications for permanent pacing in acquired AV block in adults are listed in the following:

- Class I
    (1) Third-degree AV block and advanced second-degree AV block at any anatomic level associated with:
        (a) Bradycardia with symptoms (including heart failure) or ventricular arrhythmias presumed to be due to AV block *(Level of Evidence: C)*
        (b) Arrhythmias and other medical conditions that require drug therapy that result in symptomatic bradycardia *(Level of Evidence: C)*
        (c) Documented periods of asystole greater than or equal to 3.0 s, or any escape rate less than 40 bpm, or with an escape rhythm that is below the AV node in awake, symptom-free patients *(Level of Evidence: C)*
        (d) After catheter ablation of the AV junction *(Level of Evidence: C)*
        (e) Postoperative AV block that is not expected to resolve *(Level of Evidence: C)*
        (f) Neuromuscular diseases with AV block such as myotonic muscular dystrophy, Kearns–Sayre syndrome, Kerb's dystrophy (limb-girdle), and peroneal muscular atrophy with or without symptoms *(Level of Evidence: B)*
        (g) Symptom-free patients with AF and bradycardia with 1 or more pauses of at least 5 s or longer *(Level of Evidence: C)*
    (2) Second-degree AV block regardless of type or site of block, with associated symptomatic bradycardia *(Level of Evidence: B)*
    (3) Asymptomatic persistent third-degree AV block at any anatomic site with average awake ventricular rates of 40 bpm or faster if cardiomegaly or LV dysfunction is present or if the site of block is below the AV node *(Level of Evidence: B)*
    (4) Second- or third-degree AV block during exercise in the absence of myocardial ischemia *(Level of Evidence: C)*

- Class IIa
    (1) Reasonable for persistent third-degree AV block with an escape rate greater than 40 bpm in asymptomatic adult patients without cardiomegaly *(Level of Evidence: C)*
    (2) Reasonable for asymptomatic second-degree AV block at intra- or infra-His levels found at electrophysiological study *(Level of Evidence: B)*
    (3) Reasonable for first- or second-degree AV block with symptoms similar to those of pacemaker syndrome or hemodynamic compromise *(Level of Evidence: B)*
    (4) Reasonable for asymptomatic type II second-degree AV block with a narrow QRS. When type II second-degree AV block occurs with a wide QRS, including isolated right bundle-branch block, pacing becomes a Class I recommendation *(Level of Evidence: B)*

- Class IIb
    (1) May be considered for neuromuscular diseases such as myotonic muscular dystrophy, Erb dystrophy (limb-girdle muscular dystrophy), and peroneal muscular atrophy with any degree of AV block (including first-degree AV block), with or without symptoms, because there may be unpredictable progression of AV conduction disease *(Level of Evidence: B)*

    (2)   May be considered for AV block in the setting of drug use and/or drug toxicity when the block is expected to recur even after the drug is withdrawn *(Level of Evidence: B)*

- Class III
    (1)   Asymptomatic first-degree AV block *(Level of Evidence: B)*
    (2)   Asymptomatic type I second-degree AV block at the supra-His (AV node) level or not known to be intra- or infra-Hisian *(Level of Evidence: C)*
    (3)   AV block expected to resolve and unlikely to recur (e.g., drug toxicity, Lyme disease, or transient increases in vagal tone or during hypoxia in sleep apnea syndrome in the absence of symptoms) *(Level of Evidence: B)*

CHRONIC BIFASCICULAR AND TRIFASCICULAR BLOCK

Conduction disturbances due to block below the AV node are classified on the basis of the intraventricular conduction system. Chronic bifascicular block (BFB) is defined as either a complete LBBB or a combination of a RBBB associated either with a left anterior fascicular block (LAFB) or a left posterior fascicular block (LPFB). Once a diagnosis of bifascicular block is made, maintenance of AV conduction hinges on the continuing integrity of the third remaining fascicle. The term, trifascicular block is often applied loosely to describe the ECG pattern of prolonged PR interval in association with bifascicular block. In true sense, trifascicular block is present when bifascicular block is associated with a prolonged His-Ventricular (HV) interval. A prolonged PR interval does not in itself identify patients who have prolonged HV intervals in such cases. In fact, nearly half of patients with bifascicular block and prolonged PR intervals have prolongation of the Atrial-His (AH) interval (i.e., AV nodal conduction time). A strict definition of trifascicular block is block documented in all three fascicles, whether simultaneously or at different times. Thus the term, trifascicular block should be applied only to the ECG patterns of alternating RBBB and LBBB or RBBB with intermittent LAFB and LPFB. These situations are class I indications for permanent pacing, even in asymptomatic individuals.

Although, the incidence of progression of bifascicular block to third-degree AV block is low, ranging from 2% to 6% per year, observational studies in these patients with syncope, have shown a higher mortality rate, with SCD being mainly responsible for this mortality.[11-13] Based on these data, guidelines recommend a Class IIa indication for permanent cardiac pacing in patients with bifascicular block and syncope, even if the cause of syncope cannot be determined. It must also be emphasized that though the most common cause of syncope in patients with bifascicular block is atrioventricular block, other mechanisms like reflex syncope or tachyarrhythmias (with underlying structural heart disease) may be invoked.[13,14]

Recent data in patients with more preserved left ventricular ejection fraction has shown lower total mortality rates which may accurately reflect the characteristics and clinical outcomes of patients with bifascicular block as compared to older studies.[15] This underscores the fact that increased mortality in this group of patients may be related to the presence of underlying structural heart disease than to the development of AV block. In this sense, every patient with bifascicular block and syncope should have a comprehensive cardiac evaluation to rule out underlying structural heart disease and associated impaired left ventricular function. This is essential to assess the risk of sudden death and hence the need for an implantable cardioverter-defibrillator instead of simple pacemaker. This also raises the question regarding the most optimal strategy for managing patients with bifascicular block and syncope in the absence of severe structural disease despite the above said class IIa indication. More recently, a 3-phase diagnostic strategy (initial evaluation, electrophysiologic study, and insertion of an implantable loop recorder) has been shown to be safe in patients with bifascicular block, syncope and normal left ventricular function and was able to identify the cause of syncope in majority of these patients.[16]

Future recommendations regarding management of this group of patients with normal ventricular function have to await results of an ongoing randomized trial comparing empirical permanent pacemaker versus prolonged monitoring with an implantable loop recorder.[17]

Investigators have also attempted to identify possible predictors of third-degree AV block and sudden death in the presence of underlying bifascicular block. Some have suggested that an EP study can assist in identifying patients at risk.[18] If an asymptomatic patient with bifascicular block is found to have a prolonged HV interval (greater than or equal to 100 ms) at an EP study they should be considered for permanent pacing.[18] Other maneuvers that can be performed during an EP study include atrial pacing in asymptomatic patients as a means of identifying patients at increased risk of future high grade or third-degree AV block.[19] If atrial pacing induces nonphysiologic infra-His block, this is a IIa indication for implantation of a pacemaker. Bifascicular block without AV block or symptoms is not an indication for pacing.

Indications for permanent pacing in patients with chronic bifascicular or trifascicular block are listed in the following:

- Class I
    (1) Advanced second-degree AV block or intermittent third-degree AV block (*Level of Evidence: B*)
    (2) Type II second-degree AV block (*Level of Evidence: B*)
    (3) Alternating bundle-branch block (*Level of Evidence: C*)
- Class IIa
    (1) Reasonable for syncope not demonstrated to be due to AV block when other likely causes have been excluded, specifically ventricular tachycardia (VT) (*Level of Evidence: B*)
    (2) Reasonable for an incidental finding at electrophysiologic study of markedly prolonged HV interval (greater than or equal to 100 ms) in asymptomatic patients (*Level of Evidence: B*)
    (3) Reasonable for an incidental finding at electrophysiologic study of pacing-induced infra-His block that is not physiologic (*Level of Evidence: B*)
- Class IIb
    (1) May be considered in the setting of neuromuscular diseases such as myotonic muscular dystrophy, Erb dystrophy (limb-girdle muscular dystrophy), and peroneal muscular atrophy with bifascicular block or any fascicular block, with or without symptoms (*Level of Evidence: C*)
- Class III
    (1) Fascicular block without AV block or symptoms (*Level of Evidence: B*)
    (2) Fascicular block with first-degree AV block without symptoms (*Level of Evidence: B*)

HYPERSENSITIVE CAROTID SINUS SYNDROME AND NEUROCARDIOGENIC SYNCOPE

Hypersensitive carotid sinus syndrome is an infrequent cause of syncope or presyncope. It is due to an exaggerated response to carotid sinus baroreceptor stimulation which is manifested by a cardioinhibitory response, vasodepressor response, or a combination. The cardioinhibitory response results in a decreased heart rate due to sinus bradycardia, atrioventricular block, or asystole of more than 3 s. The vasodepressor response results in a drop in blood pressure without a change in heart rate. It is important to determine the relative contribution of these two components of carotid sinus stimulation before concluding that permanent pacing is clinically indicated, because patients with symptoms due entirely to the cardioinhibitory response of carotid sinus stimulation can be effectively treated with permanent pacing. Data on benefit of pacing interventions in patients with carotid sinus syndrome is based on results from non-randomized studies suggesting a clear benefit to pacing therapy and a small number of underpowered randomized trials suggesting a reduction in symptoms.[20]

A significant number of syncopal events are due to a variety of neurally mediated syndromes, the most common being vasovagal syncope. The guidelines recommend that neurally mediated syncope with significant bradycardia reproduced by a head-up tilt with or without isoproterenol or other provocative maneuvers is a Class IIb indication for pacing. The role of cardiac pacing in neutrally mediated syncope remains controversial, with early positive results in observational and unblinded studies not being borne out consistently in randomized controlled trials.[20] Cardiac pacing may be useful in the small number of highly symptomatic patients with documented asystole on implantable loop recorder during spontaneous syncope.[21]

The guidelines for pacing in hypersensitive carotid sinus and neurally mediated syndromes are listed in the following:

- Class I
    (1) Recurrent syncope caused by spontaneously occurring carotid sinus stimulation and carotid sinus pressure that induces ventricular asystole of more than 3 s *(Level of Evidence: C)*
- Class IIa
    (1) Reasonable for syncope without clear, provocative events and with a hypersensitive cardioinhibitory response of 3 s or longer *(Level of Evidence: C)*
- Class IIb
    (1) May be considered for significantly symptomatic neurocardiogenic syncope associated with bradycardia documented spontaneously or at the time of tilt-table testing *(Level of Evidence: C)*
- Class III
    (1) Hypersensitive cardioinhibitory response to carotid sinus stimulation without symptoms or with vague symptoms *(Level of Evidence: C)*
    (2) Situational vasovagal syncope in which avoidance behavior is effective and preferred *(Level of Evidence: C)*

CARDIAC RESYNCHRONIZATION THERAPY (CRT)

CRT is an electrical treatment based on biventricular or left ventricular-only pacing that was initially applied as a last resort therapeutic solution for patients with severe heart failure (HF) associated with LBBB. In the past few years, the guidelines have been updated in such a way as to improve patient selection according to their likelihood of improvement with CRT. Notable changes in the 2012 ACCF/AHA/HRS Focused Update for CRT are based on HF severity, QRS morphology, QRS duration, and AF.

CRT has traditionally been recommended for patients in sinus rhythm with wide QRS (in most of cases associated with LBBB), left ventricular dysfunction, and moderate to severe heart failure (NYHA functional classes III–IV) despite optimal medical therapy, with proven efficacy including reduction of hospitalizations and all-cause mortality based on results of COMPANION and the CARE HF trials.[22,23] The initial indications have since evolved to include patients with mild HF and incorporate the degree of QRS prolongation, QRS morphology, and presence or absence of atrial fibrillation into clinical decision making so as to provide a more nuanced approach to patient selection. In addition, more recently CRT has been recommended in patients with depressed left ventricular function and conventional indications for permanent pacing. Finally, there is no current indication to use an echocardiographic evaluation of dyssynchrony to select patients for CRT.[24]

PATIENTS WITH SINUS RHYTHM, LEFT BUNDLE BRANCH BLOCK (LBBB), MODERATE TO SEVERE HEART FAILURE (NEW YORK HEART ASSOCIATION [NYHA] FUNCTIONAL CLASSES III–IV): QRS DURATION

In the most recent guidelines while CRT is strongly recommended in case of LBBB with QRS duration greater than or equal to 150 ms, a lower strength of recommendation is given to patients with QRS durations between 130 and 150 ms, especially if not associated with LBBB morphology.[1] These updates have been based on the evolving evidence that QRS duration greater than or equal to 150 ms and an LBBB pattern seem to correlate with the most favorable outcomes after CRT.[25] However, since the publication of these guidelines, newer evidence indicates that despite a strong impact of QRS duration on outcomes there is no clear threshold at 150 ms while no effect or adverse effect of therapy was seen only at QRS durations less than 120–130 ms.[26]

In addition, a series of recent trials (RethinQ, ESTEEM-CRT, LESSER-EARTH, and ECHO-CRT) have provided convincing evidence that the application of CRT in patients with narrow QRS complex despite evidence of dyssynchrony is not beneficial or even may lead to excess in mortality.[27–30] The recent AHA guidelines on HF have recommended a class III indication for CRT in patients with QRS duration less than 120 ms, based on the negative results of ECHO-CRT study.[31]

However, despite the lack of data suggesting benefit, in contemporary practice, a large proportion of CRT devices are still implanted in patients with a QRS duration of less than 150 ms. Pending further studies to help identify the HF patients with moderate QRS duration who are most likely to benefit from CRT; it is likely reasonable to approach management decisions for CRT use on an individual basis in patients with QRS duration 120–149 ms.

PATIENTS WITH RIGHT BUNDLE BRANCH BLOCK (RBBB): QRS MORPHOLOGY

Initial guidelines for CRT did not specify on the effectiveness of therapy between different QRS morphologies.[32] However, only approximately 10% of patients with advanced systolic HF and abnormal ventricular conduction have RBBB and another minority display nonspecific intraventricular conduction disturbance (IVCD).[33] This in turn is reflective of the fact that a majority of patients enrolled in randomized trials of CRT had LBBB. HF with LBBB is pathophysiologically different than HF with non-LBBB QRS morphology (RBBB or nonspecific IVCD). RBBB in particular is associated with relatively normal electrical activation of the LV in the absence of other disease and with less LV mechanical dyssynchrony.[34] Post hoc analysis of the MADIT-CRT and REVERSE trials has shown that subgroups with non-LBBB QRS morphology do not derive a significant benefit from CRT.[35,36] In a large cohort of Medicare patients undergoing CRT implantation, RBBB proved to be an adjusted predictor of poor outcome after CRT implant.[37] Those with nonspecific IVCD had an intermediate outcome.[37] However, there is some evidence that presence of LV mechanical dyssynchrony may identify subgroups of RBBB patients who may benefit from CRT.[38,39]

Based on the results of these recent trials, CRT is no longer recommended for non-LBBB patients with QRS duration less than 150 ms and mild HF (NYHA I or II). For more severe HF in this subgroup of patients, there are still Class IIb recommendations. For patients with non-LBBB, QRS duration more than 150 ms, the guidelines recommend class IIa recommendation for patients in NYHA functional class III or ambulatory IV and a IIb recommendation for those in NYHA functional class II.

QRS MORPHOLOGY VERSUS DURATION

Although there is considerable evidence that patients with LBBB appear to benefit most from CRT, a meta-analysis of five randomized trials suggests that QRS duration is a more powerful predictor of clinical response to CRT.[26]

TRANSCATHETER AORTIC VALVE REPLACEMENT (TAVR)-INDUCED LBBB

If CRT works in essentially all hearts with LBBB, one may wonder whether it is effective in post TAVR LBBB patients. Although the clinical implications of this new onset LBBB remains controversial, a recent study reported a high burden of arrhythmic events at 1-year follow-up in nearly one-half of patients with new onset LBBB, while significant bradyarrhythmias were detected in 20% of the patients, with a permanent pacemaker required in nearly one-half of them.[40] In addition, new onset LBBB has been shown to be associated with increased all cause and cardiovascular mortality.[41] Based on reports showing beneficial effects of CRT in patients with a low LVEF and persistent LBBB after TAVR, CRT may be reasonable among patients with preexisting LV dysfunction and new-onset LBBB persisting at 30 days after TAVR, which might put these patients at higher mortality and morbidity risk.[42,43]

PATIENTS WITH SINUS RHYTHM AND MILD HEART FAILURE

A series of trials (MADIT-CRT and REVERSE) extended the clinical use of CRT to patients with mild HF (NYHA class II) with the paradigm shift of preventing evolution of HF to more severe stages, through reverse ventricular remodeling, and reducing the burden of HF-related hospitalizations.[44,45] Although both the studies included NYHA functional class I patients, the total number of these patients included was small, and the subgroup analysis was not meaningful. Based on these data, the guidelines recommend class I indication for CRT in patients with LBBB, QRS duration more than 150 and NYHA functional class II. As discussed before, CRT is no longer recommended for non-LBBB patients with QRS duration less than 150 ms and mild HF (NYHA II) while those with QRS duration more than 150 ms, have been given a Class IIb recommendation.

PATIENTS WITH PERMANENT ATRIAL FIBRILLATION (AF), LEFT VENTRICULAR (LV) DYSFUNCTION, AND HEART FAILURE

Permanent AF is present in 25%–30% of CRT candidates, but there is little evidence from randomized studies that CRT is effective in AF. This poor outcome is attributed to suboptimal delivery of CRT because of rapid and/or irregular ventricular beats.[46,47] The indication to implant a CRT device in patients with permanent atrial fibrillation was not covered by the guidelines issued before 2007–2008. However, the results of observational studies performed on large datasets in recent years indicate that CRT implant with additional AV nodal ablation is associated with a better outcome as compared to CRT when performed in AF patients treated with rate control drugs.[47,48] These findings form the basis for a class IIa in the recent guidelines.[1]

PATIENTS WITH LV DYSFUNCTION AND CONVENTIONAL INDICATIONS FOR PACING: INDICATIONS FOR A CRT DEVICE

The premise for this indication was based on the deleterious effect of RV pacing on long-term ventricular function and outcomes.[49,50] This indication has been validated by results from BLOCK HF trial which randomized patients with left ventricular ejection fraction less than or equal to 50%, NYHA class I–III and indications for pacing for AV block to CRT or conventional right ventricular (RV) pacing, with the guidelines providing a Class IIa recommendation for these patients.[51] In addition the guidelines specify that the degree of anticipated RV pacing must be more than >40%.[50] However, it has to be considered that the benefits of CRT as an alternative to conventional pacing, in terms of absolute risk reduction of death or hospitalization for heart failure are lower than what were previously demonstrated for the classical indications to CRT. On the other hand the complications of a potential subsequent upgrade to CRT strongly suggest considering the option of biventricular pacing at the time of the first implant.[52]

PATIENTS ALREADY IMPLANTED WITH A CONVENTIONAL PACEMAKER (PM) OR IMPLANTABLE CARDIOVERTER-DEFIBRILLATOR (ICD): INDICATIONS FOR UPGRADE TO A CRT DEVICE

The use of CRT in these cases is related to patients presenting with heart failure, who have a left ventricular dysfunction and a high percentage of conventional pacing. Although no randomized studies are available to support these recommendations, the guidelines provide a Class IIa recommendation for patients with an LVEF less than or equal to 35% who are undergoing implantation of a replacement device with anticipated requirement for significant (>40%) ventricular pacing.

The following are useful guidelines to select patient for CRT therapy

- Class I
    (1) CRT is indicated for patients who have LVEF less than or equal to 35%, sinus rhythm, LBBB with a QRS duration greater than or equal to 150 ms, and NYHA class II, III, or ambulatory IV symptoms on GDMT. *(Level of Evidence: A for class III/IV. Level of Evidence: B for Class II)*
- Class IIa
    (1) CRT can be useful for patients who have LVEF less than or equal to 35%, sinus rhythm, LBBB with a QRS duration 120–149 ms, and NYHA class II, III, or ambulatory IV symptoms on GDMT. *(Level of Evidence: B)*
    (2) CRT can be useful for patients who have LVEF less than or equal to 35%, sinus rhythm, a non-LBBB pattern with a QRS duration greater than or equal to 150 ms, and NYHA class III/ambulatory class IV symptoms on GDMT. *(Level of Evidence: A)*
    (3) CRT can be useful in patients with atrial fibrillation and LVEF less than or equal to 35% on GDMT if (a) the patient requires ventricular pacing or otherwise meets CRT criteria and (b) AV nodal ablation or pharmacologic rate control will allow near 100% ventricular pacing with CRT. *(Level of Evidence: B)*
    (4) CRT can be useful for patients on GDMT who have LVEF less than or equal to 35% and are undergoing new or replacement device placement with anticipated requirement for significant (>40%) ventricular pacing. *(Level of Evidence: C)*
- Class IIb
    (1) CRT may be considered for patients who have an LVEF less than or equal to 30%, ischemic etiology of heart failure, sinus rhythm, LBBB with a QRS duration of greater than or equal to 150 ms, and NYHA class I symptoms on GDMT. *(Level of Evidence: C)*
    (2) CRT may be considered for patients who have LVEF less than or equal to 35%, sinus rhythm, a non-LBBB pattern with QRS duration 120 to 149 ms, and NYHA class III/ambulatory class IV on GDMT. *(Level of Evidence: B)*
    (3) CRT may be considered for patients who have LVEF less than or equal to 35%, sinus rhythm, a non-LBBB pattern with a QRS duration greater than or equal to 150 ms, and NYHA class II symptoms on GDMT. *(Level of Evidence: B)*
- Class III
    (1) CRT is not recommended for patients with NYHA class I or II symptoms and non-LBBB pattern with QRS duration less than 150 ms. *(Level of Evidence: B)*
    (2) CRT is not indicated for patients whose comorbidities and/or frailty limit survival with good functional capacity to less than 1 year. *(Level of Evidence: C; this is more relevant for patient with need for defibrillators)*

NEWER DEVELOPMENTS IN PACING THERAPY

TAVR CONDUCTION DISTURBANCES HIS BUNDLE PACING (HBP)

In recent years, TAVR has become a well-accepted option for treating patients with aortic stenosis at intermediate to high surgical risk.[53] However, conduction disturbances, mainly new-onset LBBB and advanced AV block requiring permanent pacemaker implantation, remain the most common complication of this procedure. Conduction disturbances in the setting of TAVR, result primarily from a direct mechanical insult to the conduction system as well as association between aortic stenosis and conduction disturbances due to calcium deposition on the conduction system because of its proximity to the aortic valve complex.[54,55] In addition, inter-individual variability of the antero-posterior relationship of the AV node with respect to the apex of the triangle of Koch, as well as the length of the non-penetrating portion of the His bundle predisposes patients to a higher risk of TAVR-induced conduction disturbances.[56] The main risk factors of conduction disturbances include the presence of baseline RBBB, the use of some self-expanding valve systems, and the depth of prosthesis implantation within the left ventricular outflow tract.[57–59]

New-onset LBBB has been reported in about one fourth of TAVR procedures using first generation valves with an increased incidence reported with implantation of self-expandable valve. Data on the occurrence of new-onset LBBB after TAVR with newer-generation devices has not shown any significant reduction with even higher incidence rates with the mechanically expanded Lotus valve (Boston Scientific, Natick, MA). As compared to surgical aortic valve replacement, the incidence of complete heart block and pacemaker implantation has been higher than expected, with rates of implantation up to 25% being reported.[60–62] The rate of pacemaker implantation after TAVR with new-generation devices is highly variable and use of newer-generation devices does not seem to reduce the risk of conduction disturbances.[63] Majority of the new-onset LBBB as well as high-risk AV block appears in the peri-procedural period.[61,64] Interestingly, up to 50% of patients have resolution of conduction disturbances during the long-term follow-up.[65,66]

The clinical implications of these conduction disturbances remains controversial with recent studies showing increased cardiac mortality and heart failure hospitalization.[41] These observations may be related to association of new-onset LBBB with risk of sudden cardiac death because of progression to high-risk AV block and long-term detrimental effects of RV pacing.[41,67] However, in one of the recent and largest meta-analysis to date, permanent pacemaker implantation was not associated with increased risk of all-cause mortality, cardiovascular mortality, stroke, or myocardial infarction both at short- and long-term follow-up.[68] Interestingly, the authors did note an impaired left ventricular ejection fraction recovery post TAVR.

To date there are no randomized data to guide management of patients with post-TAVR conduction disturbances. However, the first step in clinical decision making is proper patient selection. The presence of preexisting conduction disturbances, particularly RBBB, should probably drive the decision about selection of the transcatheter valve type.[69] Particular attention should be paid to the evolution of ECG after TAVR; a stable ECG for at least 48 h demonstrates good negative predictive value for delayed high grade AVB.[64] The timing of pacemaker implant (if indicated initially) is unclear at this time, though data from observational studies indicate that complete heart block noted in the peri-procedural period is an indication for permanent pacemaker implantation, with most studies recommending an at least 24 h, and up to 48 h, wait prior to device implant to determine reversibility.[70,71] Present ACC/HRS guidelines encourage that these decisions be left to the discretion of the physician, while European societal guidelines recommend permanent pacemaker implantation in patients with post-operative AV block only if the conduction abnormality persists at least 7 days after cardiac surgery or is not expected to resolve.[72] Management of patients with transient new-onset LBBB and those with complete heart block noted during valve deployment but no evidence of conduction disease prior to the procedure remains controversial. The role of electrophysiological studies to predict high-risk AV block is still not firmly established, though a delta-HV interval (HV interval after TAVR minus the HV interval before TAVR), with an optimal cutoff of more than equal to 13 ms has been shown to be an independent predictor of high-risk AV block in post TAVR patients including those who develop new LBBB.[73] In addition a post procedural HV interval, with an optimal cutoff of more than equal to 65 ms predicts high-risk AV block in patients with new-onset LBBB.[73]

HIS BUNDLE PACING

As evident by the role of cardiac pacing in various disorders of conduction discussed above, it will not be an understatement that RV apical pacing has been the cornerstone of ventricular pacing for decades. However, an increased burden of chronic RV apical pacing has been associated with an increased risk for heart failure (HF), and death.[49,74,75] Earlier studies had identified a pacing burden of 40% as the threshold where the risk of developing pacing induced cardiomyopathy increases substantially.[49,50] Recent data in patients with complete heart block and baseline preserved LV function have shown that pacing induced cardiomyopathy is strongly associated with RV pacing burden >20%.[76]

Most of these adverse effects stem from ventricular dyssynchrony related to perturbed ventricular depolarization as a consequence of RV apical pacing. Strategies to overcome these limitations of conventional RV apical pacing have included alternative site RV pacing and biventricular pacing. However, there are conflicting data on the potential advantages of alternative site pacing such as the RV outflow tract and RV septal pacing.[77,78] Similarly, recent trials of biventricular pacing in patients with normal/low normal LV function have shown mixed results.[79,80] Furthermore, randomized comparison of RV pacing with biventricular pacing in patients with preserved LV function have not shown any significant differences in mortality, hospitalization for HF, or quality of life despite a greater decline in LV ejection fraction and increased chamber enlargement in RV pacing group.[81,82] In addition to the well-known fact that up to one-third of patients treated with biventricular pacing do not derive clinical or echocardiographic benefit; recent evidence indicates that CRT has limited benefits in patients with non-LBBB and severely reduced ejection fraction (EF) and those with LV dysfunction and narrow QRS.[27-30,83]

With its ability to recruit the intrinsic conduction system and thereby reducing or eliminating both inter-ventricular and intraventricular dyssynchrony, HBP intuitively represents a truly physiological means of implementing ventricular pacing and CRT. Several studies in recent years have demonstrated the safety and feasibility as well as hemodynamic and clinical benefits of HBP over RV apical pacing in patients treated for AV block, though none of these were powered to detect mortality benefit. A recent meta-analysis has reported an average implant success rate of nearly 85%.[84] HBP has been shown to be feasible even in the setting of infra-nodal block.[85]

With this technology being an evolving field, there are no formal guidelines regarding indications for HBP. However based on the above-cited literature and recent multicenter collaborative group recommendations,[86] potential indications will include most patients with an anticipated high burden of ventricular pacing where recruiting the His bundle is a possibility. Though, HBP has been shown to be feasible even in the setting of infra-nodal block, reliable selection of patients who are likely to have recruitment of the left-sided conduction system is challenging. His bundle pacing in patients with AV block results in higher rates of HPS recruitment when the block is at the AV nodal level (93%–98%) compared with when it is at the infranodal level (52%–76%).[85] In light of valid concerns about the possibility of disease progression and/or lead failure, one must consider the possibility of providing a backup RV lead or intentionally targeting His bundle sites demonstrating nonselective capture with low ventricular capture thresholds (backup RV capture from the His lead).

Permanent HBP has also recently been shown to be a viable alternative to biventricular pacing in patients requiring CRT.[87,88] In the largest multicenter experience till date, using HBP as a rescue strategy in patients with failed left ventricular lead or nonresponse to biventricular pacing or as a primary strategy in CRT eligible patients, successful implantation was achieved in 90% of patients.[89] This was associated with significant narrowing of QRS duration, increase in LVEF, and improvement in NYHA functional class.

Based on the data discussed above, HBP seems feasible either as a primary option or as a rescue strategy for patients requiring CRT. Even in patients who fail LV lead placement because of complex anatomy, permanent HBP is still possible with high success rates. HBP is an alternative to achieve CRT in patients who fail biventricular pacing, usually during the index procedure. It is conceivable that in patients in whom LV lead placement is suboptimal or technically challenging, HBP may be used as an early bailout strategy. Since biventricular pacing is non-physiologic and associated with significant electrical dyssynchrony in patients with narrow QRS at baseline, HBP may be considered the primary strategy to achieve CRT in patients with AV nodal block, AV nodal ablation, and high RV pacing burden due to AV nodal disease (narrow QRS at baseline). The collaborative working group considers HBP a reasonable backup option in patients in whom biventricular pacing either cannot be performed or has failed despite ideal lead placement and optimization attempts. Given the morbidity and poor lead durability in the setting of surgical epicardial lead placement, it may be reasonable to attempt resynchronization with HBP before sending a patient for surgical LV lead placement.

Any new technology comes with its limitations and so does His bundle pacing. Although the tools and leads have become much better, the success rate and operator experience is still on the initial upslope at this time. The dislodgement rates of HBP leads in the above-cited studies are not significantly higher than conventional RV leads but they are limited to few centers and operators. The potential need for higher pacing output with permanent HBP might result in shorter battery longevity of devices, which is also a concern in some cases. Thresholds can rise progressively on follow-up and have to be monitored more carefully. In addition, there are limited data regarding extraction of leads placed on the membranous septum with a concern for iatrogenic Gerbode defect upon extraction of the lead. Although promising as a superior alternative to RV apical pacing, larger studies involving longer follow-up and wider experience is required before generalized adoption and use.

REFERENCES

1. Epstein, A.E., Darbar, D., DiMarco, J.P., et al. (2012). 2012 ACCF/AHA/HRS focused update of the 2008 guideline for device based therapy for cardiac rhythm abnormalities. *Journal of the American College of Cardiology*, 60, 1297–1313.

2. Rosenqvist M, & Obel IW. Atrial pacing and the risk for AV block: Is there a time for change in attitude? *Pacing Clin Electrophysiol* 1989;12:97–101.

3. Barold SS, Ilercil A, Leonelli F, Herweg B. First-degree atrioventricular block. Clinical manifestations, indications for pacing, pacemaker management & consequences during cardiac resynchronization. *J Interv Card Electrophysiol* 2006;17:139–152.

4. Barold SS. Lingering misconceptions about type I second-degree atrioventricular block. *Am J Cardiol* 2001;88:1018–1020.

5. Barold SS, Hayes DL. Second-degree atrioventricular block: A reappraisal. *Mayo Clin Proc* 2001;76:44–57.

6. Barold SS. 2:1 Atrioventricular block: Order from chaos. *Am J Emerg Med.* 2001;19:214–217.

7. Zeltser D, Justo D, Halkin A, et al. Drug-induced atrioventricular block: Prognosis after discontinuation of the culprit drug. *J Am Coll Cardiol* 2004;44:105–108.

8. Osmonov D, Erdinler I, Ozcan KS, et al. Management of patients with drug-induced atrioventricular block. *Pacing Clin Electrophysiol* 2012;35:804–810.

9. Feingold B, Mahle WT, Auerbach S, et al. Management of cardiac involvement associated with neuromuscular diseases: A scientific statement from the American Heart Association. *Circulation* 2017;136:e200–e231.

10. Birnie DH, Sauer DH, Bogan F, et al. HRS expert consensus statement on the diagnosis and management of arrhythmias associated with cardiac sarcoidosis. *Heart Rhythm* 2014;11:1304–1323.

11. McAnulty JH, Kauffman S, Murphy E, et al. Survival in patients with intraventricular conduction defects. *Arch Intern Med* 1978;138:30–35.

12. Dhingra RC, Denes P, Wu D, et al. Syncope in patients with chronic bifascicular block. Significance, causative mechanisms, and clinical implications. *Ann Intern Med* 1974;81:302–306.

13. McAnulty JH, Rahimtoola SH, Murphy E, et al. Natural history of "high-risk" bundle-branch block: Final report of a prospective study. *N Engl J Med* 1982;307:137–143.

14. Brignole M, Menozzi C, Moya A, et al. Mechanism of syncope in patients with bundle branch block and negative electrophysiological test. *Circulation* 2001;104:2045–2050.

15. Marti-Almor J, Cladellas M, Bazan V, et al. Long-term mortality predictors in patients with chronic bifascicular block. *Europace* 2009;11:1201–1207.

16. Moya A, García-Civera R, Croci F, et al. Diagnosis, management, and outcomes of patients with syncope and bundle branch block. *Eur Heart J* 2011;32:1535–1541.

17. Krahn AD, Morillo CA, Kus T, et al. Empiric pacemaker compared with a monitoring strategy in patients with syncope and bifascicular conduction block—Rationale and design of the syncope: Pacing or recording in the later years (SPRITELY) study. *Europace* 2012;14:1044–1048.

18. Scheinman MM, Peters RW, Suave MS, et al. Value of the H-Q interval in patients with bundle branch block and the role of prophylactic permanent pacing. *Am J Cardiol* 1982;50:1316–1322.

19. Dhingra RC, Wyndham C, Bauernfeind R, et al. Significance of block distal to the His bundle induced by atrial pacing in patients with chronic bifascicular block. *Circulation* 1979;60:1455–1464.

20. Parry SW, Matthews IG. Update on the role of pacemaker therapy in vasovagal syncope and carotid sinus syndrome. *Prog Cardiovasc Dis* 2013;55:434–442.

21. Brignole M, Menozzi C, Moya A, et al. Pacemaker therapy in patients with neutrally mediated syncope and documented asystole: Third international study on syncope of uncertain etiology (ISSUE-3): A randomized trial. *Circulation* 2012;125:2566–2571.

22. Bristow MR, Saxon LA, Boehmer J, et al. Comparison of medical therapy, pacing, and defibrillation in heart failure (COMPANION) investigators. Cardiac-resynchronization therapy with or without an implantable defibrillator in advanced chronic heart failure. *N Engl J Med* 2004;350:2140–2150.

23. Cleland JG, Daubert JC, Erdmann E, et al. The effect of cardiac resynchronization on morbidity and mortality in heart failure. *N Engl J Med* 2005;352:1539–1549.

24. Chung ES, Leon AR, Tavazzi L, et al. Results of the predictors of response to CRT (PROSPECT) trial. *Circulation* 2008;117:2608–2616.

25. Stavrakis S, Lazzara R, Thadani U. The benefit of cardiac resynchronization therapy and QRS duration: A meta-analysis. *J Cardiovasc Electrophysiol* 2012;23:163–168.

26. Cleland JG, Abraham WT, Linde C, et al. An individual patient meta-analysis of five randomized trials assessing the effects of cardiac resynchronization therapy on morbidity and mortality in patients with symptomatic heart failure. *Eur Heart J* 2013;34:3547–3556.

27. Beshai JF, Grimm RA, Nagueh SF, et al. Rethin Q study investigators. Cardiac resynchronization therapy in heart failure with narrow QRS complexes. *N Engl J Med* 2007;357:2461–2471.

28. Donahue T, Niazi I, Leon A, et al. ESTEEM-CRT investigators. Acute and chronic response to CRT in narrow QRS patients. *J Cardiovasc Transl Res* 2012;5:232–241.

29. Thibault B, Harel F, Ducharme A, et al. LESSER-EARTH investigators. Cardiac resynchronization therapy in patients with heart failure and a QRS complex <120 milliseconds: The evaluation of resynchronization therapy for heart failure (LESSER-EARTH) trial. *Circulation* 2013;127:873–881.

30. Ruschitzka F, Abraham WT, Singh JP, et al. Cardiac resynchronization therapy in heart failure with a narrow QRS complex. *N Engl J Med* 2013;369:1395–1405.

31. Yancy CW, Jessup M, Bozkurt B, et al. 2013 ACCF/AHA guideline for the management of heart failure: A report of the American College of Cardiology Foundation/American Heart Association Task Force on Practice Guidelines. *Circulation* 2013;128:e240–e327.

32. Epstein AE, DiMarco JP, Ellenbogen KA, et al. ACC/AHA/HRS 2008 guidelines for device-based therapy of cardiac rhythm abnormalities. *J Am Coll Cardiol* 2008;51:1–62.

33. Sweeney MO. Wide right. *Heart Rhythm* 2005;2:616–618.

34. Byrne MJ, Helm RH, Daya S, et al. Diminished left ventricular dyssynchrony and impact of resynchronization in failing hearts with right versus left bundle branch block. *J Am Coll Cardiol* 2007;50:1484–1490.

35. Zareba W, Klein H, Cygankiewicz I, et al. Effectiveness of cardiac resynchronization therapy by QRS morphology in the multicenter automatic defibrillator implantation trial-cardiac resynchronization therapy (MADIT-CRT). *Circulation* 2011;123:1061–1072.

36. Gold MR, Thebault C, Linde C, et al. Effect of QRS duration and morphology on cardiac resynchronization therapy outcomes in mild heart failure: Results from the resynchronization reverses remodeling in systolic left ventricular dysfunction (REVERSE) study. *Circulation* 2012;126:822–929.

37. Bilchick KC, Kamath S, DiMarco JP, Stukenborg GJ. Bundle-branch block morphology and other predictors of outcome after cardiac resynchronization therapy in medicare patients. *Circulation* 2010;122:2022–2030.

38. Gold MR, Birgersdotter-Green U, Singh JP, et al. The relationship between ventricular electrical delay and left ventricular remodelling with cardiac resynchronization therapy. *Eur Heart J* 2011;32:2516–2524.

39. Hara H, Oyenuga OA, Tanaka H, et al. The relationship of QRS morphology and mechanical dyssynchrony to long-term outcome following cardiac resynchronization therapy. *Eur Heart J* 2012;33:2680–2691.

40. Rodes-Cabau J, Urena M, Nombela-Franco L, et al. Arrhythmic burden in patients with new-onset LBBB post-TAVR. *JACC Cardiovasc Interv* 2018;11:1495–1505.

41. Fadahunsi OO, Olowoyeye A, Ukaigwe A, et al. Incidence, predictors, and outcomes of permanent pacemaker implantation following transcatheter aortic valve replacement: analysis from the U.S. Society of Thoracic Surgeons/American College of Cardiology TVT Registry. *JACC Cardiovasc Interv* 2016;9:2189–2199.

42. Meguro K, Lellouche N, Teiger E. Cardiac resynchronization therapy improved heart failure after left bundle branch block during transcatheter aortic valve implantation. *J Invasive Cardiol* 2012;24:132–133.

43. Osmancik P, Stros P, Herman D, et al. Cardiac resynchronization therapy implantation following transcatheter aortic valve implantation. *Europace* 2011;13:290–291.

44. Linde C, Abraham WT, Gold MR, et al. Randomized trial of cardiac resynchronization in mildly symptomatic heart failure patients and in asymptomatic patients with left ventricular dysfunction and previous heart failure symptoms. *J Am Coll Cardiol* 2008;52:1834–1843.

45. Moss AJ, Hall WJ, Cannom DS, et al. Cardiac-resynchronization therapy for the prevention of heart-failure events. *N Engl J Med* 2009;361:1329–1338.

46. Hayes DL, Boehmer JP, Day JD, et al. Cardiac resynchronization therapy and the relationship of percent biventricular pacing to symptoms and survival. *Heart Rhythm* 2011;8:1469–1475.

47. Gasparini MLC, Lunati M, Landolina M, et al. Cardiac resynchronization in patients with atrial fibrillation. The CERTIFY study (Cardiac Resynchronization in Atrial Fibrillation Patients Multinational Registry). *JACC: Heart Failure* 2013;1:500–507.

48. Gasparini M, Auricchio A, Metra M, et al. Multicentre longitudinal observational study (MILOS) group. Long-term survival in patients undergoing cardiac resynchronization therapy: The importance of performing atrio-ventricular junction ablation in patients with permanent atrial fibrillation. *Eur Heart J* 2008;29:1644–1652.

49. Sweeney MO, Hellkamp AS, Ellenbogen KA, et al. Adverse effect of ventricular pacing on heart failure and atrial fibrillation among patients with normal baseline QRS duration in a clinical trial of pacemaker therapy for sinus node dysfunction. *Circulation* 2003;107:2932–2937.

50. Sharma AD, Rizo-Patron C, Hallstrom AP, et al. Percent right ventricular pacing predicts outcomes in the DAVID trial. *Heart Rhythm* 2005;2:830–834.

51. Curtis AB, Worley SJ, Adamson PB, et al. Biventricular pacing for atrioventricular block and systolic dysfunction. *N Engl J Med* 2013;368:1585–1593.

52. Boriani G, Ziacchi M, Diemberger I, et al. BLOCK HF: How far does it extend indications for cardiac resynchronization therapy? *J Cardiovasc Med (Hagerstown)* 2016;17:306–308.

53. Nishimura RA, Otto CM, Bonow RO, et al. American College of Cardiology/American Heart Association Task Force on Practice Guidelines. 2014 AHA/ACC guideline for the management of patients with valvular heart disease: executive summary: A report of the American College of Cardiology/American Heart Association Task Force on Practice Guidelines. *J Am Coll Cardiol* 2014;63:2438–2488.

54. Moreno R, Dobarro D, López de Sá E, et al. Cause of complete atrioventricular block after percutaneous aortic valve implantation: Insights from a necropsy study. *Circulation* 2009;120:e29–e30.

55. Urena M, Hayek S, Cheema AN, et al. Arrhythmia burden in elderly patients with severe aortic stenosis as determined by continuous electrocardiographic recording: toward a better understanding of arrhythmic events after transcatheter aortic valve replacement. *Circulation* 2015;131:469–477.

56. Hamdan A, Guetta V, Klempfner R, et al. Inverse relationship between membranous septal length and the risk of atrioventricular block in patients undergoing transcatheter aortic valve implantation. *JACC Cardiovasc Interv* 2015;8:1218–1228.

57. van der Boon RM, Nuis RJ, Van Mieghem NM, et al. New conduction abnormalities after TAVI-frequency and causes. *Nat Rev Cardiol* 2012;9:454–463.

58. Fadahunsi OO, Olowoyeye A, Ukaigwe A, et al. Incidence, predictors, and outcomes of permanent pacemaker implantation following transcatheter aortic valve replacement: analysis from the U.S. Society of Thoracic Surgeons/American College of Cardiology TVT Registry. *JACC Cardiovasc Interv* 2016;9:2189–2199.

59. Naveh S, Perlman GY, Elitsur Y, et al. Electrocardiographic predictors of long-term cardiac pacing dependency following transcatheter aortic valve implantation. *J Cardiovasc Electrophysiol* 2017;28:216–223.

60. Houthuizen P, van der Boon RM, Urena M, et al. Occurrence, fate and consequences of ventricular conduction abnormalities after transcatheter aortic valve implantation. *Euro Intervention* 2014;9:1142–1150.

61. Nazif TM, Williams MR, Hahn RT, et al. Clinical implications of new-onset left bundle branch block after transcatheter aortic valve replacement: Analysis of the PARTNER experience. *Eur Heart J* 2014;35:1599–1607.

62. Maan A, Refaat MM, Heist EK, et al. Incidence and predictors of pacemaker implantation in patients undergoing transcatheter aortic valve replacement. *Pacing Clin Electrophysiol* 2015;38:878–886.

63. van Rosendael PJ, Delgado V, Bax JJ. Pacemaker implantation rate after transcatheter aortic valve implantation with early and new-generation devices: A systematic review. *Eur Heart J* 2018;39:2003–2013.

64. Toggweiler S, Stortecky S, Holy E, et al. The electrocardiogram after transcatheter aortic valve replacement determines the risk for post-procedural high-degree AV block and the need for telemetry monitoring. *JACC Cardiovasc Interv* 2016;9:1269–1276.

65. van der Boon RM, Van Mieghem NM, Theuns DA, et al. Pacemaker dependency after transcatheter aortic valve implantation with the selfexpanding medtronic core valve system. *Int J Cardiol* 2013;168:1269–1273.

66. Boerlage-Van Dijk K, Kooiman KM, Yong ZY, et al. Predictors and permanency of cardiac conduction disorders and necessity of pacing after transcatheter aortic valve implantation. *Pacing Clin Electrophysiol* 2014;37:1520–1529.

67. Urena M, Webb JG, Eltchaninoff H, et al. Late cardiac death in patients undergoing transcatheter aortic valve replacement: Incidence and predictors of advanced heart failure and sudden cardiac death. *J Am Coll Cardiol* 2015;65:437–448.

68. Mohananey D, Jobanputra Y, Kumar A, et al. Clinical and echocardiographic outcomes following permanent pacemaker implantation after transcatheter aortic valve replacement: Meta-analysis and meta regression. *Circ Cardiovasc Interv* 2017;10:e005046.

69. van Gils L, Tchetche D, Lhermusier T, et al. Transcatheter heart valve selection and permanent pacemaker implantation in patients with pre-existent right bundle branch block. *J Am Heart Assoc* 2017;6:e005028.

70. Hoffmann R, Herpertz R, Lotfipour S, et al. Impact of a new conduction defect after transcatheter aortic valve implantation on left ventricular function. *JACC Cardiovasc Interv* 2012;5:1257–1263.

71. Nazif TM, Dizon JM, Hahn RT, et al. Predictors and clinical outcomes of permanent pacemaker implantation after transcatheter aortic valve replacement: The PARTNER (Placement of AoRticTraNscathetER Valves) trial and registry. *JACC Cardiovasc Interv* 2015;8:60–69.

72. Brignole M, Auricchio A, Baron-Esquivias G, et al. 2013 ESC guidelines on cardiac pacing and cardiac resynchronization therapy: The task force on cardiac pacing and resynchronization therapy of the European Society of Cardiology (ESC). Developed in collaboration with the European Heart Rhythm Association (EHRA). *Eur Heart J* 2013;34:2281–2329.

73. Rivard L, Schram G, Asgar A, et al. Electrocardiographic and electrophysiological predictors of atrioventricular block after transcatheter aortic valve replacement. *Heart Rhythm* 2015;12:321–329.

74. Wilkoff BL, Cook JR, Epstein AE, et al. Dual-chamber pacing or ventricular backup pacing in patients with an implantable defibrillator: The dual chamber and VVI implantable defibrillator (DAVID) trial. *JAMA* 2002;288:3115–3123.

75. Barsheshet A, Moss AJ, Mcnitt S, et al. Long-term implications of cumulative right ventricular pacing among patients with an implantable cardioverter defibrillator. *Heart Rhythm* 2011;8:212–218.

76. Kiehl EL, Makki T, Kumar R, et al. Incidence and predictors of right ventricular pacing-induced cardiomyopathy in patients with complete atrioventricular block and preserved left ventricular systolic function. *Heart Rhythm* 2016;13:2272–2278.

77. Shimony A, Eisenberg MJ, Filion KB, Amit G. Beneficial effects of right ventricular non-apical vs. apical pacing: A systematic review and meta-analysis of randomized-controlled trials. *Europace* 2012;14:81–91.

78. Luciuk D, Luciuk M, Gajek J. Alternative right ventricular pacing sites. Advances in clinical and experimental medicine: Official organ Wroclaw Medical University. *Adv Clin Exp Med* 2015;24:349–359.

79. Curtis AB, Worley SJ, Chung ES, et al. Improvement in clinical outcomes with biventricular versus right ventricular pacing: The block HF study. *J Am Coll Cardiol* 2016;67:2148–2157.

80. BioPace Trial Preliminary Results. 2014. Available at: http://clinicaltrialresults.org/Slides/TCT%202014/Blanc_Biopace.pdf.

81. Yu CM, Chan JY, Zhang Q, et al. Biventricular pacing in patients with bradycardia and normal ejection fraction. *N Engl J Med* 2009;361:2123–2134.

82. Stockburger M, Gomez-Doblas JJ, Lamas G, et al. Preventing ventricular dysfunction in pacemaker patients without advanced heart failure: Results from a multicentre international randomized trial (PREVENT- HF). *Eur J Heart Fail* 2011;13:633–641.

83. Sipahi I, Chou JC, Hyden M, et al. Effects of QRS morphology on clinical event reduction with cardiac resynchronization therapy: Meta-analysis of randomized controlled trials. *Am Heart J* 2012;163:260–267.

84. Zanon F, Ellenbogen KA, Dandamudi G, et al. Permanent His bundle pacing: A systematic review and meta-analysis. *Europace* 2018. doi:10.1093/europace/euy058.

85. Vijayaraman P, Naperkowski A, Ellenbogen KA, et al. Electrophysiologic insights into site of atrioventricular block: Lessons from permanent His bundle pacing. *JACC Clin Electrophysiol* 2015;1:571–581.

86. Vijayaraman P, Dandamudi G, Zanon F, et al. Permanent His bundle pacing: Recommendations from a multicenter His bundle pacing collaborative working group for standardization of definitions. *Heart Rhythm* 2018;15:60–68.

87. Lustgarten DL, Crespo EM, Arkhipova-Jenkins I, et al. His bundle pacing versus biventricular pacing in cardiac resynchronization therapy patients: A crossover design comparison. *Heart Rhythm* 2015;12:1548–1557.

88. Ajijola OA, Upadhyay GA, Macias C, et al. Permanent His bundle pacing for cardiac resynchronization therapy: Initial feasibility study in lieu of left ventricular lead. *Heart Rhythm* 2017;14:1353–1361.

89. Sharma PS, Dandamudi G, Herweg B, et al. Permanent His bundle pacing as an alternative to biventricular pacing for cardiac resynchronization therapy: A multi-center experience. *Heart Rhythm* 2018;15:413–420.

SUPRAVENTRICULAR TACHYARRHYTHMIA

ATRIAL FLUTTER

Ayman A. Hussein and Oussama M. Wazni

CONTENTS

EPIDEMIOLOGY AND RISK FACTORS

The incidence of atrial flutter (AFL) in the United States is 200,000 new cases per year. Of those, 88,000 present solely as AFL.[1,2] Atrial flutter is much less frequent than atrial fibrillation in a 1 to 10 ratio.[2] It is not uncommon, however, for AFL and AF to coexist. In fact, it has been reported that over a year's follow-up, 56% of patients presenting with typical AFL develop AF.[3] Importantly, AFL is associated with an increased risk of morbidity, which is even more profound when AFL is coupled with AF.[4]

The incidence of AFL rises exponentially in relationship to advancing age but as it is for AF, is greatest with structural heart disease such as left atrial enlargement or ventricular dysfunction. Table 6.1 summarizes the risk factors for AFL.

Table 6.1 Risk factors for atrial flutter

Independent risk factors
• Advanced age
• Male gender
• Congestive heart failure
• Chronic pulmonary disease
• Prior CVA
• Myocardial infarction
Conditions associated with AFL
• Thyrotoxicosis
• Valvular heart disease (rheumatic, mitral, tricuspid)
• Pericardial disease
• Congenital heart disease
• After open heart surgery
• After major cardiac surgery (primarily in cases of congenital heart defect repair)
• Possible genetic predisposition
• Alcohol intoxication
• Pulmonary embolus
• Hypertrophic cardiomyopathy
• Cardiac tumors
• Secondarily to Na channel blocking agents to treat AF (5%)

Source: Lee, K. et al., *Curr. Probl. Cardiol.*, 30, 121–167, 2005.

CLINICAL PRESENTATION

AFL, an organized macroreentrant arrhythmia, often presents as paroxysmal, short episodes lasting from seconds to hours; but can also present as sustained and persistent.[5] The atria usually contract at a rate of 250–350 beats per minute (bpm) while in AFL.[6] The ventricular rate is generally a 2:1 ratio or slower. A 1:1 ratio can be seen in cases where the atrial rate is relatively slower or when atrioventricular (AV) nodal conduction is enhanced due to increased sympathetic tone or anticholinergic medications.[7]

Acutely, patients often complain of shortness of breath, palpitations, diaphoresis, chest discomfort, dizziness, and weakness. Patients may also complain of polyuria, which occurs as a result of increased atrial pressure from rapidly contracting atria against a closed AV valve, and the subsequent release of atrial natriuretic factor (ANF). AFL may also present as exercise-induced fatigue or worsening heart failure. Patients tend to be more symptomatic when the ventricular response rate is rapid and/or when they present with episodes of both AF and AFL. On physical examination, the peripheral pulse is generally rapid and regular (less often irregular); cannon "a" waves may be observed, and S_1 is of variable intensity.[8]

DIAGNOSIS OF AFL

The diagnosis of AFL is generally made on a 12-lead surface ECG by identifying flutter waves in leads II, III, aVF, and V1. When it is difficult to distinguish the flutter waves, slowing the ventricular rate, by using AV nodal blockers (e.g., adenosine or diltiazem) or vagal maneuvers (Valsalva or gentle carotid sinus message), may allow visualization of the flutter waves. These waves resemble the edge of a wood saw, hence the name "saw-tooth" wave. In "typical" flutter the saw-tooth waves are negative in the inferior leads and positive in V1. The negative waves can be described in succession: (i) a slowly descending segment, (ii) a rapid negative deflection, (iii) a sharp upstroke, that (iv) with a slight overshoot leads to the slowly descending segment of the next cycle (Figures 6.1 and 6.2).[9]

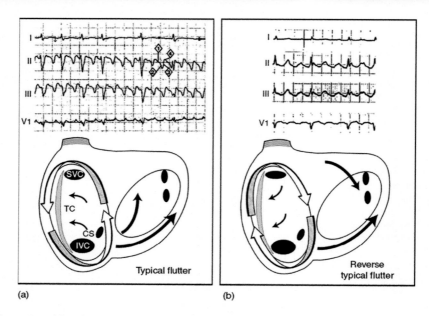

(a)   (b)

Figure 6.1 (a) 12-lead ECG of counterclockwise (CCW) atrial flutter (AFL) below which is a schematic drawing of the flutter circulating within the atrium. Note that in leads II, III, and aVF negative flutter waves and in V1 positive flutter waves are present. Negative flutter waves can be described as: (i) a slowly descending segment, (ii) a rapid negative deflection, (iii) a sharp upstroke, that (iv) with a slight overshoot leads to the slowly descending segment of the next cycle. (b) A 12-lead ECG of clockwise (CW) AFL. Note that in leads II, III, and aVF positive flutter waves and in V1 negative flutter waves are present. (Adapted from Cosio, F.G., *Card Electrophysiol. Rev.*, 6, 356–364, 2002.)

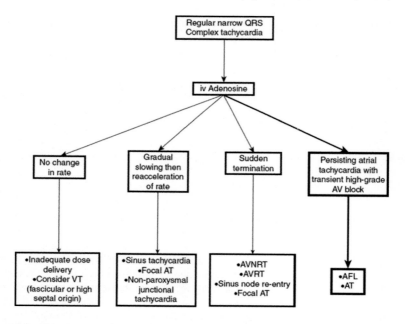

Figure 6.2 The response that a narrow complex tachycardia has to adenosine can assist in the identification of the rhythm. (Adapted from Blomstrom-Lundqvist, C. and Scheinman, M., *Circulation*, 108, 1871–1909, 2003.)

Generally speaking, re-entry occurs as a repetitive excitation of an area of the heart and transmission of that impulse around a conduction or functional barrier. In order for re-entry to occur, it would require:

1   Initiation via occurrence of unidirectional block in one limb of the circuit. This may result from an acceleration of the heart rate or a blocked premature beat that affects the refractory time of the circuit.

2   A zone of slowed conduction is required for both initiation and perpetuation (Figure 6.3).[6,9]

3   Circulation around an unexcitable anatomic or functional barrier.

In 1940, Rosenbleuth[11] demonstrated that creating a non-conducting barrier on the posterior wall of the right atrium supported AFL. The wavefront would circulate in a clockwise direction up the septum, around the roof down the free lateral wall and bounded anteriorly by the tricuspid orifice. This circulating wavefront could be extinguished by creating a lesion between the IVC and the inferior edge of the tricuspid orifice, thus providing the first basis of AFL alation.[9,12]

Re-entrant circuits include normal anatomic boundaries such as the tricuspid ring or mitral ring, and orifices of the superior vena cava (SVC) or inferior vena cava (IVC). Functional barriers are created due to an inability to conduct action potentials as rapidly as that seen

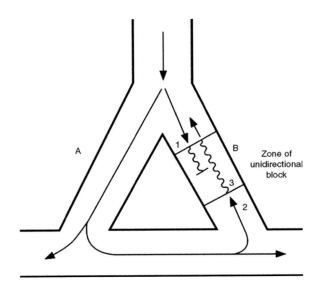

Figure 6.3   Classic re-entrant circuits with the three factors required for re-entry: an anatomic obstacle, a zone of slow conduction, and a unidirectional block. Limbs A and B are independent units that are formed by the anatomic obstacle and are capable of electrical conduction. Because the two pathways have different electrophysiologic properties (e.g., a refractory period longer in one pathway than the other), the impulse (1) is blocked in one pathway (B) and (2) propagates slowly in the adjacent pathway (A). If conduction in this alternative route is sufficiently depressed, especially when a premature impulse occurs, the slowly propagating impulse excites tissue beyond the blocked pathway and returns in a reversed direction along the pathway initially blocked to (3) zone of unidirectional block. (Reproduced from Topol, E.J. (ed.), *Textbook of Cardiovascular Medicine*, 2nd edn., Lippincott, Williams and Wilkins, Philadelphia, PA, 2002. With permission.)

in AFL. In 1980, Spach[13] suggested that the right atrium is able to support re-entry due to anisotropic conduction. The crista terminalis (CT) is a thick bundle of myocardial fibers that run in a superior/inferior direction, extending from the roof of the right atrium adjacent to the SVC opening laterally and inferiorly to the IVC. This band of tissue is able to conduct rapidly in the longitudinal direction but very slowly in the transverse direction, which is due to relative abundance of gap junctions in the longitudinal versus transverse direction, in a 10:1 ratio. This property allows for a functional transverse barrier. The openings of the IVC and the SVC linked by the CT provide a posterior obstacle to conduction, the tricuspid orifice (TR) provides an anterior obstacle; and this creates a ring that is able to support re-entry in either a clockwise or counterclockwise direction.[9,11] The isthmus between the IVC and TR, called the cavotricuspid isthmus (CTI) is often targeted with ablation and flutters which use this critical isthmus are often referred to as CTI-dependent AFLs and are the most commonly encountered AFLs in clinical practice, especially in patients with no prior history of cardiac surgery or ablation procedures.

TOOLS FOR DIAGNOSING ATRIAL FLUTTER

A multi-polar diagnostic catheter that covers the septal and anterior walls of the right atrium allows recording of almost the entire circuit of typical AFL (Figure 6.4). An electrogram of the CTI, recorded with a mapping/ablation catheter, will provide information on the remaining circuit. A characteristic ECG pattern along a typical "circular" endocardial activation map is diagnostic without further need for entrainment. It is important, however, to perform pacing and entrainment maneuvers, especially in patients with documented atypical AFL morphology and in those with any history of cardiac surgery or structural damage. During entrainment, the length of the pacing cycle should be slightly shorter than the AFL cycle length thus not to disturb the arrhythmia. This is especially true if there are multiple potential circuits such as in cases of scar-dependent macro-re-entry.[9]

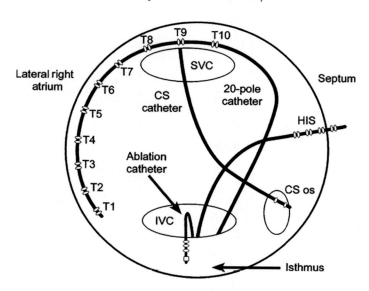

Figure 6.4 A diagram of a 20-pole "halo" catheter in the right atrium which is used to analyze the activation sequence during the tachycardia. IVC, inferior vena cava; SVC, superior vena cava; CS, coronary sinus; os, ostium; HIS, His bundle region. (Reproduced from Lee, K. et al., *Curr. Probl. Cardiol.*, 30, 121–167, 2005. With permission.)

AFLs are classified based on their location and mechanism (Figure 6.5 and Table 6.2).[5,6]

RIGHT ATRIAL CAVOTRISCUSPID-ISTHMUS-DEPENDENT FLUTTER
COUNTERCLOCKWISE (CCW) ATRIAL FLUTTER

This represents 90% of clinical AFL cases.[14] ECG findings include negative saw-tooth waves in the inferior leads and positive waves in V1 that transition to negative in V6 (Figure 6.1). The wavefront of the CCW–AFL circuit propagates up the posterior and septal wall of the right atrium (RA) and down the RA anterior and lateral walls when viewed from left atrial oblique (LAO) perspective. The predominant flutter wave negativity in the inferior leads largely reflects low to high activation of the atrial septum. This wavefront perpetuates in

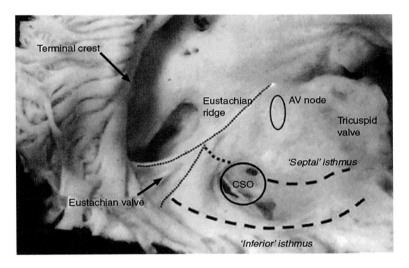

Figure 6.5 Photograph of the key anatomic structures involved in cavotricuspid isthmus-dependent AFLs. (Reproduced from Lee, K. et al., *Curr. Probl. Cardiol.*, 30, 121–167, 2005. With permission.)

Table 6.2 Classification of atrial flutter

Right atrial CTI-dependent flutter
• Counterclockwise flutter
• Clockwise flutter
• Double-wave re-entry
• Lower loop re-entry
• Intra-isthmus re-entry
Right atrial non-CTI-dependent flutter
• Scar-related flutter
• Upper loop flutter
Left atrial flutter
• Mitral annular flutter
• Scar and pulmonary vein related flutter
• Coronary sinus flutter
• Left septal flutter

Source: Lee, K. et al., *Curr. Probl. Cardiol.*, 30, 121–167, 2005.
Abbreviation: CTI: cavotricuspid isthmus.

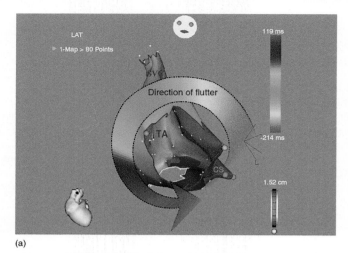

(a)

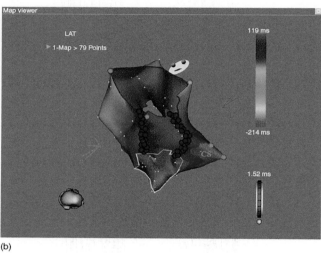

(b)

Figure 6.6 Electro-anatomic activation map of the right atrium during flutter. (a) In the AP view, the activation wave is seen propagating up the septum and down the lateral wall, where "early meets late" at the inferior wall (CCW direction). (b) Inferior view of the right atrium showing the CT isthmus. Two ablation lines are designed to encompass the broad CTI; line A joins the Tricuspid annulus to the CS os and further down to the IVC (septal isthmus), while line B joins the lateral tricuspid annulus to the IVC (lateral annulus).

a circular CCW direction around the tricuspid annulus until it is interrupted (Figure 6.6). Anatomically, the circuit is anteriorly bound by the tricuspid orifice, and posteriorly bound by the vena cava orifices, Eustachian ridge, and the coronary sinus (cs).[15–19] This flutter can be successfully ablated with a line which connects the tricuspid annulus and the IVC (i.e., CTI line).

CLOCKWISE (CW) ATRIAL FLUTTER
This represents 10% of clinical AFL cases. ECG findings include positive saw-tooth waves in the inferior leads and negative waves in V1. The wavefront of the CW–AFL circuit propagates down the posterior and septal wall of the RA and up the RA anterior and lateral walls when

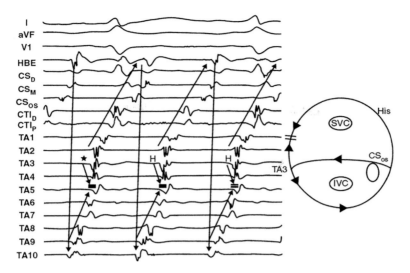

Figure 6.7 Lower loop re-entry. The left panel shows simultaneous recordings of a surface ECG (I, aVF, and V1), and intracardiac electrogram recorded from the His bundle region (HBE), the ostium of coronary sinus (CS$_{OS}$), and the middle and distal of the coronary sinus (CS$_M$ and CS$_D$) during lower loop re-entry. Note the early breakthrough at the low lateral tricuspid annulus (TA3) (marked by an asterisk) and wavefront collision at the high lateral annulus (TA5). The right panel is an illustration of lower loop re-entry. Note that the activation pattern circles the IVC rather than the tricuspid annulus, but still uses the CTI. The arrow denotes a CCW direction of activation around the IVC. His, HIS; SVC, superior vena cava; IVC, inferior vena cava; CS$_{OS}$, coronary sinus os; TA3, low lateral tricuspid annulus. (From Lee, K. et al., *Curr. Probl. Cardiol.*, 30, 121–167, 2005. With permission.)

viewed from the LAO perspective. The predominant flutter wave positivity in the inferior leads largely reflects high to low activation of the atrial septum. This wavefront propagates in a circular CW direction around the tricuspid annulus until it is interrupted (Figure 6.7). The CW–AFL circuit has the same anatomic boundaries as CCW–AFL.[5] Similar to typical AFL, this flutter can be successfully ablated with a CTI line.

DOUBLE-WAVE RE-ENTRY (DWR)

DWR flutter occurs when a carefully timed stimulus is delivered to the isthmus between the tricuspid annulus and the Eustachian ridge, resulting in a unidirectional antidromic block of the paced impulse and acceleration of the CCW–AFL. The acceleration of the tachycardia is due to two successive activation fronts traveling in the same direction in the re-entrant circuit. DWR flutter is not sustained and typically degenerates into AF.[5,20,21] This flutter is successfully ablated with a CTI line.

LOWER LOOP RE-ENTRY

Lower loop re-entry AFL propagates around the IVC in either a CW or CCW direction or around the IVC and tricuspid annulus in a figure of 8 double-loop configuration (Figure 6.7).[5,22,23] The isthmus is critical for this flutter and a CTI line results in successful ablation (Figure 6.8).

INTRA-ISTHMUS RE-ENTRY

The intra-isthmus re-entry AFL circuit is localized to the CTI. The circuit is bound by medial CTI and the coronary sinus ostium. The lateral CTI is not involved. Fractionated or double

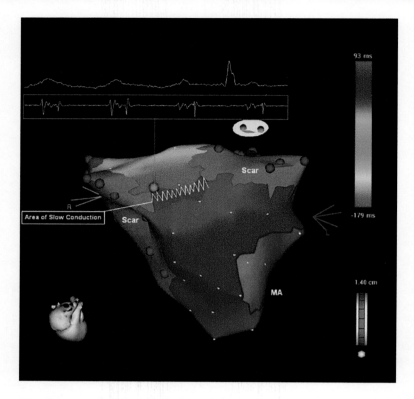

Figure 6.8 Electro-anatomic map of the left atrium in a previously ablated patient. Two scars at the location of the PVs on both sides provide anatomic obstacles around which a flutter propagates. The flutter activation wave is seen traveling down the posterior wall, around the mitral annulus, and up the anterior wall. An area of slow conduction is shown between the two scars anteriorly where fractionated potentials are recorded. MA, mitral annulus.

potentials can be recorded at the CTI just outside the coronary sinus ostium and the circuit can be entrained.[5,24,25] Successful ablation is possible with a CTI line which involves the medial isthmus.

RIGHT ATRIAL NON-CAVOTRICUSPID-ISTHMUS-DEPENDENT FLUTTER
SCAR-RELATED ATRIAL FLUTTER
Macro-re-entrant circuits can occur at sites other than the CTI. Areas of scar or low voltage provide an anatomic obstacle and favor macro-re-entry, such as in patients with prior cardiac surgery. These scars could be related to the surgical intervention itself, such as in patients with repair of congenital heart defects, or to right atriotomy for cannulation in case of on-pump cardiac surgery. Re-entrant circuits in scar-related AFL would use for re-entry either the non-conducting scar tissue, areas with slow conduction within scar tissue, as well as areas of anatomic boundaries.[5,26–28] Successful ablation could be achieved with an ablation line, which connects the scar to an anatomical non-conducting structure, which creates a block to propagation of the re-entrant wave.

UPPER LOOP RE-ENTRY
Upper loop re-entry circuits are due to functional barriers to propagation of electrical impulses rather than anatomic barriers. Upper loop re-entry circuits are localized to the

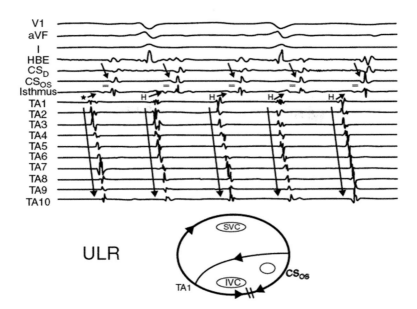

Figure 6.9 Upper loop re-entry (ULR). Upper panel shows simultaneous recordings of a surface ECG and intracardiac electrogram in a patient with sustained ULR flutter. The lower schematic illustrates the re-entrant circuit in the upper part of the right atrium. The cavotricuspid isthmus is *not* a critical part of the circuit. His, recording from the His bundle region; CS_D, distal coronary sinus; CS_{OS}, ostium of coronary sinus; TA, recordings from the 20-pole, "halo" electrode catheter positioned along the tricuspid annulus with its distal pole (TA1) at 7 o'clock in the left anterior oblique projection, and proximal at the high right atrium (TA5); SVC, superior vena cava; IVC, inferior vena cava. (Reproduced from Lee, K. et al., *Curr. Probl. Cardiol.*, 30, 121–167, 2005. With permission.)

upper portion of the right atrium with the crista terminalis and its slowed conduction serving as the functional obstacle. Maintenance of the conduction gap across the area of slow conduction is vital for the perpetuation of the circuit. This allows time for tissue to recover conduction before its activation by the propagating wavefront. The circuit can travel in either a clockwise or counterclockwise direction (Figure 6.9).[5,29] Successful ablation requires ablation at the critical isthmus, which needs to be extended to an anatomical non-conducting structure.

LEFT ATRIAL FLUTTER
Left atrial flutter occurs less frequently than right atrial CTI-dependent AFLs and often co-exists with AF. Left atrial flutters arise in structurally damaged left atria such as in patients with prior cardiac surgery of left atrial ablation procedures. The re-entry mechanism, as it is the case of right-sided AFLs, involves areas of block as well as areas with slow conduction, which sustain AFL. ECG findings of CCW left atrial circuits include low amplitude flutter waves and positive waves in leads V1 and V2 (Figure 6.7).[5]

MITRAL ANNULAR ATRIAL FLUTTER
The anatomic boundaries of the circuit include the mitral annulus and low-voltage area or scar in the posterior wall of the left atrium. The circuit rotates around the mitral annulus in either a CW or CCW direction (Figure 6.10).[5,30,31] Typical ablation lines to successfully treat this flutter include a right superior pulmonary vein to mitral annulus ablation or a line of ablation

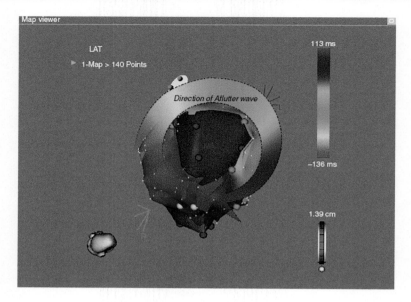

Figure 6.10 Electro-anatomic map of the left atrium. Sequential activation around the mitral annulus in a clockwise fashion.

between the left inferior pulmonary vein and the mitral annulus. The latter often involves need for ablation within the coronary sinus to achieve bidirectional block.

SCAR AND PULMONARY VEIN RELATED ATRIAL FLUTTER

This circuit rotates around one or more of the pulmonary veins or scar in the posterior wall.[5,30,31] Re-entry may also involve both entrance and exit into a pulmonary vein in patients with prior pulmonary vein isolation who had pulmonary venous conduction recovery. Generally speaking, once the flutter circuit and critical isthmus are identified, successful ablation requires either isolation of the veins or linear ablation to connect non-conducting structures and therefore creating a structural barrier to re-entry.

CORONARY SINUS ATRIAL FLUTTER

The circuit travels from the coronary sinus to the lateral left atrium, up to the roof and anterior wall and down the interatrial septum and back to the CS. This typically occurs in patients with prior atrial damage but very rarely can occur the absence of structural abnormality.[32] This flutter could be ablated by creating a conduction block across the coronary sinus.

LEFT SEPTAL ATRIAL FLUTTER

The circuit rotates in either a CW or CCW manner around the left septum primum. ECG findings include dominant positive waves in V1. The critical isthmus is located between the septum primum and pulmonary veins or between the septum primum to the right inferior pulmonary vein and the mitral annular ring. The creation of block across the critical isthmus results in successful ablation. To be noted that in the absence of prior cardiac surgery, these flutters seem to depend on low-voltage areas of the posterior wall and left atrial roof. It is hypothesized that atrial conduction slowing in these cases is secondary to either atrial dilated cardiomyopathy or anti-arrhythmics (sotalol, amiodarone).[33]

REFERENCES

1. DeStafano F, Eaker ED, Broste SK et al. Epidemiologic research in an integrated regional medical care system: The marshfield epidemiologic study area. *J Clin Epidemiol* 1996; 49: 643–652.

2. Granada J, Uribe W, Chyou PF et al. Incidence and predictors of atrial flutter in the general population. *J Am Coll Cardiol* 2000; 36: 2242–2246.

3. Halligan SC, Gersch BJ, Brown RD Jr. The natural history of lone atrial flutter. *Ann Intern Med* 2004; 140: 265–268.

4. Vidaillet H, Granada JF, Chyou PH et al. A population-based study of mortality among patients with atrial fibrillation or flutter. *Am J Med* 2002; 113(5): 365–370.

5. Lee K, Yang Y, Scheinman MM. Atrial flutter: A review of its history, mechanisms, clinical features, and current therapy. *Curr Probl Cardiol* 2005; 30(3): 121–167.

6. Blomstrom-Lundqvist C, Scheinman M. ACC/AHA/ESC guidelines for the management of patients with supraventricular arrhythmias—Executive summary. *Circulation* 2003; 108: 1871–1909.

7. Niebauer M, Chung M. Management of atrial flutter. *Cardiol Rev* 2001; 9(5): 253–258.

8. Harvey WP, Ronan JA Jr. Bedside diagnosis of arrhythmias. *Prog Cardiovasc Dis* 1966; 8: 419–445.

9. Cosio FG. Atrial flutter update. *Card Electrophysiol Rev* 2002; 6: 356–364.

10. Topol EJ (ed.). *Textbook of Cardiovascular Medicine*, 2nd edn. Philadelphia, PA: Lippincott, Williams and Wilkins, 2002.

11. Rosenbleuth A, Garcia-Ramos J. Studies on flutter and fibrillation II. The influence of artificial obstacles on experimental auricular flutter. *Am Heart J* 1947; 33: 677–684.

12. Spach MS, Miller WT, Geselowitz DB et al. The discontinuous nature of propagation in normal canine cardiac muscle. Evidence for recurrent discontinuities of intracellular resistance that affect the membrane currents. *Circ Res* 1981; 48: 39–54.

13. Spach MS, Dolber PC. Relating extracellular potentials and their derivatives to anisotropic propagation at a microscopic level in human cardiac muscle. Evidence for electrical uncoupling of side-to-side fiber connections with increasing age. *Circ Res* 1986; 58(3): 356–371.

14. Saoudi N, Cosio F, Waldo A et al. A classification of atrial flutter and regular atrial tachycardia according to electrophysiological mechanisms and anatomical bases; a statement from a joint expert group from the working group of arrhythmias of the European Society of Cardiology and the North American Society of Pacing and Electrophysiology. *Eur Heart J* 2001; 22: 1162–1182.

15. Olgin JE, Kalman JM, Fitzpatrick AP, Lesh MD. Role of right atrial endocardial structures as barriers to conduction during human type I atrial flutter. Activation and entrainment mapping guided by intracardiac echocardiography. *Circulation* 1995; 92: 1839–1848.

16. Nakagwa H, Lazzara R, Khastgir T et al. Role of tricuspid annulus and the Eustachian valve/ridge on atrial flutter. Relevance to catheter ablation of the septal isthmus and a new technique for rapid identification of ablation success. *Circulation* 1996; 94: 398–406.

17. Kalman JM, Olgin JE, Saxon LA et al. Activation and entrainment mapping defines the tricuspid annulus as the anterior barrier in typical atrial flutter. *Circulation* 1996; 94: 398–406.

18. Arribas F, Lopez-Gil M, Cosio FG, Nunez A. The upper link of human common atrial flutter circuit: Definition by multiple endocardial recordings during entrainment. *Pacing Clin Electrophysiol* 1997; 20: 2924–2929.

19. Tsuchiya T, Okumura K, Tabuchi T et al. The upper turnover site in the reentry circuit of common atrial flutter. *Am J Cardiol* 1996; 78: 1439–1442.

20. Cheng J, Scheinman MM. Acceleration of typical atrial flutter due to double-wave reentry induced by programmed electrical stimulation. *Circulation* 1998; 97: 1589–1596.

21. Yang Y, Mangat I, Glatter KA et al. Mechanism of conversion of atypical right atrial flutter to atrial fibrillation. *Am J Cardiol* 2003; 1: 46–52.

22. Cheng J, Cabeen JWR, Scheinman MM. Right atrial flutter due to lower loop reentry mechanisms and anatomic substrates. *Circulation* 1999; 99: 1700–1705.

23. Zhang S, Younis G, Hariharan R et al. Lower loop reentry as a mechanism of clockwise right atrial flutter. *Circulation* 2004; 109: 1630–1635.

24. Yang Y, Varma N, Scheinman MM. Reentry within the cavotricuspid isthmus: A novel isthmus dependent circuit (abstract). *J Am Coll Cardiol* 2003; 41: 119A.

25. Yang Y, Varma N, Keung EC, Scheinman MM. Surface ECG characteristics of intra-isthmus reentry. *Pacing Clin Electrophysiol* 2003; 26: 1032.

26. Feld GK, Shahandeh-Rad F. Activation patterns in experimental canine atrial flutter produced by right atrial crush injury. *J Am Coll Cardiol* 1992; 20: 441–451.

27. Nakagawa H, Shah N, Matsudaira K et al. Characterization of reentrant circuit in macroentrant right atrial tachycardia after surgical repair of congenital heart disease: Isolated channels between scar allow "focal" ablation. *Circulation* 2001; 103(5): 669–709.

28. Kalman JM, Olgin JE, Saxon LA et al. Electrocardiographic and electrophysiologic characterization of atypical atrial flutter in man: Use of activation and entrainment mapping and implications for catheter ablation. *J Cardiovasc Electrophysiol* 1997; 8(2): 121–144.

29. Tai CT, Huang JL, Lin YK et al. Noncontact three-dimensional mapping and ablation of upper loop re-entry originating in the right atrium. *J Am Coll Cardiol* 2002; 40: 746–753.

30. Jais P, Shah DC, Haissaguerre M et al. Mapping and ablation of left atrial flutters. *Circulation* 2000; 101: 2928–2934.

31. Ouyang F, Ernst S, Vogtmann T et al. Characterization of reentrant circuits in left atrial macroreentrant tachycardia: Critical isthmus block can prevent atrial tachycardia recurrence. *Circulation* 2002; 105: 1934–1942.

32. Olgin JE, Jayachandran JV, Engesstein E et al. Atrial macroreentry involving the myocardium of the coronary sinus: A unique mechanism for atypical flutter. *J Cardiovasc Electrophysiol* 1998; 9: 1094–1099.

33. Marrouche NF, Natale A, Wazni O et al. Left septal atrial flutter: Electrophysiology, anatomy, and results of ablation. *Circulation* 2004; 109: 2240–2247.

ATRIAL FIBRILLATION

Rong Bai, Mohamed Salim, Luigi Di Biase, Robert Schweikert, and Walid Saliba

CONTENTS

INTRODUCTION

Atrial fibrillation (AF) is the most common sustained cardiac arrhythmia in clinical practice. In 2010, the prevalence of diagnosed AF in the United States was 5.2 million and predicted to increase to 12.1 million by 2030. Similar increases are also seen in other countries in Europe, Asia, and Africa. Compared to those with sinus rhythm, AF is associated with an increased risk of death in both men and women. Hence a further understanding on the risk factors, classification, and mechanism is essential in the management of patients with AF.

RISK FACTORS

• Male gender	• Obesity
• Age	• Obstructive sleep apnea
• Diabetes	• Smoking
• Hypertension	• Exercise
• Heart failure	• Alcohol use
• Valvular heart disease	• Hyperthyroidism
• Myocardial infarction	• Increased pulse pressure
• Left ventricular hypertrophy	

CLASSIFICATION AND DEFINITION

- *Paroxysmal*: AF is self-terminating within 7 days of recognized onset. Most episodes last less than 24 h.
- *Persistent*: Continuous AF that is sustained >7 days or is terminated electrically or pharmacologically.
- *Long standing persistent*: Continuous AF > 12 months.
- *Permanent*: Cardioversion failed or not attempted.

PATHOGENESIS

Currently, the mechanism of AF has not been conclusively understood. The most common theory is that AF is mostly triggered and driven by rapid firing from a focal source like pulmonary veins, and less common from the superior vena cava, ligament of Marshall, and coronary sinus. Sometimes the triggering mechanism may also be the driving mechanism sustaining AF. It has been reported that dilated atria, scar, and electrical remodeling provide the substrate for AF.

CLINICAL PRESENTATION

Patients frequently present with palpitation, fatigue, dizziness, presyncope, dyspnea, and less commonly with chest pain and syncope. However, some patients with permanent AF are asymptomatic. Factors affecting patients' clinical presentation include the pattern of AF break out, duration of AF episode, ventricular response (heart rate), and the status of underlying cardiac disease. Irregularly irregular pulse, pulse deficits, and varying intensity of the first heart sound may be observed during physical examination (Table 7.1).

Table 7.1 Minimum and additional clinical evaluation in patients with atrial fibrillation

Minimum evaluation
1. *History and physical examination, to define*
   Presence and nature of symptoms associated with AF
   Clinical type of AF (first episode, paroxysmal, persistent, or permanent)
   Onset of the first symptomatic attack or date of discovery of AF
   Frequency, duration, precipitating factors, and modes of termination of AF
   Response to any pharmacologic agents that have been administered
   Presence of any underlying heart disease or other reversible conditions (e.g.,
      hyperthyroidism or alcohol consumption)
2. *Electrocardiogram, to identify*
   Rhythm (verify AF)
   LV hypertrophy
   P-wave duration and morphology or fibrillatory waves
   Pre-excitation
   Bundle-branch block
   Prior MI
   Other atrial arrhythmias
   To measure and follow the RR, QRS, and QT intervals in conjunction with anti-arrhythmic
      drug therapy
3. *Transthoracic echocardiogram, to identify*
   Valvular heart disease
   LA and RA size
   LV size and function
   Peak RV pressure (pulmonary hypertension)
   LV hypertrophy
   LA thrombus (low sensitivity)
   Pericardial disease
4. *Blood tests of thyroid, renal, and hepatic function*
   For a first episode of AF, when the ventricular rate is difficult to control

Additional testing
One or several tests may be necessary.
1. *Six-minute walk test*
   If the adequacy of rate control is in question
2. *Exercise testing*
   If the adequacy of rate control is in question (permanent AF)
   To reproduce exercise-induced AF
   To exclude Ischemia before treatment of selected patients with a type IC anti-arrhythmic drug
3. *Holter monitoring or event recording*
   If diagnosis of the type of arrhythmia is in question
   As a means of evaluating rate control
4. *Transesophageal echocardiography*
   To identify LA thrombus (in the LA appendage)
   To guide cardioversion
5. *Electrophysiologic study*
   To clarify the mechanism of wide-QRS-complex tachycardia
   To identify a predisposing arrhythmia such as atrial flutter or paroxysmal supraventricular
      tachycardia
   To seek sites for curative ablation or AV conduction block/modification
6. *Chest radiograph, to evaluate*
   Lung parenchyma, when clinical findings suggest an abnormality pulmonary vasculature,
      when clinical findings suggest an abnormality

Once AF episode is confirmed by ECG recording (Figure 7.1), further medical evaluations may be required (Table 7.1). Treatment strategies for AF patients depend on the type of AF, cause, comorbidities, and patient preference. The management of AF includes: (i) rate control, (ii) rhythm control, and (iii) stroke prevention.

RATE CONTROL DURING AF

The target rate in AF patient is <80 bpm at rest and <110 bpm on moderate exercise. This is usually assessed by 24-h or 48-h Holter monitoring. Atrioventricular nodal ablation with permanent pacing is recommended for patients who are unable to meet rate control targets. Rate control strategy is suitable for asymptomatic patients or those with mild symptoms and normal ejection fraction (Table 7.2):

Rate controlling medications include: beta-blockers, non-hydropyridine calcium-channel blockers, and Class I and III anti-arrhythmic drugs (Sotalol, amiodarone propafenone, and flecanide).

RESTORATION AND MAINTENANCE OF SINUS RHYTHM

- *Restoration of sinus rhythm*: A rhythm control strategy should probably be the first-line strategy in newly diagnosed AF, symptomatic AF with poor rate control, young patient age, tachycardia-mediated cardiomyopathy, AF precipitated by an acute illness, and patient preference. Depending on the agent of choice and on the type of AF this could be performed in the hospital or on an outpatient basis. Anticoagulation should be optimized as discussed in the next section before attempting to restore sinus rhythm, especially if AF has been present for longer than 48 h.
- *Pharmacologic conversion*: Medications may convert the AF into sinus rhythm and their recommended doses are shown in Table 7.3.

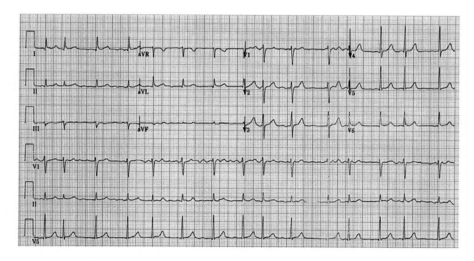

Figure 7.1   AF episode is confirmed by ECG recording.

Table 7.2 Pharmacologic rate control for atrial arrhythmias

Agent	Loading dose	Maintenance dose	Side-effects/toxicity	Comments
Digoxin	0.25–0.5 mg iv or po, then 0.25 mg q 4–6 to 1 mg in 1st 24 h	0.125–0.25 mg po or iv qd	Anorexia, nausea; AV block; ventricular arrhythmias; accumulates in renal failure	Used in CHF; vagotonic effects on the AVN; delayed onset of action; narrow therapeutic window; less effective in postoperative, paroxysmal AF with high adrenergic states
Beta-blockers				
Propranolol	1 mg iv q 2–5' to 0.1–0.2 mg/kg	10–80 mg po tid-qid	Bronchospasm; CHF; ↓ BP	Effective in heart rate control; rapid onset of action; esmolol short acting
Metoprolol Esmolol	5 mg iv q 5' to 15 mg 500 µg/kg iv over 1'	25–100 mg po bid-tid 50 µg/kg iv for 4'; repeat load prn; and ↑ maintenance 20–50 µg/kg/min q 5–10'		
Calcium-channel blockers				
Verapamil	2.5–10 mg iv over 2'	5–10 mg iv q 30–60' or 40–160 mg po tid or 120–480 mg/day, sustained release	↓ BP, CHF ↑ digoxin lev	Rapid onset, can be used safely in COPD and DM
Diltiazem	0.25 mg/kg over 2', repeat prn p 15' at 0.35 mg/kg	5–15 mg/h iv or 30–90 mg po qid or 120–360 mg sustained release qd		Often well tolerated with low LVEF pts

Table 7.3 Pharmacologic conversion regimens

Drug	Route	Dose	Success rate (%)
Quinidine	po	200–324 mg tid to 1.5 g/day	48–86
Procainamide	iv	1 g over 20–30 min	48–65
Propafenone	po	600 mg	55–87
	iv	2 mg/kg over 10 min	40–90
Flecainide	po	300 mg	90
	iv	2 mg/kg over 10 min	65–90
Amiodarone	iv	1.2 g over 24 h	45–85
Sotalol	po	80–160 mg, then 160–360 mg/day	52
Dofetilide	po	125–500 µg bid, based on CrCl	30
Ibutilide	iv	1 mg over 10 min, repeat in 10 min as required	31

In patient with no structural heart disease, Class IC drugs (propafenone and flecanide) can be used as "pill-in-the-pocket" strategy. Usually beta-blockers and nonhydropyridine calcium-channel blockers are given for AVN blockade.

- *Electrical cardioversion*
- Most effective method of restoring sinus rhythm.
- Performed when AF duration <48 h.
- Anticoagulation is undertaken in those with AF > 48 h with 3 weeks before and 4 weeks after cardioversion.
- Performed when AF with rapid ventricular rate does not respond to pharmacological therapy.
- Recommended when AF is associated with hemodynamic instability.
- Requires conscious sedation with a short-acting anesthetic.
- Monophasic (200–360 J) and biphasic (50–200 J) external cardioversion.
- This may be enhanced with anti-arrhythmic medications such as amiodarone, flecainide, or ibutilide.
- May be guided by transesophageal echocardiography. It can help rule out left atrial clot and expedite cardioversion in patients who are tolerating AF poorly. In this strategy, anticoagulation should be started with unfractionated heparin or low molecular weight heparin before cardioversion and continued until a therapeutic international normalized ratio (INR) is achieved with warfarin therapy.

MAINTENANCE OF SINUS RHYTHM (TABLE 7.4)

After cardioversion, maintenance of sinus rhythm is by anti-arrhythmic drugs like flecanide, propafenone, sotalol, dofetilide, dronedarone, or amiodarone.

Catheter ablation is considered in those who failed to maintain sinus rhythm with at least one drug. Cryoballoon ablation is an alternative to radiofrequency ablation to achieve pulmonary vein isolation.

Table 7.4 Drugs for maintenance of sinus rhythm

Anti-arrhythmic drug	Dose	% Maintenance SR (6–12 mos)	Side-effects/comments
Class IA			
Quinidine	200–400 mg po tid-qid	30–79	↑ QT, pro-arrhythmia/ TdP, potential ↑ AVN conduction, diarrhea, nausea, ↑ digoxin levels, thrombocytopenia
Procainamide	10–15 mg/kg iv at ≤50 mg/min or 2–6 g/day po in bid or qid sustained release	N/A	↑ BP, CHF, drug-induced lupus, agranulocytosis; active metabolite NAPA with class III activity accumulates in renal failure
Disopyramide	100–300 mg po tid	44–67	Anticholinergic effects (e.g., urinary retention, dry eyes/mouth), CHF
Class IC			
Flecainide	50–200 mg po bid	34–81	Pro-arrhythmia, visual disturbance, dizziness, CHF, avoid in CAD, or LV dysfunction
Propafenone	150–300 mg tid	30–76	CHF, avoid in CAD/LV dysfunction
Class IA/B/C			
Moricizine	200–300 mg tid	N/A	Pro-arrhythmia, dizziness, GI/nausea, headache, caution in CAD/LV dysfunction
Class III			
Sotalol	80–240 mg bid	37–70	CHF, bronchospasm, bradycardia, ↑ QT proarrhythmia/TdP
Amiodarone	600–1600 mg/day loading in divided doses, 100–400 mg qd maintenance	40–79	Pulmonary toxicity, bradycardia, hyper- or hypothyroidism, hepatic toxicity, GI (nausea, constipation), neurologic, dermatologic, and ophthalmologic side effects, drug interactions
Dofetilide	CrCl (mL/min) >60: 500 µg bid 40–60: 250 µg bid 20–40: 125 µg bid	58–71	Exclude CrCl < 20 mL/min. ↑ QT, pro-arrhythmia/TdP, headache, muscle cramps

AF is associated with a 5-fold increase of stroke. AF-induced strokes are secondary to emboli probably originating from left atrial appendage or fibrillating atria, and are known to be more severe than non-AF-related stroke. Antithrombotic therapy is based on shared decision making, understanding of the risks of stroke and bleeding with patients' preferences. CHA_2DS_2-VaSC is used for stroke risk assessment.

RISK FACTORS FOR STROKE WITH AF

- TIA or previous stroke
- Diabetes
- Hypertension
- Age
- Left ventricular dysfunction
- Increased left atrial size
- Rheumatic mitral valve disease
- Prosthetic valves
- Women age 75
- Mitral annular calcification
- Increased wall thickness
- Thyrotoxicosis

GUIDELINES FOR ANTITHROMBOTIC THERAPY FOR AF

PHARMACOLOGICAL STROKE PREVENTION

- Anticoagulation is recommended if AF persists longer than 48 h, particularly if cardioversion is anticipated after this time or AF continues to recur after cardioversion.
- Anticoagulation with warfarin (target INR 2.5, range 2.0–3.0 for AF) or novel oral anti-coagulants (dabigatran, rivaroxaban, apixaban) should be recommended for all anticoagulation-eligible patients (Table 7.5). Risk factors include:
  - Prior transient ischemic attack, systemic embolus or stroke
  - Hypertension
  - Age
  - Poor left ventricular function
  - Rheumatic mitral valve disease
  - Prosthetic heart valves
- Patients aged 65–75 years with no risk factors can be treated with aspirin or warfarin.
- Aspirin is recommended for patients, 65 years old and who have no risk factors.
- Anticoagulation therapy with warfarin might be contraindicated for patients who have one of the following risk factors of bleeding complication:
  - Advanced age: 80 years old.
  - Uncontrolled hypertension, particularly when systolic is 160 mmHg.
  - Prior history of cerebrovascular disease.
  - Prior history of subdural hematoma.
  - These recommendations apply to paroxysmal as well as persistent and permanent AF.

Table 7.5 Dose selection of oral anticoagulants

Renal function	Warfarin	Dabigatran	Rivaroxaban	Apixaban
Normal/Mild impairment	Dose adjusted INR 2.0–3.0	150 mg BID (CrCl > 30 mL/min)	20 mg QD with evening meal (CrCl > 50 mL/min)	5.0 or 2.5 mg BID
Moderate impairment	Dose adjusted INR 2.0–3.0	150 mg BID (CrCl > 30 mL/min)	15 mg QD with evening meal (CrCl 30–50 mL/min)	5.0 or 2.5 mg BID
Severe impairment	Dose adjusted INR 2.0–3.0	75 mg BID (CrCl 15–30 mL/min)	15 mg QD with evening meal (CrCl > 15–30 mL/min)	No recommendation
End-stage CKD not on dialysis	Dose adjusted INR 2.0–3.0	Not recommended (CrCl < 15 mL/min)	Not recommended (CrCl < 15 mL/min)	No recommendation
End-stage CKD on dialysis	Dose adjusted INR 2.0–3.0	Not recommended (CrCl < 15 mL/min)	Not recommended (CrCl < 15 mL/min)	No recommendation

NON-PHARMACOLOGICAL STROKE PREVENTION

Exclusion of the LAA is performed since LAA is the primary source for thromboembolism in AF. This involves percutaneous insertion of WATCHMAN device, Amplatzer cardiac plug, or LARIAT.

SUMMARY

The overall strategies of AF management are summarized in Figure 7.2.

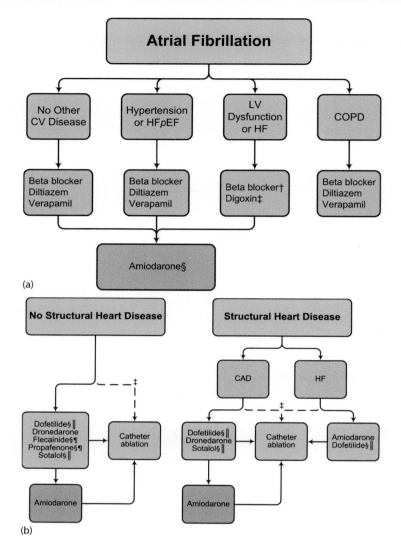

Figure 7.2 A flowchart of AF management strategies (a) Approach to selecting drug therapy for ventricular rate control. † Beta blockers should be instituted following stabilization of patients with decompensated HF. The choice of beta blocker (e.g., cardioselective) depends on the patient's clinical condition. ‡ Digoxin is not usually first-line therapy. It may be combined with a beta blocker and/or a non-dihydropyridine calcium-channel blocker when ventricular rate control is insufficient and may be useful in patients with HF. § In part because of concern over its side-effect profile, use of amiodarone for chronic control of ventricular rate should be reserved for patients who do not respond to or are intolerant of beta blockers or non-dihydropyridine calcium antagonists. COPD: chronic obstructive pulmonary disease; CV: cardiovascular; HF: heart failure; HFpEF: heart failure with preserved ejection fraction; LV: left ventricular. (b) Strategies for rhythm control in patients with paroxysmal* and persistent AF. * Catheter ablation is only recommended as first-line therapy for patients with paroxysmal AF (Class IIa recommendation). ‡ Depending on patient preference when performed in experienced centers. § Not recommended with severe LVH (wall thickness >1.5 cm). ‖ Should be used with caution in patients at risk for Torsades de pointes (Tdp) ventricular tachycardia. ¶ Should be combined with AV nodal blocking agents. AF: atrial fibrillation; AV: atrioventricular; CAD: coronary artery disease; HF: heart failure; and LVH: left ventricular hypertrophy.

ADDITIONAL READING

1. January CT, Wann LS, Alpert JS, et al. 2014 AHA/ACC/HRS guideline for the management of patients with atrial fibrillation: A report of the American College of Cardiology/ American Heart Association Task Force on Practice Guidelines and the Heart Rhythm Society. *J Am Coll Cardiol.* 2014;64(21):2305–2307.

VENTRICULAR TACHYARRHYTHMIA

GENETICALLY DETERMINED VENTRICULAR ARRHYTHMIAS

Houman Khakpour and Jason S. Bradfield

CONTENTS

The discovery of the genetic basis of inherited arrhythmogenic syndromes over the past two decades has led to significant advancement in our understanding of diseases with predisposition towards sudden cardiac death (SCD) in patients with "normal" hearts.

This chapter will focus on the current understanding of what are now distinct and well-understood genetically determined disorders/syndromes, which predispose patients to ventricular arrhythmias.

LONG QT SYNDROME

Congenital long QT syndrome (LQTS) is a heterogeneous channelopathy that is characterized by ECG alterations—with prolongation of the QT interval as its hallmark—and risk of arrhythmic events. Clinical manifestations of LQTS include syncope due to torsade de pointes (TdP), cardiac arrest, and SCD. The estimated prevalence of LQTS is 1:2000 persons among caucasians, though this does not take into account mutation-positive patients with normal QTc.[1] This discussion excludes secondary causes of QT prolongation that can occur with drugs, electrolyte imbalance, and acquired cardiac conditions.

GENETIC CHARACTERISTICS

To date, 13 genes have been linked to congenital LQTS encoding for potassium, sodium, and calcium channel-related proteins, as well as membrane adaptor proteins.[2,3] However, the first 3 genes discovered in 1995, encompassing the patients with *LQT1*, *LQT2*, and *LQT3* genotypes with mutations involving *KCNQ1*, *KCNH2*, and *SCN5A* make up over 92% of patients with genetically confirmed LQTS.[3-6] Notably, up to 20% of patients with LQTS remain genetically undiagnosed after comprehensive genetic testing.[7] The majority of LQTS has an autosomal dominant inheritance (Romano–Ward syndrome). The autosomal recessive form (Jervell and Lange-Nielsen syndrome) is rare, more virulent, and associated with deafness. Other rare phenotypes, Anderson–Tawil syndrome and Timothy syndrome, have been classified as LQT7 and LQT8 and are associated with QT prolongation in addition to other distinct clinical manifestations (Table 8.1).[7,8]

Table 8.1 Genes associated with LQTS

Channelopathy	Gene
LQT 1	KCNQ1
LQT 2	KCNH2
LQT 3	SCN5A
LQT 4	ANK2
LQT 5	KCNE1
LQT 6	KCNE2
LQT 7	KCNJ2
LQT 8	CACNA1C
LQT 9	CAV3
LQT 10	SCN4B
LQT 11	AKAP9
LQT 12	SNTA1
LQT 13	KCNJ5

Source: Webster, G. and Berul, C.I., *Circulation*, 127, 126–140, 2013.

CLINICAL PRESENTATION

Symptoms of LQTS are due to arrhythmic events caused by TdP and its deterioration into VF, leading to possible syncope, cardiac arrest, and even SCD. Common precipitants of an arrhythmic event are often specific to the particular genotype[9]:

- In LQT1 most events occur during physical or emotional stress.
- In LQT2 most events occur at rest or in association with abrupt auditory stimulation.
- In LQT3 most events occur at rest or during sleep.
- The risk of overall cardiac events is significantly higher in patients with LQT1 or LQT2, but the percentage of lethal cardiac events is significantly higher in patients with LQT3.[10]

ECG IN LONG QT SYNDROME

The 12-lead ECG alterations are important and helpful:

- To confirm the suspicion of LQTS
- To provide clues to the possible underlying channel defect
- To assist risk stratification
- To guide effective and safe therapy

Though not always present at rest, QT prolongation is the hallmark of LQTS.[11] The accurate measurement of the QT interval may be challenging in patients with underlying atrial fibrillation, "U" waves, paced ventricular rhythms, pre-excitation syndromes, or low amplitude waves on the ECG. Variability in QT interval measurement is mainly at the end of the T-wave, rather than the onset of the QRS complex. It is important to measure the longest QT interval observed in any lead of the 12 ECG leads.[12,13] The Bazett's formula ($QT/RR^{1/2}$) is the recommended heart rate correction formula (QTc) by the most recent expert consensus statement.[3]

T-wave morphology can provide important additional diagnostic and prognostic clues (Figures 8.1 and 8.2):

- Macroscopic T-wave alternans—a marker of cardiac electrical instability—though infrequently seen, should prompt an evaluation for LQTS.[14]
- Extremely broad-based T-wave are seen in LQT1.
- Notches on the T-wave are typical of LQT2 and their presence (compared to genetically proven LQT2 without notching) is a marker for higher risk of arrhythmic events.[15]
- LQT3 show peaked T-waves preceded by a long, isoelectric ST segment.

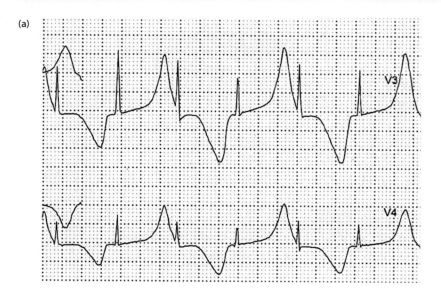

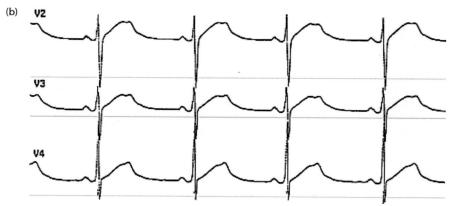

Figure 8.1 Notched T-wave and T-wave alternans in two patients with LQTS. (a) Macroscopic T-wave alternans in a 2-year-old LQTS patient with multiple episodes of cardiac arrest. (b) Notched T-waves in a 37-year-old man with LQTS. (From Schwartz, P.J. and Ackerman, M.J., *Eur. Heart J.*, 34, 3109–3116, 2013.)

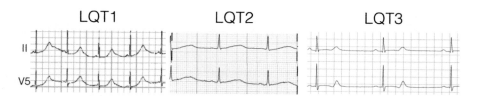

Figure 8.2 LQT1, LQT2, and LQT3 ECG patterns.

DIAGNOSIS

Congenital LQTS is diagnosed mainly based on the measurement of QTc interval (Bazett's formula) after excluding acquired causes of QT prolongation. A scoring system, taking into account the patient's age, symptoms, medical and family history, and ECG features including QTc has been developed which provides a probability of the diagnosis of LQTS.[16] LQTS can also be diagnosed in the presence of an unequivocally pathogenic mutation.[3] Approximately 20%–25% of patients with LQTS confirmed by genetic testing may have a normal QTc (concealed LQTS).[17] To unmask QT prolongation, the use of provocative testing, including during infusion of epinephrine,[18,19] in the recovery phase of exercise testing,[20] or during position change from supine to standing,[21] has been proposed. These techniques may be used in uncertain cases, though more clinical validation is needed.[3] Based on the 2013 expert consensus recommendations (Table 8.2)[3]:

1   LQTS is diagnosed:
   (a)   In the presence of an LQTS risk score of ≥3.5 in the absence of a secondary cause for QT prolongation, and/or
   (b)   In the presence of an unequivocally pathologic mutation in one of the LQTS genes, or
   (c)   In the presence of a QTc ≥ 500 ms on repeated 12-lead ECGs and in the absence of a secondary cause for QT prolongation.
2   LQTS can be diagnosed in the presence of QTc between 480 and 499 ms on repeated 12-lead ECGs in a patient with unexplained syncope in the absence of a secondary cause for QT prolongation and in the absence of a pathogenic mutation.

PROGNOSIS AND RISK STRATIFICATION

Genotype and certain clinical findings can be helpful in risk stratification of patients with LQTS. Jervell and Lange-Nielsen syndrome and Timothy syndrome (LQT8) are highly virulent and manifest with arrhythmic events early on.[8] Within the common variants, the location,

Table 8.2   LQTS scoring

			Points
Electrocardiographic findings[a]			
A OTc[b]		≥480 ms	3
		460–479 ms	2
		450–459 (male) ms	1
B QTc[b] 4th minute of recovery from exercise stress test ≥480 ms			1
C Torsade de pointes[c]			2
D T-wave alternans			1
E Notched T-wave in three leads			1
F Low heart rate for age[d]			0.5
Clinical history			
A Syncope[c]		With stress	2
		Without stress	1
B Congenital deafness			0.5
Family history			
A Family members with definite LQTS[e]			1
B Unexplained sudden cardiac death below age 30 among immediate family members[e]			0.5

Source: Schwartz, P.J. and Ackerman, M.J., *Eur. Heart J.*, 34, 3109–3116, 2013. With permission.
SCORE: ≤1 point: low possibility of LQTS. 1.5–3 points: intermediate probability LQTS. ≥3.5 points high probability.
[a]   In the absence of medications of disorders known to affect these electrocardiographic features.
[b]   QTc calculated by Bazett's formula where QTc = QT/√RR.
[c]   Mutually exclusive.
[d]   Resting heart rate below the 2nd percentile for age.
[e]   The same family member cannot be counted in A and B.

type, and degree of mutation are associated with different risks.[22] High-risk variants include mutations in the cytoplasmic loop of LQT1 and mutations in the pore region of LQT2.[22]

Clinical findings associated with high-risk include:

- QTc > 500 ms (extremely high if QTc > 600 ms)[23]
- Overt T-wave alternans
- Arrhythmic event before age 7 (extremely high if in the first year)[24,25]
- Arrhythmic events on full medical therapy

THERAPY FOR LQTS

Treatment of asymptomatic patients is justified by the occurrence of SCD as a first clinical manifestation in some patients. All patients with LQTS should avoid QT-prolonging drugs (www. qtdrugs.org). Lifestyle modifications should include correction of factors that may cause QT prolongation such as imbalanced diets, avoidance of strenuous exercises, especially unsupervised swimming, in LQT1 patients, and avoidance of exposure to abrupt loud noises in LQT2 patients.[26]

Therapies for prevention of sudden death in patients with LQTS include use of beta-blockers, implantable cardioverter-defibrillator (ICD), and left cardiac sympathetic denervation (LCSD).

BETA-BLOCKERS

Several large studies have shown that beta-blocker therapy reduces fatal arrhythmic events in LQTS patients.[27,28] Beta-blockers are therefore indicated for all patients with LQTS, including asymptomatic patients and those with a genetic diagnosis and normal QTc, unless there is a clear contraindication.[3,24,25] Beta-blocker therapy is most effective in LQT1 and may be less effective in LQT3.[2,24] To date, there is no substantial evidence favoring cardioselective versus non-cardioselective beta-blockers or for determining the most effective dosage.

Prospective studies comparing the efficacy of different β-blockers have not been performed and the conclusions rely on retrospective analysis of cohorts. Cardioselective beta-blockers are recommended in patients with active asthma and long-acting beta-blockers such as nadolol or sustained-released propranolol are favored to avoid blood level fluctuation.[3] A retrospective analysis in 207 patients with LQT1 and 176 patients with LQTS2 showed equal prophylactic efficacy of nadolol, propranolol, and metoprolol in asymptomatic patients.

Among symptomatic patients, nadolol and propranolol performed better than metoprolol. The risk of cardiac events was 3.9-fold greater when patients were treated with metoprolol.[29] However, in another recent large retrospective study assessing the efficacy of the 4 most commonly prescribed β-blockers (atenolol, metoprolol, nadolol, and propranolol) in 1530 patients, all β-blockers were equally effective in reducing the risk of a first cardiac event. In the subcohort of patients with LQT1 ($n = 379$), no β-blocker was superior, whereas in LQT2 ($n = 406$), nadolol was slightly more effective than other β-blockers. In patients with at least one cardiac event while taking β-blockers, propranolol appeared to be the least effective drug.[30] The data from the retrospective studies clearly underline the beneficial effect of β-blocker therapy in LQTS but caution should be exercised before drawing conclusions about their relative efficacy. There is agreement that nadolol is probably one of the more effective drugs for this condition.[31] Abrupt discontinuation of beta-blockers should be avoided.

GENE-SPECIFIC THERAPIES

Sodium-channel blockers including mexiletine, flecaindine, and ranolazine have been used in high-risk patients with SCN5A mutation (LQT3) refractory to beta-blocker therapy or with recurrent events despite ICD and LCSD therapies.[32-34] The follow-up experience has been limited; the 2013 expert consensus endorses their use as a potential add-on therapy for LQT3 patients with QTc > 500 ms who shorten their QTc by >40 ms following an acute oral drug test with one of the above compounds (class IIa).[3]

ICD

ICD implantation is recommended for patients who are survivors of SCD and those with recurrent syncopal episodes despite beta-blocker therapy.[35,36] In very-high-risk patients, such as those with two or more gene mutations with symptoms as well as Jervell and Lange-Nielsen variant, prophylactic ICD should be considered.[8] However, given the life-time implication/potential complications of ICDs, particularly in the younger population, careful consideration of risk–benefit ratio and the patient's preferences are required. ICD therapy is not recommended in asymptomatic LQTS patients as a first-line therapy except for those deemed to be at very-high-risk for arrhythmic events.[3]

LEFT CARDIAC SYMPATHETIC DENERVATION (LCSD)

Left cardiac sympathetic denervation (LCSD) is another modality that has been reported to reduce the risk of SCD in very-high-risk patients. Through a left supraclavicular incision or as a minimally invasive procedure in experienced centers, the lower half of the left stellate ganglion as well as the T2–T4 thoracic ganglia are resected leading to a reduction in the adrenergic stimulation from the left cardiac sympathetic network.[37-39] In a study of 147 symptomatic high-risk patients with LQTS who underwent LCSD, cardiac event rates per patient decreased by 91%.[40] LCSD is recommended for high-risk patients in whom ICD therapy is refused or contraindicated and/or beta-blocker therapy is ineffective or cannot be used, and in LQTS patients who experience breakthrough events with ICD or beta-blocker therapy (Table 8.3).[3,26]

Table 8.3 2013 Expert consensus for treatment of LQTS

2013 Expert consensus recommendations on LQTS therapies
Class I

1. The following lifestyle changes are recommended in all patients with a diagnosis of LQTS:
  a. Avoidance of QT-prolonging drugs (www.qtdrugs.org)
  b. Identification and correction of electrolyte abnormalities that may occur during diarrhea, vomiting, metabolic conditions, or imbalanced diets for weight loss.
2. Beta-blockers are recommended for patients with a diagnosis of LQTS who are:
  a. Asymptomatic with QTc ≥ 470 ms *and/or*
  b. Symptomatic for syncope or documented ventricular tachycardia/ventricular fibrillation (VT/VF).
3. Left cardiac sympathetic denervation (LCSD) is recommended for high-risk patients with a diagnosis of LQTS in whom:
  a. Implantable cardioverter-defibrillator (ICD) therapy is contraindicated or refused *and/or*
  b. Beta-blockers are either not effective in preventing syncope/arrhythmias, not tolerated, not accepted, or contraindicated.
4. ICD implantation is recommended for patients with a diagnosis of LQTS who are survivors of a cardiac arrest.
5. All LQTS patients who wish to engage in competitive sports should be referred to a clinical expert for evaluation of risk.

Class IIa
1. Beta-blockers can be useful in patients with a diagnosis of LQTS who are asymptomatic with QTc ≤ 470 ms. 2. ICD implantation can be useful in patients with a diagnosis of LQTS who experience recurrent syncopal events while on beta-blocker therapy. 3. LCSD can be useful in patients with a diagnosis of LQTS who experience breakthrough events while on therapy with beta-blockers/ICD. 4. Sodium channel blockers can be useful, as add-on therapy, for LQT3 patients with a QTc > 500 ms who shorten their QTc by >40 ms following an acute oral drug test with one of these compounds.
Class III
1. Except under special circumstances, ICD implantation is *not* indicated in asymptomatic LQTS patients who have not been tried on beta-blocker therapy.

Source: Priori, S.G. et al., *Heart Rhythm*, 10, 1932–1963, 2013.

SHORT QT SYNDROME (SQTS)

Short QT syndrome, first described by Gussak et al.[41] is one of the rarer channelopathies associated with atrial and ventricular fibrillation and SCD.[42] SQTS patients present with recurrent syncope, atrial fibrillation, and SCD.

GENETIC CHARACTERISTICS

To date, gain of function mutations in 3 potassium channel genes have been associated with SQTS (KCNH2, KCNQ1, KCNJ2).[43,44] Mutations in the *CACNA1C* and *CACNB2* genes, which encode the alpha- and beta-subunits of the L-type cardiac calcium channels have been described as well.[2] These mutations result in an abnormally rapid repolarization.

ECG IN SQTS

QTc should be calculated avoiding tachycardia and bradycardia as use of Bazett's formula at these rates is not linear and it may lead to underestimation or overestimation of QTc. Aside from the short QT interval, the following ECG findings are associated with SQTS (Figure 8.3):

- Symmetric tall T-waves in V1–6
- Early repolarization with near absence of the ST segment

DIAGNOSIS

The cut-off value at the lower end of the QTc used to diagnose SQTS remains a point of discussion. The following was recommended by the 2013 expert consensus[3]:

1 SQTS is diagnosed in the presence of a QTc ≤ 330 ms.
2 SQTS can be diagnosed in the presence of a QTc < 360 ms and one or more of the following: a pathologic mutation, family history of SQTS, family history of SCD at age ≤40, survival of a VT/VF episode in the absence of heart disease.

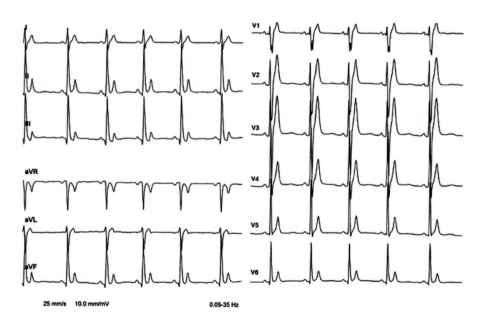

25 mm/s   10.0 mm/mV   0.05-35 Hz

Figure 8.3 SQTS ECG Pattern. (From Rudic, B. et al., *Arrhythm. Electrophysiol. Rev.*, 3, 76–79, 2014.)

Table 8.4 2013 Expert consensus for treatment of SQTS

2013 Expert consensus recommendations on SQTS therapies
Class I
1. ICD implantation *is recommended* in symptomatic patients with a diagnosis of SQTS who
a. Are survivors of a cardiac arrest *and/or*
b. Have documented spontaneous sustained VT with or without syncope.
Class IIb
1. ICD implantation *may be considered* in asymptomatic patients with a diagnosis of SQTS and a family history of SCD.
2. Quinidine *may be considered* in asymptomatic patients with a diagnosis of SQTS and a family history of SCD.
3. Sotalol *may be considered* in asymptomatic patients with a diagnosis of SQTS and a family history of SCD.

Source: Priori, S.G. et al., *Heart Rhythm*, 10, 1932–1963, 2013.

THERAPY IN SQTS

ICD implantation is recommended in patients with SQTS who are survivors of a cardiac arrest or have a documented spontaneous sustained VT/VF.[45] However, optimal risk stratification strategy for primary prevention of SCD in patients with SQTS is not yet clear given lack of independent risk factors for cardiac arrest.[3] There is no clear role for an ICD in asymptomatic patients, as data from Finland revealed no risk of arrhythmic events in asymptomatic patients with QTc < 340 ms after an average follow-up of 29 years.[46] An ICD may be considered in SQTS patients with a strong family history of SCD.[3] Attention should be paid to appropriate programming of ICD to avoid T-wave oversensing in patients with SQTS.

Quinidine, which has been reported as more potent in prolonging the QT interval compared to class IC and III agents, might have a role in primary prevention of cardiac arrest but confirmatory data is needed.[2,3] Larger cohorts of patients and longer follow-up is needed for better patient identification, risk stratification, and management of this complex but rare electrical disorder (Table 8.4).

BRUGADA SYNDROME

Brugada syndrome (BrS) is another heterogeneous channelopathy characterized by a specific ECG pattern and predisposition to SCD. The syndrome was first formally described by the Brugada brothers in 1992 in a series of eight patients with aborted SCD.[47] The ECG during sinus rhythm in these patients showed right bundle branch block, normal QT interval, and persistent ST segment elevation in precordial leads V1 to V2–V3.[13] In all series, approximately 80% of the affected individuals are men. The prevalence of BrS is much higher in Asia and Southeast Asia including in Thailand, the Philippines, and Japan.[48]

GENETICS CHARACTERISTICS

Disease inheritance is by an autosomal dominant mode of transmission. Loss-of-function mutations in the SCN5A sodium channel were the first and the most well-known cause of BrS, but it only account for about 20% of phenotypic disease. Twelve genes, including mutations in the sodium channel beta subunits, the potassium channel encoded by *KCNE3* and the I-type calcium channel (*CACNA1C* and *CACNB2B*), have been identified so far.[3]

There is no widely accepted proposed mechanism for sudden death in BrS. The repolarization hypothesis, which is based largely on the results from an arterially perfused wedge preparation of the canine right ventricle implicates electrical heterogeneity in the subepicardium and subendocardium during repolarization—caused by unequal transient outward current (I_{to})—and increased risk of arrhythmia due to phase 2 re-entry in development of sudden death.[49] The depolarization hypothesis contends that in BrS, the RVOT is the last to depolarize and implicates the delayed activation of the RVOT in the development of arrhythmia. This is consistent with mutations in the sodium channel causing slow conduction and reentry and is supported by electrophysiological studies with endo- and epicardial mapping of patients with BrS showing extremely slow conduction of the electrical impulse at the right ventricular outflow tract area.[50]

CLINICAL PRESENTATION

Clinical manifestation of BrS include[3]:

- Palpitations
- Syncope
- VF or aborted SCD

Symptoms usually occur during sleep or at rest (periods with increased vagal tone), or during febrile states, but rarely during exercise. Age of presentation is usually in adulthood with mean of around 40 years. BrS is not definitively associated with structural heart disease,[3] however, there are numerous studies showing imaging, biopsy, and electrogram evidence of RV abnormalities including findings of RV fibrosis,[51] delayed activation of the RVOT,[52–54] and epicardial RVOT abnormal electrograms including low voltage and delayed depolarization.[55] These finding suggest possible RVOT structural abnormalities in BrS, but further data is needed.

ECG IN BRUGADA SYNDROME

The second Consensus Conference on Brugada Syndrome recognized 3 types of ECG patterns. Type 1 is the only diagnostic pattern and the other two may suggest the disease.[48]

- *Type 1* : Characterized by coved ST-segment elevation $\geq$2 mm (0.2 mV) followed by a negative T-wave in >1 lead from V_1 to V_3.
- *Type 2* : Has $\geq$2 mm J-point elevation, $\geq$1 mm ST-segment elevation and a saddleback appearance, followed by a positive or biphasic T-wave.
- *Type 3* : Has either a saddleback or coved appearance with an ST-segment elevation of <1 mm.

In uncertain cases, modifying the placement of right precordial leads and recording the ECG from higher intercostal spaces (2nd and 3rd) has been recommended to increase the sensitivity for a type 1 pattern (Figure 8.4).[56]

Several studies have demonstrated that the ECG findings in BrS can be dynamic and that class I antiarrhythmic drugs could reproduce the diagnostic pattern in those whose ECG had normalized.[57,58] These observations have formed the rationale for provocative drug testing using sodium-channel blockers for "unmasking" type 1 ECG pattern, in cases in which the disease is suspected, but the ECG is non-diagnostic (Figure 8.5).

(1) Ajmaline, procainamide, flecaindine, dispyramide, propafenone, and pilsicainide have been used to unmask the ECG pattern.[58,59]

(2) Drug challenge is only considered positive when a conversion to the diagnostic type 1 occurs.

DIAGNOSIS

The second Consensus Conference on Brugada Syndrome defined Brugada Syndrome as a type 1 ST-segment elevation in $\geq$1 right precordial lead (V1–V3) in conjunction with one of the following: documented VF, polymorphic VT, family history of SCD at <45 years of age, coved-type ECGs in family members, inducibility of VT with programmed electrical stimulation, syncope, or nocturnal agonal respiration.[48] The 2013 expert consensus extended the definition of Brugada Syndrome to anyone with spontaneous or provoked Brugada type 1 pattern in at least one right precordial lead (V1 or V2) placed in a standard or superior position without any additional requirement.[3]

PROGNOSIS AND RISK STRATIFICATION

Several clinical findings are associated with a higher risk of arrhythmic events and worse outcomes. There is a high-risk of recurrent cardiac arrest in survivors of SCD with BrS. Patients with syncope with a spontaneous type 1 ECG at baseline have high-risk of arrhythmic

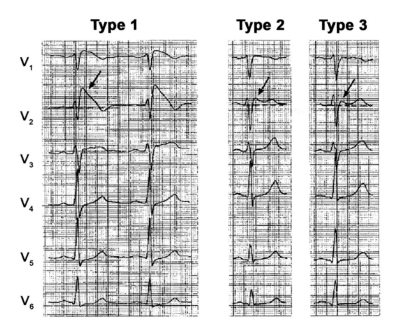

Figure 8.4 Brugda ECG pattern. (From Khasnis, A., Genetically determined ventricular arrhythmias, In Natale A, ed., *Handbook of Cardiac Electrophysiology*, 1st ed., London, UK, CRC Press, 113–132, 2007; figure 10.4.)

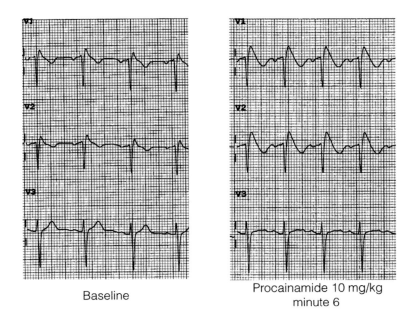

Baseline

Procainamide 10 mg/kg
minute 6

Figure 8.5 Procainamide challenge unmasking Brugada 1 pattern.

events.[60] The presence of fragmented QRS,[60] male gender,[61] and spontaneous atrial fibrillation[62] have been shown to be associated with more arrhythmic events. In Patients with BrS, neither family history of SCD nor a SCN5A mutation have been shown to be a risk marker for worse outcomes in the larger studies.[61,63,64]

There is currently no consensus on the utility of EPS for risk stratification and outcome prediction. Inducibility during EPS was shown to be an independent predictor of SCD by Brugada et al.[65] and an excellent negative predictive value of EPS was reported in a community-based prospective study.[66] However, in the PRELUDE registry lack of inducibility did not have a strong negative predictive value.[60] In the FINGER registry, inducibility was associated with a shorter time to first arrhythmic event in the univariate analysis but did not predict arrhythmic events in the multivariate analysis.[67] Therefore, at best the data is mixed.

THERAPY FOR BRUGADA SYNDROME

In all patients with BrS, avoidance of drugs that can worsen the ST-segment elevation in the precordial leads (brugadadrugs.org), immediate treatment of fever, and avoidance of excessive alcohol intake are recommended. The following specific therapies apply to certain groups of patients who are at an increased risk of arrhythmic events.

ICD

ICD implantation is the only definitive therapy for patients with BrS who are survivors of SCD. The 2013 expert consensus makes the following recommendations regarding ICD use for patients with BrS[3]:

- ICD implantation is recommended in patients with BrS and aborted SCD or with documented spontaneous sustained VT (class I).
- ICD implantation can be useful in patients with BrS (spontaneous diagnostic type I) who have a history of syncope felt to be caused by ventricular arrhythmias (class IIa).
- ICD implantation may be considered in patients with BrS who develop VF during programmed electrical stimulation (class IIb).
- ICD implantation is not indicated in asymptomatic BrS patients and on the basis of a family history of SCD alone (class III).

DRUG AND ABLATIVE THERAPIES

Quinidine is effective in preventing spontaneous and induced ventricular arrhythmias in patients with BrS[68] though no randomized studies are available. Quinidine is not available in many countries and its use may be limited by patient intolerance and development of serious side-effects such as thrombocytopenia.[69] Furthermore, a recent study failed to demonstrate a beneficial effect of quinidine treatment in asymptomatic Brugada patients with inducible VF.[70] Current guidelines endorse the use of quinidine in patients with BrS who qualify for an ICD but refuse it or have contraindications and in those with VT/VF storm (class IIa). Quinidine may be considered in asymptomatic patients with BrS with a spontaneous type I ECG (class IIb).[3]

Isoproterenol has also been shown to suppress VT/VF storm in BrS and may be considered in this group but controlled studies are lacking.[71] Beta-adrenergic stimulation by isoproterenol increases the I_{CAL}, and thereby decreases the local and transmural heterogeneity, which may be sufficient to decrease the degree of ST elevation and VF initiation.[72]

The free wall of the RVOT appears to be the site of origin of PVCs that trigger VF in BrS; it also is the most successful site for arrhythmia induction.[73] RF ablation of ventricular ectopy in high-risk patients with BrS in a number of cases has shown short-term freedom from recurrence of arrhythmic events.[74] Epicardial substrate ablation in the RVOT has also been shown to prevent VF inducibility and eliminate Brugada phenotype on ECG.[55,75] There is no data regarding the long-term outcome of ablation in this group of patients (Figure 8.6 and Table 8.5).

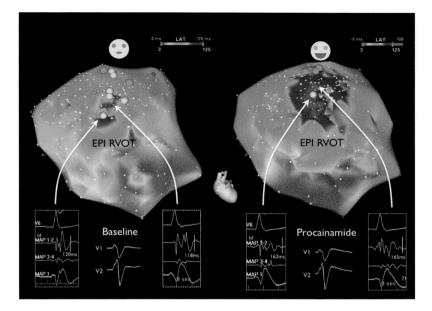

Figure 8.6 Epicardial RVOT ablation of a patient with BrS. Baseline activation and local electrograms (left panel) and activation and electrograms after procainamide infusion (right panel) in a patient with BrS. Local electrograms become more fractionated and the region of late activation increases after procainamide infusion and induction of a type I BrS pattern.

Table 8.5 Expert consensus for treatment of Brugada syndrome

2013 Expert Consensus Recommendations on Brugada Syndrome Therapies
Class I
1. The following lifestyle changes *are recommended* in all patients with diagnosis of BrS:
a. Avoidance of drugs that may induce or aggravate ST-segment elevation in right precordial leads (Brugadadrugs.org).
b. Avoidance of excessive alcohol intake.
c. Immediate treatment of fever with antipyretic drugs.
2. ICD implantation *is recommended* in patients with a diagnosis of BrS who:
a. Are survivors of a cardiac arrest and/or
b. Have documented spontaneous sustained VT with or without syncope.
Class IIa
1. ICD implantation *can be useful* in patients with a spontaneous diagnostic type I ECG who have a history of syncope judged to be likely caused by ventricular arrhythmias.
2. Quinidine *can be useful* in patients with a diagnosis of BrS and history of arrhythmic storms defined as more than two episodes of VT/VF in 24 hours.
3. Quinidine *can be useful* in patients with a diagnosis of BrS:
a. Who qualify for an ICD but present a contraindication to the ICD or refuse it *and/or*
b. Have a history of documented supraventricular arrhythmias that require treatment.
4. Isoproterenol infusion can be useful in suppressing arrhythmic storms in BrS patients.

(Continued)

Table 8.5 (*Continued*)   Expert consensus for treatment of Brugada syndrome

2013 Expert Consensus Recommendations on Brugada Syndrome Therapies
Class IIb 1. ICD implantation *may be considered* in patients with a diagnosis of BrS who develop VF during programmed electrical stimulation (Inducible patients). 2. Quinidine *may be considered* in asymptomatic patients with a diagnosis of BrS with a spontaneous typo 1 ECG. 3. Catheter ablation *may be considered* in patients with a diagnosis of BrS and history of arrhythmic storms or repeated appropriate ICD shocks.
Class III 1. ICD implantation is not indicated in asymptomatic BrS patients with a drug-induced type 1 ECG and on the basis of a family history of SCD alone.

Source: Priori, S.G. et al., *Heart Rhythm*, 10, 1932–1963, 2013.

CATECHOLAMINERGIC POLYMORPHIC VENTRICULAR TACHYCARDIA (CPVT)

CPVT is a rare idiopathic ventricular arrhythmia that arises as a consequence of mutation in genes responsible for myocardial calcium handling and is characterized by bidirectional and polymorphic VT. Ventricular arrhythmias are usually triggered by exercise or adrenergic stimuli.[13]

GENETIC CHARACTERISTICS

Two variants of CPVT have been described based on their genetic mutation and mode of transmission. CPVT1 has a mutation in the ryanodine 2 receptor gene (*RyR2*) which leads to delayed afterdepolarization (DAD)-induced extrasystolic activity from defective calcium handling. The resulting transmural dispersion of repolarization provides the substrate for the development of re-entrant tachyarrhythmias.[13,76] The RyR2 gene shows autosomal dominant inheritance. CPVT2 is defined by a mutation in the calsequestrin (*CASQ2*) gene and has an autosomal recessive inheritance. Other unidentified genes are also believed to result in CPVT. The ryanodine receptor is located on the sarcoplasmic reticulum and allows the release of calcium into the cell, thus facilitating excitation contraction coupling in the myocardium. Calsequestrin gene mutations interfere with sarcoplasmic calcium storage.[13]

CLINICAL PRESENTATION

CPVT has an ominous course, with approximately 30% of affected individuals experiencing symptoms before the age of 10 years and the majority (60%–80%) of patients experiencing one or more symptomatic arrhythmia episodes before age 40. The typical history is that of syncope or SCD induced by exercise or emotional stress.[13,77,78]

DIAGNOSIS

Patients with CPVT have a normal resting ECG and no specific structural heart abnormalities.[77] Exercise testing, either on a treadmill or using Holter monitoring, is often sufficient to document the arrhythmia. Findings during exercise testing initially include frequent monomorphic PVCs followed by polymorphic PVCs and bidirectional or polymorphic VT. On cessation of exercise, there is typically prompt termination of the arrhythmia. For patients who are unable to exercise, drug challenge with epinephrine or isoproterenol

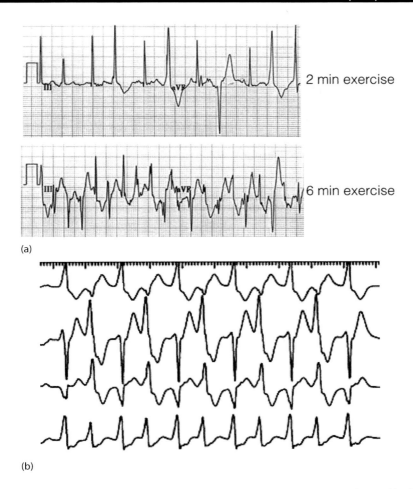

(a)

(b)

Figure 8.7 (a) Stress testing showing PVC and bidirectional VT in a patient with CPVT. (b) Bidirectional VT in a patient with CPVT.

may induce arrhythmias.[13] EPS has limited value in CPVT, as the tachycardia is seldom inducible by programmed stimulation. No specific electrophysiologic abnormality has been demonstrated.[13,79]

The 2013 expert consensus recommends the following for the diagnosis of CPVT[3] (Figure 8.7):

(1) CPVT is diagnosed in the presence of a structurally normal heart, normal ECG, and unexplained exercise or catecholamine-induced bidirectional VT or polymorphic PVCs or VT in an individual <40 years.

(2) CPVT is diagnosed in patients who have a pathogenic mutation (index case or family member).

(3) CPVT is diagnosed in family members of a CPVT index case with a normal heart who manifest exercise-induced bidirectional VT or polymorphic PVCs or VT.

PROGNOSIS AND RISK STRATIFICATION

Predictors of worse outcomes include: early/childhood presentation, occurrence of cardiac arrest as the initial presentation, persistence of complex ectopy during exercise, lack of beta-blocker therapy, and use of beta-blocker other than nadolol after diagnosis.[80]

THERAPY FOR CPVT
DRUG THERAPY

Combined with exercise restriction, beta-blockers are the first-line therapy for patients with CPVT. Nadolol, titrated to maximum tolerated dose has been shown to be clinically effective.[3] The annual arrhythmic event rate is 3%–11% on beta-blocker therapy.[80] Flecainide inhibits *RyR2* activity and has shown to significantly reduce ventricular arrhythmia in a limited number of CPVT patients and is regarded as the second-line drug therapy when beta-blocker is ineffective in controlling the arrhythmia.[3,81] Verapamil has been shown to reduce the ventricular arrhythmia burden on top of beta-blockers in some patients,[82] although long-term efficacy is unclear.

LEFT CARDIAC SYMPATHETIC DENERVATION (LCSD)

A significant reduction of arrhythmic events with LCSD in CPVT patients have been reported in a number of small series.[83,84] Though larger studies and longer-term outcomes are needed, LCSD seems to be a promising intervention for select patients refractory to drug therapy.

ICD

ICD implantation should be considered in patients with CPVT who experience recurrent arrhythmic events despite optimal medical therapy and when LCSD is not an option.[3] ICD should be programmed with high cut-off rates and long delays before delivery of shock, as ICD shocks may trigger further arrhythmic events by increasing the sympathetic tone (Table 8.6).

Table 8.6 Expert consensus for treatment of CPVT

2013 Expert Consensus Recommendations on CPVT Therapies
Class I
1. The following lifestyle changes *are recommended* in all patients with diagnosis of CPVT: a. Limit/avoid competitive sports b. Limit/avoid strenuous exercise c. Limit exposure to stressful environments.
2. Beta-blockers *are recommended* in all symptomatic patients with a diagnosis of CPVT.
3. ICD implantation *is recommended* in patients with a diagnosis of CPVT who experience cardiac arrest, recurrent syncope, or polymorphic/bidirectional VT despite optimal medical management, and/or LCSD.
Class IIa
1. Flecainide *can be a useful* addition to beta-blockers in patients with a diagnosis of CPVT who experience recurrent syncope or polymorphic/bidirectional VT while on beta-blockers.
2. Beta-blockers *can be useful* in carriers of a pathogenic CPVT mutation without clinical manifestabons of CPVT (concealed mutation-positive patients).
Class IIb
1. LCSD *may be considered* in patients with a diagnosis of CPVT who experience recurrent syncope or polymorphic/bidirectional VT/several appropriate ICD shocks while on beta-blockers and in patients who are intolerant or with contraindication to beta-blockers.
Class III
1. ICD as a standalone therapy *is not indicated* in an asymptomatic patient with a diagnosis of CPVT.
2. Programmed electrical stimulation *is not indicated* in CPVT patients.

Source: Priori, S.G. et al., *Heart Rhythm*, 10, 1932–1963, 2013.

IDIOPATHIC VENTRICULAR FIBRILLATION (IVF)

Idiopathic ventricular fibrillation (IVF) is defined as resuscitated cardiac arrest that remains unexplained despite a comprehensive investigation.[3] It is therefore a diagnosis of exclusion, which potentially includes a heterogeneous group of disorders. In a meta-analysis, most patients with idiopathic VF shared several characteristics: (1) the first arrhythmic event occurred during young adulthood with a mean presenting age of 36 years; (2) the majority of the patients were male; and (3) the primary documented arrhythmia was VF triggered by a short-coupled PVC.[85] The is a paucity of systemic data on the prevalence of IVF. In the CASPER registry of cardiac arrest survivors without overt coronary or structural heat disease, 44% of patients presenting patients remained without a diagnosis after a comprehensive evaluation.[86]

DIAGNOSIS

In survivors of a cardiac arrest, IVF is defined after exclusion of known or suspected etiologies—cardiac, respiratory, metabolic, or toxic—that may lead to cardiac arrest. Ideally VF should be documented.[3] Systematic clinical testing in the CASPER registry unmasked the cause of apparently unexplained cardiac arrest in >50% of patients and should be considered as part of the evaluation prior to making the diagnosis of IVF[86]: (1) ECG, signal-averaged ECG and telemetry; (2) imaging (ECHO, MRI with and without contrast); (3) provocative tests (exercise stress test, epinephrine infusion, procainamide); (4) EPS and voltage map; (5) ventricular biopsy if indicated; and (6) targeted genetic testing.

MANAGEMENT

The natural history of IVF is not well defined. Most patients are advised to undergo an ICD implantation at the index hospitalization. Data from small series showed that at 2.8 years of follow-up after the initial diagnosis, 10% of patients had a recurrence of VT but none had an ICD shock or died.[87] Quinidine has been shown to have antiarrhythmic efficacy in idiopathic VF. Belhassen et al. showed that the majority of idiopathic VF patients with inducible VF during programmed electrical stimulation become non-inducible after initiation of quinidine therapy. These patients remained without VF or death during mean follow-up ranging between 14 and 216 months while being treated with quinidine.[88] Use of quinidine is a class IIb indication based on the 2013 expert consensus in patients with a diagnosis of IVF in conjunction with ICD implantation or when ICD is contraindicated or refused.[3] In patients with recurrent IVF (refractory to median to of 2 antiarrhythmic drugs) initiated by short-coupled PVCs, who underwent catheter ablation of PVCs, Knecht et al. showed that the majority (36/38) were free of VF at 52 months of follow-up.[89] PVC ablation may therefore be considered for patients with IVF and uniform morphology PVCs (Class IIb).[3]

CONCLUSIONS AND FUTURE DIRECTIONS

Major advances in the field of genetics over the past 20 years have vastly expanded our understanding of inherited ventricular arrhythmias. Available genetic testing can aid in screening family members of affected individuals, and in certain conditions such as LQTS, may provide therapy and prognostic guidance. Our basic science and clinical knowledge of these channelopathies nonetheless remain imperfect and detailed pathogenetic mechanisms of inherited ventricular arrhythmias are poorly understood. This is partly due to the heterogeneous nature of these disorders and partly because of lack of large patient populations and appropriate experimental models. Further advances in the field of genetics and translational research is expected to enhance these genotype–phenotype correlations, provide better risk stratification tools, and outline new therapies including target or gene-directed treatment strategies.

REFERENCES

1. Schwartz PJ, Stramba-Badiale M, Crotti L, et al. Prevalence of the congenital long-QT syndrome. *Circulation*. 2009;120(18):1761–1767. doi:10.1161/CIRCULATIONAHA.109.863209.

2. Webster G, Berul CI. An update on channelopathies: From mechanisms to management. *Circulation*. 2013;127(1):126–140. doi:10.1161/CIRCULATIONAHA.111.060343.

3. Priori SG, Wilde AA, Horie M, et al. HRS/EHRA/APHRS expert consensus statement on the diagnosis and management of patients with inherited primary arrhythmia syndromes: Document endorsed by HRS, EHRA, and APHRS in May 2013 and by ACCF, AHA, PACES, and AEPC in June 2013. *Heart Rhythm*. 2013;10(12):1932–1963. doi:10.1016/j.hrthm.2013.05.014.

4. Curran ME, Splawski I, Timothy KW, et al. A molecular basis for cardiac arrhythmia: HERG mutations cause long QT syndrome. *Cell*. 1995;80(5):795–803. http://www.ncbi.nlm.nih.gov/pubmed/7889573. Accessed January 25, 2016.

5. Wang Q, Shen J, Splawski I, et al. SCN5A mutations associated with an inherited cardiac arrhythmia, long QT syndrome. *Cell*. 1995;80(5):805–811. http://www.ncbi.nlm.nih.gov/pubmed/7889574. Accessed November 27, 2015.

6. Wang Q, Curran ME, Splawski I, et al. Positional cloning of a novel potassium channel gene: KVLQT1 mutations cause cardiac arrhythmias. *Nat Genet*. 1996;12(1):17–23. doi:10.1038/ng0196-17.

7. Ackerman MJ, Priori SG, Willems S, et al. HRS/EHRA expert consensus statement on the state of genetic testing for the channelopathies and cardiomyopathies: This document was developed as a partnership between the Heart Rhythm Society (HRS) and the European Heart Rhythm Association (EHRA). *Europace*. 2011;13(8):1077–1109. doi:10.1093/europace/eur245.

8. Schwartz PJ, Spazzolini C, Crotti L, et al. The Jervell and Lange-Nielsen syndrome: Natural history, molecular basis, and clinical outcome. *Circulation*. 2006;113(6):783–790. doi:10.1161/CIRCULATIONAHA.105.592899.

9. Schwartz PJ, Priori SG, Spazzolini C, et al. Genotype-phenotype correlation in the long-QT syndrome: Gene-specific triggers for life-threatening arrhythmias. *Circulation*. 2001;103(1):89–95. http://www.ncbi.nlm.nih.gov/pubmed/11136691. Accessed January 8, 2016.

10. Zareba W, Moss AJ, Schwartz PJ, et al. Influence of genotype on the clinical course of the long-QT syndrome. International Long-QT Syndrome Registry Research Group. *N Engl J Med*. 1998;339(14):960–965. doi:10.1056/NEJM199810013391404.

11. Priori SG, Schwartz PJ, Napolitano C, et al. Risk stratification in the long-QT syndrome. *N Engl J Med*. 2003;348(19):1866–1874. doi:10.1056/NEJMoa022147.

12. Cowan JC, Yusoff K, Moore M, et al. Importance of lead selection in QT interval measurement. *Am J Cardiol*. 1988;61(1):83–87. http://www.ncbi.nlm.nih.gov/pubmed/3337022. Accessed January 25, 2016.

13. Khasnis A. Genetically determined ventricular arrhythmias. In: Natale A, editor. *Handbook of Cardiac Electrophysiology*. 1st ed., London: CRC Press, 2007:113–132.

14. Schwartz PJ, Malliani A. Electrical alternation of the T-wave: Clinical and experimental evidence of its relationship with the sympathetic nervous system and with the long Q-T syndrome. *Am Heart J*. 1975;89(1):45–50. http://www.ncbi.nlm.nih.gov/pubmed/1109551. Accessed December 6, 2015.

15. Malfatto G, Beria G, Sala S, et al. Quantitative analysis of T wave abnormalities and their prognostic implications in the idiopathic long QT syndrome. *J Am Coll Cardiol*. 1994;23(2):296–301. http://www.ncbi.nlm.nih.gov/pubmed/7905012. Accessed January 25, 2016.

16. Schwartz PJ, Moss AJ, Vincent GM, Crampton RS. Diagnostic criteria for the long QT syndrome. An update. *Circulation*. 1993;88(2):782–784. http://www.ncbi.nlm.nih.gov/pubmed/8339437. Accessed January 25, 2016.

17. Goldenberg I, Horr S, Moss AJ, et al. Risk for life-threatening cardiac events in patients with genotype-confirmed long-QT syndrome and normal-range corrected QT intervals. *J Am Coll Cardiol*. 2011;57(1):51–59. doi:10.1016/j.jacc.2010.07.038.

18. Vyas H, Hejlik J, Ackerman MJ. Epinephrine QT stress testing in the evaluation of congenital long-QT syndrome: Diagnostic accuracy of the paradoxical QT response. *Circulation*. 2006;113(11):1385–1392. doi:10.1161/CIRCULATIONAHA.105.600445.

19. Shimizu W, Noda T, Takaki H, et al. Diagnostic value of epinephrine test for genotyping LQT1, LQT2, and LQT3 forms of congenital long QT syndrome. *Heart Rhythm*. 2004;1(3):276–283. doi:10.1016/j.hrthm.2004.04.021.

20. Horner JM, Horner MM, Ackerman MJ. The diagnostic utility of recovery phase QTc during treadmill exercise stress testing in the evaluation of long QT syndrome. *Heart Rhythm*. 2011;8(11):1698–1704. doi:10.1016/j.hrthm.2011.05.018.

21. Viskin S, Postema PG, Bhuiyan ZA, et al. The response of the QT interval to the brief tachycardia provoked by standing: A bedside test for diagnosing long QT syndrome. *J Am Coll Cardiol*. 2010;55(18):1955–1961. doi:10.1016/j.jacc.2009.12.015.

22. Moss AJ, Zareba W, Kaufman ES, et al. Increased risk of arrhythmic events in long-QT syndrome with mutations in the pore region of the human ether-a-go-go-related gene potassium channel. *Circulation*. 2002;105(7):794–799. http://www.ncbi.nlm.nih.gov/pubmed/11854117. Accessed January 26, 2016.

23. Goldenberg I, Moss AJ, Peterson DR, et al. Risk factors for aborted cardiac arrest and sudden cardiac death in children with the congenital long-QT syndrome. *Circulation*. 2008;117(17):2184–2191. doi:10.1161/CIRCULATIONAHA.107.701243.

24. Priori SG. Association of long QT syndrome loci and cardiac events among patients treated with β-blockers. *JAMA*. 2004;292(11):1341. doi:10.1001/jama.292.11.1341.

25. Schwartz PJ, Spazzolini C, Crotti L. All LQT3 patients need an ICD: True or false? *Heart Rhythm*. 2009;6(1):113–120. doi:10.1016/j.hrthm.2008.10.017.

26. Zipes DP, Camm AJ, Borggrefe M, et al. ACC/AHA/ESC 2006 guidelines for management of patients with ventricular arrhythmias and the prevention of sudden cardiac death: A report of the American College of Cardiology/American Heart Association Task Force and the European Society of Cardiology Com. *J Am Coll Cardiol*. 2006;48(5):e247–e346. doi:10.1016/j.jacc.2006.07.010.

27. Garson A, Dick M, Fournier A, et al. The long QT syndrome in children. An international study of 287 patients. *Circulation*. 1993;87(6):1866–1872. http://www.ncbi.nlm.nih.gov/pubmed/8099317. Accessed January 26, 2016.

28. Sauer AJ, Moss AJ, McNitt S, et al. Long QT syndrome in adults. *J Am Coll Cardiol*. 2007;49(3):329–337. doi:10.1016/j.jacc.2006.08.057.

29. Chockalingam P, Crotti L, Girardengo G, et al. Not all beta-blockers are equal in the management of long QT syndrome types 1 and 2: Higher recurrence of events under metoprolol. *J Am Coll Cardiol*. 2012;60(20):2092–2099. doi:10.1016/j.jacc.2012.07.046.

30. Abu-Zeitone A, Peterson DR, Polonsky B, et al. Efficacy of different beta-blockers in the treatment of long QT syndrome. *J Am Coll Cardiol*. 2014;64(13):1352–1358. doi:10.1016/j.jacc.2014.05.068.

31. Wilde AAM, Ackerman MJ. Beta-blockers in the treatment of congenital long QT syndrome: Is one beta-blocker superior to another? *J Am Coll Cardiol*. 2014;64(13):1359–1361. doi:10.1016/j.jacc.2014.06.1192.

32. Schwartz PJ, Priori SG, Locati EH, et al. Long QT syndrome patients with mutations of the SCN5A and HERG genes have differential responses to Na⁺ channel blockade and to increases in heart rate. Implications for gene-specific therapy. *Circulation.* 1995;92(12):3381–3386. http://www.ncbi.nlm.nih.gov/pubmed/8521555. Accessed December 23, 2015.

33. Moss AJ, Windle JR, Hall WJ, et al. Safety and efficacy of flecainide in subjects with Long QT-3 syndrome (DeltaKPQ mutation): A randomized, double-blind, placebo-controlled clinical trial. *Ann Noninvasive Electrocardiol.* 2005;10(4 Suppl):59–66. doi:10.1111/j.1542-474X.2005.00077.x.

34. Moss AJ, Zareba W, Schwarz KQ, et al. Ranolazine shortens repolarization in patients with sustained inward sodium current due to type-3 long-QT syndrome. *J Cardiovasc Electrophysiol.* 2008;19(12):1289–1293. doi:10.1111/j.1540-8167.2008.01246.x.

35. Jons C, Moss AJ, Goldenberg I, et al. Risk of fatal arrhythmic events in long QT syndrome patients after syncope. *J Am Coll Cardiol.* 2010;55(8):783–788. doi:10.1016/j.jacc.2009.11.042.

36. Zareba W, Moss AJ, Daubert JP, et al. Implantable cardioverter defibrillator in high-risk long QT syndrome patients. *J Cardiovasc Electrophysiol.* 2003;14(4):337–341. http://www.ncbi.nlm.nih.gov/pubmed/12741701. Accessed January 26, 2016.

37. Moss AJ, McDonald J. Unilateral cervicothoracic sympathetic ganglionectomy for the treatment of long QT interval syndrome. *N Engl J Med.* 1971;285(16):903–904. doi:10.1056/NEJM197110142851607.

38. Odero A, Bozzani A, De Ferrari GM, et al. Left cardiac sympathetic denervation for the prevention of life-threatening arrhythmias: The surgical supraclavicular approach to cervicothoracic sympathectomy. *Heart Rhythm.* 2010;7(8):1161–1165. doi:10.1016/j.hrthm.2010.03.046.

39. Collura CA, Johnson JN, Moir C, et al. Left cardiac sympathetic denervation for the treatment of long QT syndrome and catecholaminergic polymorphic ventricular tachycardia using video-assisted thoracic surgery. *Heart Rhythm.* 2009;6(6):752–759. doi:10.1016/j.hrthm.2009.03.024.

40. Schwartz PJ, Priori SG, Cerrone M, et al. Left cardiac sympathetic denervation in the management of high-risk patients affected by the long-QT syndrome. *Circulation.* 2004;109(15):1826–1833. doi:10.1161/01.CIR.0000125523.14403.1E.

41. Gussak I, Brugada P, Brugada J, et al. Idiopathic short QT interval: A new clinical syndrome? *Cardiology.* 2000;94(2):99–102.

42. Gaita F, Giustetto C, Bianchi F, et al. Short QT syndrome: A familial cause of sudden death. *Circulation.* 2003;108(8):965–970. doi:10.1161/01.CIR.0000085071.28695.C4.

43. Bellocq C, van Ginneken ACG, Bezzina CR, et al. Mutation in the KCNQ1 gene leading to the short QT-interval syndrome. *Circulation.* 2004;109(20):2394–2397. doi:10.1161/01.CIR.0000130409.72142.FE.

44. Priori SG, Pandit SV, Rivolta I, et al. A novel form of short QT syndrome (SQT3) is caused by a mutation in the KCNJ2 gene. *Circ Res.* 2005;96(7):800–807. doi:10.1161/01.RES.0000162101.76263.8c.

45. Giustetto C, Schimpf R, Mazzanti A, et al. Long-term follow-up of patients with short QT syndrome. *J Am Coll Cardiol.* 2011;58(6):587–595. doi:10.1016/j.jacc.2011.03.038.

46. Anttonen O, Junttila MJ, Rissanen H, et al. Prevalence and prognostic significance of short QT interval in a middle-aged Finnish population. *Circulation.* 2007;116(7):714–720. doi:10.1161/CIRCULATIONAHA.106.676551.

47. Brugada P, Brugada J. Right bundle branch block, persistent ST segment elevation and sudden cardiac death: A distinct clinical and electrocardiographic syndrome. A multicenter report. *J Am Coll Cardiol.* 1992;20(6):1391–1396. http://www.ncbi.nlm.nih.gov/pubmed/1309182. Accessed December 5, 2015.

48. Antzelevitch C, Brugada P, Borggrefe M, et al. Brugada syndrome: Report of the second consensus conference. *Heart Rhythm.* 2005;2(4):429–440. http://www.ncbi.nlm.nih.gov/pubmed/15898165. Accessed December 5, 2015.

49. Antzelevitch C. The Brugada syndrome: Ionic basis and arrhythmia mechanisms. *J Cardiovasc Electrophysiol.* 2001;12(2):268–272. http://www.ncbi.nlm.nih.gov/pubmed/11232628. Accessed March 13, 2016.

50. Coronel R, Casini S, Koopmann TT, et al. Right ventricular fibrosis and conduction delay in a patient with clinical signs of Brugada syndrome: A combined electrophysiological, genetic, histopathologic, and computational study. *Circulation.* 2005;112(18):2769–2777. doi:10.1161/CIRCULATIONAHA.105.532614.

51. Frustaci A, Priori SG, Pieroni M, et al. Cardiac histological substrate in patients with clinical phenotype of Brugada syndrome. *Circulation.* 2005;112(24):3680–3687. doi:10.1161/CIRCULATIONAHA.105.520999.

52. Tukkie R. Delay in right ventricular activation contributes to brugada syndrome. *Circulation.* 2004;109(10):1272–1277. doi:10.1161/01.CIR.0000118467.53182.D1.

53. Postema PG, van Dessel PFHM, de Bakker JMT, et al. Slow and discontinuous conduction conspire in Brugada syndrome: A right ventricular mapping and stimulation study. *Circ Arrhythm Electrophysiol.* 2008;1(5):379–386. doi:10.1161/CIRCEP.108.790543.

54. Lambiase PD, Ahmed AK, Ciaccio EJ, et al. High-density substrate mapping in Brugada syndrome: Combined role of conduction and repolarization heterogeneities in arrhythmogenesis. *Circulation.* 2009;120(2):106–117, 1–4. doi:10.1161/CIRCULATIONAHA.108.771401.

55. Nademanee K, Veerakul G, Chandanamattha P, et al. Prevention of ventricular fibrillation episodes in Brugada syndrome by catheter ablation over the anterior right ventricular outflow tract epicardium. *Circulation.* 2011;123(12):1270–1279. doi:10.1161/CIRCULATIONAHA.110.972612.

56. Nakazawa K, Sakurai T, Takagi A, et al. Clinical significance of electrocardiography recordings from a higher intercostal space for detection of the brugada sign. *Circ J.* 2004;68(11):1018–1022. http://www.ncbi.nlm.nih.gov/pubmed/15502382. Accessed January 28, 2016.

57. Veltmann C, Schimpf R, Echternach C, et al. A prospective study on spontaneous fluctuations between diagnostic and non-diagnostic ECGs in Brugada syndrome: Implications for correct phenotyping and risk stratification. *Eur Heart J.* 2006;27(21):2544–2552. doi:10.1093/eurheartj/ehl205.

58. Brugada R, Brugada J, Antzelevitch C, et al. Sodium channel blockers identify risk for sudden death in patients with ST-segment elevation and right bundle branch block but structurally normal hearts. *Circulation.* 2000;101(5):510–515. http://www.ncbi.nlm.nih.gov/pubmed/10662748. Accessed January 28, 2016.

59. Morita H, Takenaka-Morita S, Fukushima-Kusano K, et al. Risk stratification for asymptomatic patients with Brugada syndrome. *Circ J.* 2003;67(4):312–316. http://www.ncbi.nlm.nih.gov/pubmed/12655161. Accessed January 28, 2016.

60. Priori SG, Gasparini M, Napolitano C, et al. Risk stratification in brugada syndrome: Results of the PRELUDE (Programmed Electrical stimUlation Predictive value) registry. *J Am Coll Cardiol.* 2012;59(1):37–45. doi:10.1016/j.jacc.2011.08.064.

61. Gehi AK, Duong TD, Metz LD, et al. Risk stratification of individuals with the Brugada electrocardiogram: A meta-analysis. *J Cardiovasc Electrophysiol.* 2006;17(6):577–583. doi:10.1111/j.1540-8167.2006.00455.x.

62. Morita H, Kusano-Fukushima K, Nagase S, et al. Atrial fibrillation and atrial vulnerability in patients with brugada syndrome. *J Am Coll Cardiol.* 2002;40(8):1437–1444. http://www.ncbi.nlm.nih.gov/pubmed/12392834. Accessed January 28, 2016.

63. Priori SG, Napolitano C, Gasparini M, et al. Natural history of Brugada syndrome: Insights for risk stratification and management. *Circulation*. 2002;105(11):1342–1347. http://www.ncbi.nlm.nih.gov/pubmed/11901046. Accessed January 28, 2016.

64. Eckardt L, Probst V, Smits JPP, et al. Long-term prognosis of individuals with right precordial ST-segment-elevation brugada syndrome. *Circulation*. 2005;111(3):257–263. doi:10.1161/01.CIR.0000153267.21278.8D.

65. Brugada J, Brugada R, Brugada P. Determinants of sudden cardiac death in individuals with the electrocardiographic pattern of brugada syndrome and no previous cardiac arrest. *Circulation*. 2003;108(25):3092–3096. doi:10.1161/01.CIR.0000104568.13957.4F.

66. Giustetto C, Drago S, Demarchi PG, et al. Risk stratification of the patients with brugada type electrocardiogram: A community-based prospective study. *Europace*. 2009;11(4):507–513. doi:10.1093/europace/eup006.

67. Probst V, Veltmann C, Eckardt L, et al. Long-term prognosis of patients diagnosed with Brugada syndrome: Results from the FINGER brugada syndrome registry. *Circulation*. 2010;121(5):635–643. doi:10.1161/CIRCULATIONAHA.109.887026.

68. Belhassen B, Glick A, Viskin S. Efficacy of quinidine in high-risk patients with Brugada syndrome. *Circulation*. 2004;110(13):1731–1737. doi:10.1161/01.CIR.0000143159.30585.90.

69. Veerakul G, Nademanee K. Brugada syndrome: Two decades of progress. *Circ J*. 2012;76(12):2713–2722. http://www.ncbi.nlm.nih.gov/pubmed/23149437. Accessed March 13, 2016.

70. Bouzeman A, Traulle S, Messali A, et al. Long-term follow-up of asymptomatic brugada patients with inducible ventricular fibrillation under hydroquinidine. *Europace*. 2014;16(4):572–577. doi:10.1093/europace/eut279.

71. Maury P, Hocini M, Haïssaguerre M. Electrical storms in Brugada syndrome: Review of pharmacologic and ablative therapeutic options. *Indian Pacing Electrophysiol J*. 2005;5(1):25–34. http://www.pubmedcentral.nih.gov/articlerender.fcgi?artid=1502067&tool=pmcentrez&rendertype=abstract. Accessed February 1, 2016.

72. Alings M, Wilde A. "Brugada" syndrome: Clinical data and suggested pathophysiological mechanism. *Circulation*. 1999;99(5):666–673. http://www.ncbi.nlm.nih.gov/pubmed/9950665. Accessed March 13, 2016.

73. Morita H, Fukushima-Kusano K, Nagase S, et al. Site-specific arrhythmogenesis in patients with Brugada syndrome. *J Cardiovasc Electrophysiol*. 2003;14(4):373–379. http://www.ncbi.nlm.nih.gov/pubmed/12741708. Accessed February 1, 2016.

74. Haïssaguerre M, Extramiana F, Hocini M, et al. Mapping and ablation of ventricular fibrillation associated with long-QT and brugada syndromes. *Circulation*. 2003;108(8):925–928. doi:10.1161/01.CIR.0000088781.99943.95.

75. Brugada J, Pappone C, Berruezo A, et al. Brugada syndrome phenotype elimination by epicardial substrate ablation. *Circ Arrhythm Electrophysiol*. 2015;8(6):1373–1381. doi:10.1161/CIRCEP.115.003220.

76. Nam G-B. Cellular mechanisms underlying the development of catecholaminergic ventricular tachycardia. *Circulation*. 2005;111(21):2727–2733. doi:10.1161/CIRCULATIONAHA.104.479295.

77. Leenhardt A, Lucet V, Denjoy I, et al. Catecholaminergic polymorphic ventricular tachycardia in children. A 7-year follow-up of 21 patients. *Circulation*. 1995;91(5):1512–1519. http://www.ncbi.nlm.nih.gov/pubmed/7867192. Accessed February 1, 2016.

78. Priori SG, Napolitano C, Memmi M, et al. Clinical and molecular characterization of patients with catecholaminergic polymorphic ventricular tachycardia. *Circulation*. 2002;106(1):69–74. http://www.ncbi.nlm.nih.gov/pubmed/12093772. Accessed February 1, 2016.

79. Bauce B, Rampazzo A, Basso C, et al. Screening for ryanodine receptor type 2 mutations in families with effort-induced polymorphic ventricular arrhythmias and sudden death: Early diagnosis of asymptomatic carriers. *J Am Coll Cardiol.* 2002;40(2):341–349. http://www.ncbi.nlm.nih.gov/pubmed/12106942. Accessed February 1, 2016.

80. Hayashi M, Denjoy I, Extramiana F, et al. Incidence and risk factors of arrhythmic events in catecholaminergic polymorphic ventricular tachycardia. *Circulation.* 2009;119(18):2426–2434. doi:10.1161/CIRCULATIONAHA.108.829267.

81. van der Werf C, Kannankeril PJ, Sacher F, et al. Flecainide therapy reduces exercise-induced ventricular arrhythmias in patients with catecholaminergic polymorphic ventricular tachycardia. *J Am Coll Cardiol.* 2011;57(22):2244–2254. doi:10.1016/j.jacc.2011.01.026.

82. Rosso R, Kalman JM, Rogowski O, et al. Calcium channel blockers and beta-blockers versus beta-blockers alone for preventing exercise-induced arrhythmias in catecholaminergic polymorphic ventricular tachycardia. *Heart Rhythm.* 2007;4(9):1149–1154. doi:10.1016/j.hrthm.2007.05.017.

83. Wilde AAM, Bhuiyan ZA, Crotti L, et al. Left cardiac sympathetic denervation for catecholaminergic polymorphic ventricular tachycardia. *N Engl J Med.* 2008;358(19):2024–2029. doi:10.1056/NEJMoa0708006.

84. Coleman MA, Bos JM, Johnson JN, et al. Videoscopic left cardiac sympathetic denervation for patients with recurrent ventricular fibrillation/malignant ventricular arrhythmia syndromes besides congenital long-QT syndrome. *Circ Arrhythm Electrophysiol.* 2012;5(4):782–788. doi:10.1161/CIRCEP.112.971754.

85. Viskin S, Belhassen B. Idiopathic ventricular fibrillation. *Am Heart J.* 1990;120(3):661–671. http://www.ncbi.nlm.nih.gov/pubmed/2202193. Accessed February 20, 2016.

86. Krahn AD, Healey JS, Chauhan V, et al. Systematic assessment of patients with unexplained cardiac arrest: Cardiac arrest survivors with preserved ejection fraction registry (CASPER). *Circulation.* 2009;120(4):278–285. doi:10.1161/CIRCULATIONAHA.109.853143.

87. Crijns HJ, Wiesfeld AC, Posma JL, Lie KI. Favourable outcome in idiopathic ventricular fibrillation with treatment aimed at prevention of high sympathetic tone and suppression of inducible arrhythmias. *Br Heart J.* 1995;74(4):408–412. http://www.pubmedcentral.nih.gov/articlerender.fcgi?artid=484048&tool=pmcentrez&rendertype=abstract. Accessed February 21, 2016.

88. Belhassen B, Viskin S, Fish R, et al. Effects of electrophysiologic-guided therapy with Class IA antiarrhythmic drugs on the long-term outcome of patients with idiopathic ventricular fibrillation with or without the Brugada syndrome. *J Cardiovasc Electrophysiol.* 1999;10(10):1301–1312. http://www.ncbi.nlm.nih.gov/pubmed/10515552. Accessed February 21, 2016.

89. Knecht S, Sacher F, Wright M, et al. Long-term follow-up of idiopathic ventricular fibrillation ablation: A multicenter study. *J Am Coll Cardiol.* 2009;54(6):522–528. doi:10.1016/j.jacc.2009.03.065.

90. Schwartz PJ, Ackerman MJ. The long QT syndrome A transatlantic clinical approach to diagnosis and therapy. *Eur Heart J.* 2013;34:3109–3116.

91. Rudic B, Schimpf R, Borggrefe M. Short QT syndrome–review of diagnosis and treatment. *Arrhythm Electrophysiol Rev.* 2014;3(2):76–79.

IDIOPATHIC VENTRICULAR TACHYCARDIA

Jackson J. Liang and David S. Frankel

CONTENTS

INTRODUCTION

Ventricular tachycardia (VT) most frequently occurs in the setting of structural heart disease. However, the minority (10%) of patients with VT have structurally normal hearts. VT is considered to be "idiopathic" in these patients. While patients with idiopathic VT have a benign long-term prognosis, they often are troubled by symptoms such as palpitations and syncope.

Extensive diagnostic evaluation should be performed in all patients presenting with sustained VT to rule out structural heart disease. Imaging with echocardiography, magnetic resonance imaging, coronary angiography, and positron emission tomography are most helpful.

This chapter will focus on idiopathic VT including outflow tract VT (OTVT) and fascicular VT, also sometimes referred to as Idiopathic Left Ventricular Tachycardia (ILVT). We will describe the epidemiology, clinical presentation, mechanisms, relevant anatomy, diagnosis, and treatment of idiopathic VT. Radiofrequency catheter ablation is a highly effective treatment option to cure idiopathic VT. Ablation will be introduced in this chapter and treated more extensively in Chapter 25. Additionally, electrocardiographic (ECG) features will be discussed in detail in Chapter 32.

OUTFLOW TRACT VENTRICULAR TACHYCARDIA

Outflow tract VT comprises the largest subgroup of idiopathic VT. These arrhythmias are sensitive to adenosine and originate from the right and left ventricular outflow tracts (RVOT and LVOT), pulmonary artery, aortic root, and epicardial LV summit.

EPIDEMIOLOGY AND CLINICAL PRESENTATION
- While there is a wide range, patients most commonly present in the 3rd to 5th decade of life.[1]
- RVOT VT is more common in women while LVOT VT is more common in men.[2-4]
- Typically presents as isolated premature ventricular complexes (PVCs) or salvos of nonsustained VT (NSVT). Sustained VT occurs less commonly.
- Palpitations, chest discomfort, and lightheadedness are common presenting symptoms.

- Syncope uncommon (10%) and sudden cardiac death is extremely rare
  - When syncope or sudden cardiac death occurs, may be due to early form of undiagnosed cardiomyopathy such as arrhythmogenic right ventricular cardiomyopathy (ARVC), sarcoidosis, etc.
- Heart failure due to PVC or tachycardia-induced cardiomyopathy
  - >20% PVC burden at highest risk for cardiomyopathy, although cardiomyopathy can still occur in those with 10%–20% PVC burden.[5–8]
- Sex-specific triggers may be present. For example, RVOT VT triggers are more commonly related to exercise, stress and caffeine in men, while hormonal changes (i.e., premenstrual, gestational, perimenopausal) are more likely to be triggers in women.[9]

MECHANISMS

- Arrhythmia mechanism is most commonly triggered activity.
  - Delayed after depolarizations due to cAMP-mediated calcium overload.
- Decreasing intracellular cAMP results in inhibition of arrhythmia.
  - Adenosine, beta blockers, calcium channel blockers, acetylcholine, vagal maneuvers (carotid sinus massage, Valsalva).
- Increasing intracellular cAMP promotes arrhythmia.
  - Beta agonists such as isoproterenol.
  - Increased heart rate (such as with rapid pacing) and increased catecholamine states.

ANATOMIC CONSIDERATIONS

- RVOT VT
  - RVOT region extends from top of tricuspid valve to the pulmonic valve and is comprised of septal and free wall aspects.
  - RVOT lies anterior to the LVOT and courses more leftward as it rises superiorly such that the distal RVOT and pulmonary artery are anatomically leftward and anterior to the LVOT and aortic root.
  - Pulmonic valve lies anterior and 1–2 cm superior to the aortic valve.
  - Sleeves of muscle extend above the pulmonic valve into the pulmonary artery and may be the VT site of origin.
  - Most commonly ventricular arrhythmias originate along the septal aspect, just beneath the pulmonic valve.
- LVOT VT
  - Includes areas surrounding aortic valve and top of mitral valve.
  - The epicardial LV summit is located between the bifurcation of the left anterior descending and circumflex coronary arteries. It is bisected by the great cardiac vein/anterior interventricular vein. Ventricular arrhythmias originating from the LV summit are challenging to ablate secondary to proximity to coronary arteries and significant amounts of epicardial fat.
  - Sleeves of ventricular muscle extend into the right and left coronary cusps (RCC and LCC). These muscular sleeves may be the site of origin of LVOT VT.
  - The RCC is the anterior-most cusp, lying directly adjacent to the posterior aspect of the RVOT. The RCC abuts the top of the LV septum. The LCC is leftward and posterior to the RCC, while the NCC lies rightward and posterior to the RCC.
  - The RCC and NCC lie inferior to the LCC due to the rightward tilt of the aortic valve.
  - The NCC articulates with both atria and the interatrial septum. Atrial arrhythmias can sometimes be ablated from the NCC. Ventricular arrhythmias are very rarely ablated from the NCC.

DIAGNOSIS

- ECG
    - OTVT is positive in the inferior leads (II, III, aVF).
    - The free wall of the RVOT is most anterior within the chest, and thus the activation wavefront moves away from the precordial leads, generating a left bundle configuration in lead V1 and precordial transition ≥V4 (Figure 9.1).[10]
    - As one progresses posteriorly within the outflow tracts (septal RVOT, RCC, LCC, aortomitral continuity [AMC], superior mitral annulus), the wavefront shifts progressively towards the precordial leads, with greater degrees of positivity in lead V1 and earlier precordial transition.
    - V2 transition ratio can be helpful to predict RVOT vs. LVOT site of origin for ventricular arrhythmias with left bundle configuration in lead V1 and V3 transition (Figure 9.2).[11]
    - LV summit has pattern break in lead V2, with more net negativity than lead V1 or V3.
    - VT originating from the junction of the RCC and LCC typically has notch in downstroke or W pattern in lead V1.
    - AMC origin typically manifests a qR pattern in lead V1.

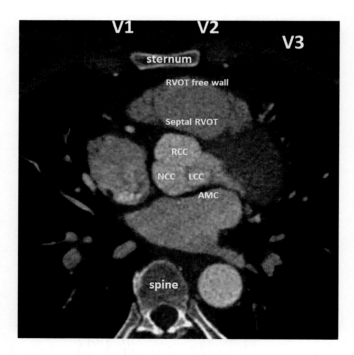

Figure 9.1 Anatomy of the outflow tracts. The free wall of the right ventricular outflow tract lies directly beneath the sternum and the precordial ECG leads. Thus VT originating from the free wall of the RVOT is negative in lead V1 and has a late precordial transition (≥V4). As the site of VT origin shifts posteriorly within the chest, from the septal RVOT, to the right coronary cusp, left coronary cups, aortomitral continuity and superior mitral annulus, the degree of positivity in lead V1 increases and the precordial transition becomes progressively earlier. (Adapted from Liang, J.J. et al., *Curr. Treat Options Cardiovasc. Med.*, 17, 363, 2015. With permission.)

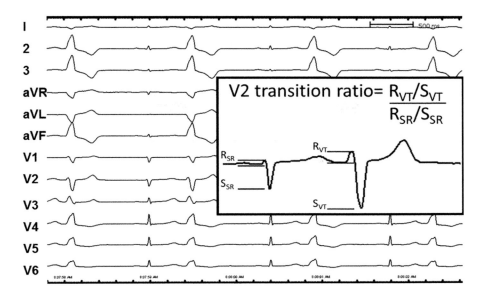

Figure 9.2 Electrocardiogram of outflow tract VT. 12-lead electrocardiogram of VT originating from the left coronary cusp. Like all outflow tract VT, the complex is positive in the inferior leads. The VT has a left bundle configuration in lead V1 and transitions in lead V3. Outflow tract VT that transitions before V3 originates from the LVOT. Outflow tract VT that transitions after V3 originates from the RVOT. Outflow tract VT that transitions in lead V3 can originate from the RVOT or LVOT. In such cases, the VT precordial transition can be normalized to the sinus rhythm precordial transition by calculating a V2 transition ratio, as is shown in the inset. Interestingly, the V3 transition ratio is not as useful for distinguishing RVOT from LVOT sites of origin.

TREATMENT

- Medications
  - Adenosine, beta blocker, calcium channel blocker for acute treatment
  - For long-term suppression, beta blocker, calcium channel blocker, sodium channel blocker, less commonly potassium channel blocker.
- Catheter ablation is generally safe and effective. When successful, it eliminates the need for long-term medication use. Can be considered first-line treatment in many patients.
- Activation and pace mapping are techniques to localize the VT site of origin.
- Activation mapping
  - Identifies the site of earliest activation, which should be well before the onset of the QRS complex
  - The unipolar electrogram at the site of origin should have a qS pattern
  - The preferred technique when PVCs are frequent enough
- Pace mapping
  - Method to map when VT/PVCs are too infrequent for activation mapping
  - Pacing at threshold output to identify a perfect (12/12) QRS morphology match
  - Pace mapping alone results in lower success rates compared with activation mapping
- A detailed description of mapping and ablation strategies for OTVT is presented in Chapter 25.

Verapamil-sensitive ILVT (fascicular VT) is a macroreentrant arrhythmia, which is generally characterized by the following: (1) Inducibility with atrial or ventricular pacing; (2) ECG during VT demonstrating narrow, typical right bundle branch block configuration in lead V1; (3) Termination with administration of verapamil.

EPIDEMIOLOGY AND CLINICAL PRESENTATION

- Occurs more commonly in men (60%–80%).
- Typically presents in younger patients (<40 years of age) and is uncommon in patients older than 55.
- Similar to OTVT, patients usually present with palpitations or lightheadedness. Syncope and sudden death are rare.
- When incessant, may result in tachycardia-mediated cardiomyopathy.[12,13] There are three major types of fascicular VT: (1) Left posterior fascicular (90%); (2) Left anterior fascicular (10%); (3) Upper septal (<1%).

MECHANISMS

- The most common mechanism of fascicular VT is macroreentry and the following characteristics are observed:
  - Reproducible initiation and termination of VT with both atrial and ventricular stimulation
  - Ability to entrain and reset with fusion
  - Inverse relationship between coupling interval of initiating extrastimulus and first VT beat
- The reentry circuit is sizable and uses the left posterior fascicle as the retrograde limb and abnormal Purkinje tissue or adjacent ventricular myocardium with decremental properties as the anterograde limb (Figure 9.3).
- During sinus rhythm, anterograde conduction occurs over both the left posterior fascicle as well as the slowly conducting Purkinje/adjacent ventricular tissue. Anterograde and retrograde wavefronts collide within this area of slow conduction. During macroreentrant fascicular VT, retrograde conduction occurs over the left posterior fascicle while anterograde conduction proceeds over the abnormal Purkinje fibers.[14–17]
- The association that has been observed between false tendons and fascicular VT has been largely disproven. False tendons are commonly observed in patients without fascicular VT.

ANATOMIC CONSIDERATIONS

- Below the AV node, the conduction axis continues through the central fibrous body as the insulated Bundle of His penetrating the membranous ventricular septum. It bifurcates at the level of the junction between the membranous and muscular ventricular septum, entering the ventricles as the left and right bundle branches.
- The left bundle branch is a broad, fan-like structure, which continues along the subendocardial aspect of the LV septum and branches into two fascicles.
- The left anterior fascicle innervates the anterolateral papillary muscle and gives off terminal Purkinje fibers which supply the anterolateral LV.
- The left posterior fascicle innervates the posteromedial papillary muscle and gives off terminal Purkinje fibers which supply the inferoseptal LV.

Sinus Rhythm

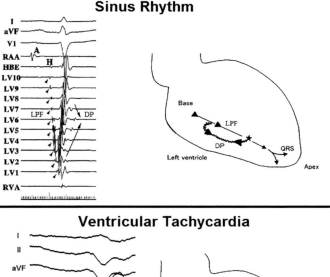

Ventricular Tachycardia

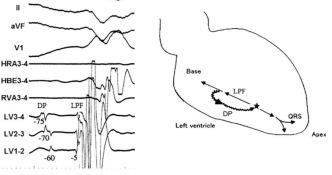

Figure 9.3 Macroreentrant circuit of fascicular VT. During sinus rhythm (top panel), anterograde conduction occurs over the left posterior fascicle (LPF), as well as the abnormal, decremental, Purkinje tissue (DP). The activation wavefront also proceeds retrograde over the DP, resulting in a collision within the DP. During fascicular VT (bottom panel), retrograde conduction is over the LPF, with anterograde conduction over the DP. (Adapted from Maruyama, M. et al., *J. Cardiovasc. Electrophysiol.*, 12, 968–972, 2001; Nogami, A. et al., *J Am. Coll. Cardiol.*, 36, 811–823, 2000; and Aiba, T. et al., *Pacing Clin. Electrophysiol.*, 24, 333–344, 2001. With permission.)

DIAGNOSIS

- ECG is consistent with exit from one of the fascicles of the left bundle (Figure 9.4)
  - Typical right bundle branch block configuration in lead V1.
  - Rapid intrinsic deflection (RS interval in precordial leads of 60–80 ms).
  - QRS duration is narrow (<150 ms).
  - Major differential diagnosis is papillary muscle VT, which tends to be wider with qS pattern in lead V1, rather than RSR'.
  - Left posterior fascicular VT has qS pattern in leads 1 and aVL, consistent with early, unopposed left to right activation of ventricular septum. qS pattern in leads 1 and aVL is not observed with posteromedial papillary muscle VT, as exit is not directly on septum.
  - Fascicular VT must also be distinguished from supraventricular tachycardia with aberrant conduction.

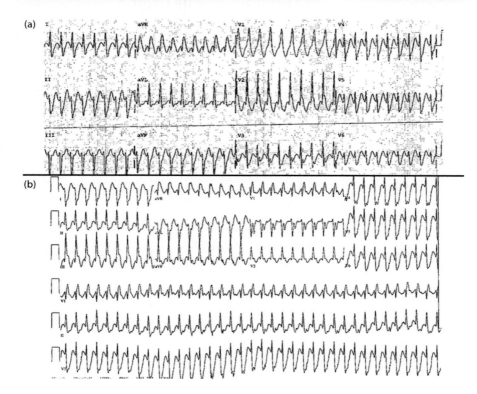

Figure 9.4 Electrocardiogram of fascicular VT. Example of 12-lead electrocardiograms of left posterior fascicular VT (panel A) and left anterior fascicular VT (panel B). In panel A, note the sharp intrinsic deflection and q waves in leads 1 and aVL. In panel B, note the RSR' configuration in lead V1 (typical of right bundle branch block), as well as the sharp intrinsic deflection.

TREATMENT

- Acute management
  - For patients with hemodynamically unstable VT, electrical cardioversion should be performed promptly.
  - Intravenous verapamil is usually effective in terminating VT[18]
  - For the most part, vagal maneuvers and adenosine are ineffective.
- Long-term medical management
  - Calcium channel blockers are most effective, followed by beta blockers and potassium channel blockers. Sodium channel blockers are least effective.
- Catheter ablation
  - Highly effective (90% success rate).[17,19–21]
  - Often considered first line treatment, particularly in younger patients.
  - Some target the abnormal, slowly conducting Purkinje tissue/adjacent ventricular tissue, which forms the diastolic limb of the VT circuit, preceding the QRS complex by 40–110 ms.[17,20]
  - Others target the left posterior fascicle itself, which is the systolic limb of the VT circuit. During VT, they ablate the earliest Purkinje potential along the apical half of the inferoseptum, typically preceding the QRS complex by 15–40 ms at successful sites.[19] These sites will also record Purkinje potentials in sinus rhythm, after the His recording and preceding the QRS.

- Best to transect the left posterior fascicle midway from base to apex. If too basal, risk of causing left bundle branch block or complete heart block. If too apical, may be ineffective as the left posterior fascicle arborizes.
- Pace mapping is challenging, as one must capture the fascicle without capturing the surrounding myocardium. Thus it is only useful if a perfect 12 of 12 match is obtained.
- Mechanical suppression with catheter bump of superficial components of the circuit not uncommonly makes VT non-inducible. In this situation, an anatomic ablation can be performed, with a line of ablation perpendicular to the left posterior fascicle, transecting it midway from base to apex. The line is typically <2 cm.[22]
- Similar ablation strategies can be used to target left anterior fascicular VT.

CONCLUSIONS

Idiopathic OTVT and fascicular VT occur in patients with structurally normal hearts and are generally associated with a benign long-term prognosis, but can result in significant symptoms or cardiomyopathy. Long-term treatment options include medications and catheter ablation. Catheter ablation is generally effective and safe for abolishing idiopathic VT. A detailed understanding of the relevant anatomy and electrocardiography is vital to success.

REFERENCES

1. Lerman BB, Stein KM, Markowitz SM. Idiopathic right ventricular outflow tract tachycardia: A clinical approach. *Pacing Clin Electrophysiol* 1996;19:2120–2137.
2. Callans DJ, Menz V, Schwartzman D et al. Repetitive monomorphic tachycardia from the left ventricular outflow tract: Electrocardiographic patterns consistent with a left ventricular site of origin. *J Am Coll Cardiol* 1997;29:1023–1027.
3. Dixit S, Gerstenfeld EP, Lin D et al. Identification of distinct electrocardiographic patterns from the basal left ventricle: Distinguishing medial and lateral sites of origin in patients with idiopathic ventricular tachycardia. *Heart Rhythm* 2005;2:485–491.
4. Nakagawa M, Takahashi N, Nobe S et al. Gender differences in various types of idiopathic ventricular tachycardia. *J Cardiovasc Electrophysiol* 2002;13:633–638.
5. Lee GK, Klarich KW, Grogan M, Cha YM. Premature ventricular contraction-induced cardiomyopathy: A treatable condition. *Circ Arrhythm Electrophysiol* 2012;5:229–236.
6. Baman TS, Lange DC, Ilg KJ et al. Relationship between burden of premature ventricular complexes and left ventricular function. *Heart Rhythm* 2010;7:865–869.
7. Takemoto M, Yoshimura H, Ohba Y et al. Radiofrequency catheter ablation of premature ventricular complexes from right ventricular outflow tract improves left ventricular dilation and clinical status in patients without structural heart disease. *J Am Coll Cardiol* 2005;45:1259–1265.
8. Yarlagadda RK, Iwai S, Stein KM et al. Reversal of cardiomyopathy in patients with repetitive monomorphic ventricular ectopy originating from the right ventricular outflow tract. *Circulation* 2005;112:1092–1097.

9. Marchlinski FE, Deely MP, Zado ES. Sex-specific triggers for right ventricular outflow tract tachycardia. *Am Heart J* 2000;139:1009–1013.

10. Liang JJ, Han Y, Frankel DS. Ablation of outflow tract ventricular tachycardia. *Curr Treat Options Cardiovasc Med* 2015;17:363.

11. Betensky BP, Park RE, Marchlinski FE et al. The V(2) transition ratio: A new electrocardiographic criterion for distinguishing left from right ventricular outflow tract tachycardia origin. *J Am Coll Cardiol* 2011;57:2255–2262.

12. Toivonen L, Nieminen M. Persistent ventricular tachycardia resulting in left ventricular dilatation treated with verapamil. *Int J Cardiol* 1986;13:361–365.

13. Castro-Rodriguez J, Verbeet T, Morissens M et al. Complicated forms of tachycardia-mediated cardiomyopathy associated with idiopathic left ventricular tachycardia. *Pacing Clin Electrophysiol* 2011;34:e52–e55.

14. Frankel DS, Marchlinski FE. Chapter 82—Fascicular ventricular arrhythmias. In: Zipes DP, Jalife J, editors. *Cardiac Electrophysiology: From Cell to Bedside* (6th ed.). Philadelphia: W.B. Saunders, 2014:827–833.

15. Maruyama M, Tadera T, Miyamoto S, Ino T. Demonstration of the reentrant circuit of verapamil-sensitive idiopathic left ventricular tachycardia: Direct evidence for macro-reentry as the underlying mechanism. *J Cardiovasc Electrophysiol* 2001;12:968–972.

16. Aiba T, Suyama K, Aihara N et al. The role of Purkinje and pre-Purkinje potentials in the reentrant circuit of verapamil-sensitive idiopathic LV tachycardia. *Pacing Clin Electrophysiol* 2001;24:333–344.

17. Nogami A, Naito S, Tada H et al. Demonstration of diastolic and presystolic Purkinje potentials as critical potentials in a macroreentry circuit of verapamil-sensitive idiopathic left ventricular tachycardia. *J Am Coll Cardiol* 2000;36:811–823.

18. Iwai S, Lerman BB. Management of ventricular tachycardia in patients with clinically normal hearts. *Curr Cardiol Rep* 2000;2:515–521.

19. Nakagawa H, Beckman KJ, McClelland JH et al. Radiofrequency catheter ablation of idiopathic left ventricular tachycardia guided by a Purkinje potential. *Circulation* 1993;88:2607–2617.

20. Tsuchiya T, Okumura K, Honda T et al. Significance of late diastolic potential preceding Purkinje potential in verapamil-sensitive idiopathic left ventricular tachycardia. *Circulation* 1999;99:2408–2413.

21. Wen MS, Yeh SJ, Wang CC et al. Radiofrequency ablation therapy in idiopathic left ventricular tachycardia with no obvious structural heart disease. *Circulation* 1994;89:1690–1696.

22. Lin D, Hsia HH, Gerstenfeld EP et al. Idiopathic fascicular left ventricular tachycardia: Linear ablation lesion strategy for noninducible or nonsustained tachycardia. *Heart Rhythm* 2005;2:934–939.

SYNCOPE

SYNCOPE EVENTS, DEFINITIONS, CAUSES, AND FEATURES

Subramanya Prasad, Oussama M. Wazni, Mina K. Chung, Kenneth Mayuga, and Robert Schweikert

CONTENTS

INTRODUCTION

- Syncope is a common clinical problem both in the outpatient and the in-hospital setting.[1] It has been estimated that approximately one-third of individuals experience a syncopal episode during their lifetime,[2] with a 30% recurrence rate.[3]
- Though most syncopal episodes are benign and self-limiting, it can be a presenting symptom of organic heart disease, and accounts for significant injuries in 35% of patients.[4]
- This chapter provides a comprehensive overview of the definition, pathophysiology, classification/causes including clinical features, and initial management.

DEFINITION

- The 2009 European Society of Cardiology (ESC) guidelines[40] define syncope as a transient loss of consciousness due to transient global cerebral hypoperfusion characterized by rapid onset, short duration, and spontaneous complete recovery.
- The 2015 Heart Rhythm Society (HRS) Consensus Document[39] defines syncope as a transient loss of consciousness, associated with an inability to maintain postural tone, rapid and spontaneous recovery, and the absence of clinical features specific for another form of transient loss of consciousness such as epileptic seizure.
- Presyncope or near-syncope generally refers to a condition in which syncope is felt to be imminent without LOC.

- A lack of consensus in syncope-related terminology makes the interpretation of early syncope literature confusing. Table 10.1 lists the guidelines regarding acceptable terminology in syncope issued by the ESC[5] and ACC.

Table 10.1 Acceptable syncope terminology with explanation

Term	Description/recommended terminology
Breath holding spells/reflex anoxic seizure	They represent a form of VVS in infants. "Infantile vasovagal syncope" is preferred.
Classical vasovagal syncope	Should be reserved for neurally mediated/reflex syncope initiated by triggers (pain, emotional, or orthostatic stress, instrumentation)
Convulsive syncope	This term should be used as an abbreviated description of "syncope accompanied by myoclonic jerks and other involuntary movements"; the term does not imply epilepsy.
Drop attacks	Should be strictly restricted to sudden loss of lower extremity tone without LOC
Dysautonomia/dysautonomic	Should be reserved for Riley-day syndrome
Hyperventilation syncope	Currently it is unclear if hyperventilation can cause syncope
	Syncopal symptoms attributable to hyperventilation fall under "panic attacks" in DSM-IV.
Neurally mediated syncope (NMS)	NMS and reflex syncope are synonyms.
Neurogenic syncope	NMS is preferred.
Neurocardiogenic syncope	Since the term emphasizes the origin of reflex in the heart, it should be strictly used for a putative type of reflex syncope where the trigger is in the heart.
Orthostatic intolerance	Erroneously used as synonyms for POH and POTS. Strict restriction of the term to describe patient complaints only is advised.
Presyncope	Should be used to describe a collective constellation of symptoms due to compromised CBF, and diminished cortical functioning (dizziness, lightheadedness, blurred vision). Though headache and shoulder pain, sweating and nausea, and paresthesias can occur before syncopal onset, they are not linked to LOC.
Psychogenic syncope	Pseudosyncope or psychogenic pseudosyncope is preferred, implying the lack of cerebral hypoperfusion among these patients (factitious disorders, malingering, and conversion).
Seizures	Strictly restricted for epilepsy
Transient LOC (TLOC)	Should be used when 4 criteria are satisfied: LOC Transient Self-limited Absence of head or brain injury
Vasodepressor syncope	Should be used in syncope when a vasodepressor response is seen without an associated cardioinhibitory response

Abbreviations: VVS, vasovagal syncope; LOC, loss of consciousness; DSM-IV, Diagnostic and Statistical Manual of Mental Disorders, Fourth Edition; POH, postural orthostatic hypotension; POTS, postural orthostatic tachycardia syndrome; CBF, cerebral blood flow.

SCOPE OF THE PROBLEM

- Syncope is a common presenting problem accounting for 3%–5% of emergency room visits and 1%–3% of hospital admissions,[2] with an incidence of 3% (men) and 3.5% (women) in the general population.[2]
- Susceptibility to syncope increases with advancing age,[2,6] with a 6% annual incidence and a recurrence rate of 30% among the institutionalized elderly.
- The annual cost of evaluating and treating patients with syncope in the USA is estimated to be 800 million dollars.[7]
- Patients at high risk of recurrent syncope require hospitalization, with diagnostic studies averaging $5281 per patient (1993 dollars).[7] Table 10.2 shows the cost of investigations in syncopal patients.

Table 10.2 Clinical features of true syncope and syncope mimics

Type of syncope	Specific syndromes	Clinical features/comments	Diagnostic criteria
DISORDERS WITH True LOC			

Neurally mediated (reflex)¶	Vasovagal syncope* (common faint)
	  Classic
	  Non-classic
	Carotid sinus syncope
	Situational syncope
	  Acute hemorrhage
	  Cough*, sneeze
	  Gastrointestinal and/or genitourinary
	  stimulation (swallowing*, defecation#, visceral
	  pain, endoscopy, bladder catheterization)
	  Micturition (post-micturition)*
	  Postexercise
	  Postprandial#
	  Others (e.g., brass instrument playing,
	  weightlifting)
	  Glossopharyngeal neuralgia#
		NMS:
		Absence of cardiac disease
		Long history of syncope
		After unpleasant sight, sound, smell, or pain
		Prolonged standing or crowded, hot places
		Nausea, vomiting associated with syncope
		During or in the absorptive state after a meal
		With head rotation, pressure on carotid sinus
		(as in tumors, shaving, tight collars)
		After exertion
			VVS is diagnosed if precipitating events such as fear, severe pain, emotional distress, instrumentation, or prolonged standing are associated with typical prodromal symptoms.
			Situational syncope is diagnosed if syncope occurs during or immediately after urination, defecation, cough, or swallowing.

Orthostatic hypotension¶	Autonomic failure Primary autonomic failure syndromes (e.g., pure autonomic failure, multiple system atrophy, Parkinson's disease with autonomic failure) Secondary autonomic failure syndromes (e.g., diabetic neuropathy*, amyloid neuropathy) Postexercise Postprandial Drug (and alcohol)-induced orthostatic syncope	After standing up Temporal relationship with start of medication leading to hypotension or changes of dosage Prolonged standing, especially in crowded, hot places Presence of autonomic neuropathy or Parkinsonism After exertion	POH is diagnosed when there is documentation of POH associated with syncope/presyncope. Orthostatic BP measurements are recommended after 5 min of lying supine, followed by measurements each minute, or more often, after 3 min of standing. Measurements may be continued longer if BP is still falling at 3 min.

(Continued)

Table 10.2 (Continued) Clinical features of true syncope and syncope mimics

Type of syncope	Specific syndromes	Clinical features/comments	Diagnostic criteria
	Volume depletion* Hemorrhage, diarrhea, Addison's disease		If the patient does not tolerate standing for this period, the lowest BP in the upright posture is recorded. A decrease in SBP ≥ 20 mmHg or a decrease in SBP to <90 mmHg is defined as POH, regardless of occurrence of symptoms.[41]
Cardiac arrhythmias as primary cause (see Table 10.5)	Sinus node dysfunction (including bradycardia/tachycardia syndrome)* Atrioventricular conduction system disease (AV block)*, myocardial ischemia, medications* (digoxin, beta-blockers, verapamil), hypertension, valvular heart disease, cardiomyopathy Paroxysmal supraventricular (accessory pathways) (SVT) and ventricular tachycardias (VT) Inherited syndromes (e.g., long QT syndrome#, Brugada syndrome, ARVD#) Implanted device (pacemaker, ICD) malfunction Drug-induced pro-arrhythmias (digoxin, inotropes, drugs causing QT prolongation)	Presence of severe structural heart disease During exertion, or supine Preceded by palpitation or accompanied by chest pain Family history of sudden death	Arrhythmia-related syncope is diagnosed by ECG when there is • Sinus bradycardia <40 beats/min or repetitive sinoatrial blocks or sinus pauses >3s. • Mobitz II 2nd or 3rd degree AV block. • Alternating LBBB and RBBB. • Rapid paroxysmal SVT or VT. • Pacemaker malfunction with cardiac pauses.
Structural cardiac or cardiopulmonary disease (see Table 10.5)	Arrhythmias, supraventricular# and ventricular tachycardia* Acute myocardial infarction/ischemia Obstructive cardiac valvular disease (aortic stenosis*, mitral stenosis) Hypertrophic obstructive cardiomyopathy* non-ischemic cardiomyopathy with low EF Atrial myxoma# Acute aortic dissection Pericardial disease/tamponade Pulmonary embolus#/pulmonary hypertension#	Presence of severe structural heart disease During exertion, or supine Preceded by palpitation or accompanied by chest pain Family history of sudden death	Myocardial ischemia-related syncope is diagnosed when symptoms are present with ECG evidence of acute ischemia with or without myocardial infarction, independently of its mechanism.

(Continued)

Table 10.2 (*Continued*) Clinical features of true syncope and syncope mimics

Type of syncope	Specific syndromes	Clinical features/comments	Diagnostic criteria
Cerebrovascular disease	Vascular steal syndromes#, migraine# Vertebrobasilar TIA	With arm exercise. Differences in blood pressure or pulse in the two arms. Vertebrobasilar system TIAs (vertigo, ocular palsy, and dysarthria) caused by atherosclerotic narrowing or extrinsic compression (cervical spondylosis, cervical rib) should be considered if syncope/presyncope is associated with extension or lateral rotation of the neck. Subclavian steal syndrome (subclavian artery narrowing at its origin, accounts for <0.1% of all syncopal episodes†) or severe carotid artery disease (atherosclerotic disease, Takayasu's disease) can cause syncope. Syncope or dizziness can be seen during upper extremity exercise due to shunting of blood from the brain via the vertebral artery system to the affected limb. Extracranial vasospasm seen during migraine can cause NMS.	

Note: * Major common causes; # major uncommon causes; † NMS and POH account for 33% of all syncopal episodes.

PATHOPHYSIOLOGY

- The pathophysiology of syncope is complex and incompletely understood.
- *In healthy humans*, assumption of the upright posture causes peripheral venous and splanchnic pooling, displacing 500–800 mL of blood (within the first 10 s), thus reducing preload.[5,8]
- The reducing preload stimulates the central arterial baroreceptor system (carotid body, aortic arch) and cardiopulmonary mechanoreceptors.[9,10]
- The cardiopulmonary mechanoreceptors (inferoposterior wall of the left ventricle and the chest wall) stimulate the brainstem (nucleus ambiguous and dorsal vagal nucleus), causing augmented sympathetic activity and parasympathetic withdrawal.[9,10]
- The resulting increase in circulating catecholamines causes compensatory vasoconstriction of the splanchnic, musculocutaneous, and renal vascular beds, thus maintaining systemic arterial pressure and cerebral perfusion.[10]
- *In neurally mediated syncope (NMS) susceptible individuals*, hypoactive neurocardiovascular reflexes along with a diminished central blood volume result in a reduced preload.
- A reduced preload triggers a paradoxic reflex vasodilatation and bradycardia, mediated by enhanced parasympathetic activity and sympathetic withdrawal.[11] Inadequate vasoconstriction or inappropriate vasodilatation may play a critical role in mediating hypotension seen in the reflex syncopal syndromes.[5]
- Vasomotor center (VMC) stimulation is believed to cause most of the prodromal symptoms (diaphoresis, nausea, vomiting) accompanying NMS.
- The mechanism of syncope in an individual patient could be multi-factorial. In addition to venous pooling and decreased central volume, decreased cardiac output and an inability to increase vascular resistance during upright posture can play significant roles in the causation of syncope.
- In contrast to other viscera, the metabolism of the brain is largely dependent on adequate perfusion. In healthy young to middle-aged individuals, the average cerebral blood flow (CBF) is 50–60 mL/min/100 g tissue.
- In the young healthy cerebrovascular bed, cerebral autoregulation maintains the average CBF over a wide range of blood pressures, thus maintaining adequate cerebral O_2 requirements (3.0–3.5 mL O_2/100 g tissue/min).
- An abrupt reduction in CBF for 6–8 s is enough to produce reduced blood flow to the reticular activating system, resulting in complete loss of consciousness.[14] Lesser periods of reduced CBF result in presyncope or near-syncope.
- Cerebral autoregulation can be compromised due to increasing age or underlying disease, thus reducing the safety margin for oxygen delivery. Aging alone causes a 25% reduction in CBF, among individuals aged 20–70 years.[15] Hence a small drop (as low as 20%) in cerebral oxygen delivery is sufficient to cause loss of consciousness.[4]

CEREBRAL AUTOREGULATION

- Adequate cerebral perfusion is largely dependent on systemic arterial pressure and cerebral autoregulation (maintenance of cerebral blood flow over a relatively wide range of mean arterial pressures).
- In the presence of hypertension, the autoregulatory curve is shifted higher, requiring higher arterial pressures to maintain perfusion. A decrease in systolic blood pressure #60 mmHg is associated with syncope.[16]

- Though cerebrovascular autoregulation is largely controlled by local metabolic and chemical mediators (pCO_2, 20 mmHg and 80 mmHg, pH, and pO_2, 50 mmHg), baroreceptor responses to changes in systemic arterial pressure play a minor role. These mechanisms are deregulated among the elderly or critically ill patients.[16]
- Presyncope/syncope seen during panic attacks/hyperventilation syndromes is due to reduced CBF, probably secondary to low pCO_2-induced vasoconstriction.

CAUSES AND CLINICAL FEATURES OF TRANSIENT LOSS OF CONSCIOUSNESS (TLOC)[5]

- Clinicians approaching patients with TLOC have to differentiate true syncope from "non-syncopal" conditions (syncope mimics) to help decide further management.
- A thorough history and a focused physical examination (orthostatic blood pressure measurements and a standard ECG) are usually sufficient to identify the probable cause of syncope in 75% of patients.[17,18]
- In the outpatient/emergency setting, non-cardiac syncope is the commonest cause. In the in-hospital setting, cardiac causes are the most common. A list of the causes and clinical features of true syncope and syncope mimics is seen in Table 10.2.

TRUE SYNCOPE

NEURALLY MEDIATED SYNCOPAL SYNDROMES (NMSs)
- NMS is the most common variety of syncope among all age groups.
- Though NMS occurs in response to a variety of triggers they share a common pathophysiologic basis.
- Among NMS, vasovagal syncope (VVS) and carotid sinus hypersensitivity (CSH) are the most common types.

VASOVAGAL SYNCOPE
- VVS is the most common form of syncope among the young and the elderly, with a benign and self-limited course.
- Various triggers induce VVS through
  - Neural (Bezold–Jarisch and carotid sinus) reflexes.
  - Neuroendocrine (chemical) pathways.

NEURAL REFLEXES
- *Bezold–Jarisch reflex*: Mechanoreceptors located in the atria, great veins, left ventricle, and thoracic wall are activated in response to pressure or volume loading, which stimulates afferent C fibers.[19] This activates vagal efferents to induce a cardioinhibitory response and reduce BP.
- *Carotid sinus reflex*: As above, mechanical stimulation (CSM) or increased BP increases baroreceptor firing (carotid sinus and aortic arch), activating vagal efferents.

NEURAL MECHANISMS OF VVS

- Afferent neural signals originating centrally (CNS in anxiety) or peripherally (barore-ceptors, mechanoreceptors, and chemoreceptors) stimulate the VMC.[11,19]
- The vagal efferents mediate bradycardia whereas sympathetic withdrawal mediates vasodepression.[20]
- In classic VVS, prodromal symptoms followed by a vasodepressor and cardio-inhibitory (sinus bradycardia to AV block to asystole) response are seen in that order.
- Clinically, atypical VVS (absent prodrome with a mixed response) is more common. Interestingly, all three response patterns can be seen in the same patient at different times, and the clinical pattern may differ from the head-up tilt (HUT) response.

NEUROENDOCRINE MECHANISMS OF VVS

- *Central serotoninergic pathways*: These appear to have a role in the pathogenesis of neu-rocardiogenic syncope. Animal studies have shown that elevated extracellular sero-tonin levels can inhibit central sympathetic activity responsible for the cardioinhibitory and vasodepressor response of VVS.[21]
- *Adenosine (ATP)*: ATP is a potent AV node depressant with significant negative ino-tropic and vasodepressor effects.[22] Intravenous administration of ATP can induce VVS and has been used as a pharmacologic adjunct in HUT testing.
- Though recent studies measuring multiple neurohumoral markers (norepinephrine, endothelin, prolactin, cortisol, renin, vasopressin, beta-endorphins, and substance P) have reported differential changes in serum levels during HUT testing, their patho-physiologic significance is unclear at the present time.[23,24]

CLINICAL FEATURES

- VVS is commonly encountered in crowded warm places. A typical history includes pro-dromal symptoms (absent in elderly) followed by partial or complete LOC.
- With the exception of pallor, the physical exam is usually benign. Complete recovery is usual although fatigue and nausea may persist for several minutes. Table 10.2 lists the salient clinical features of the various causes of syncope.

SITUATIONAL SYNCOPE

- This applies to the group of NMSs initiated by specific triggers. The most common types are cough, deglutition, defecation, and postprandial syncope. Table 10.3 lists their salient features and pertinent management.
- Most of them result in a cardioinhibitory response (sinus bradycardia, sinus arrest, and AV block). Treatment involves removal or avoidance of the trigger responsible for syn-cope. When anticipated (e.g., diagnostic endoscopy), prophylactic atropine administra-tion can prevent syncope.

CAROTID SINUS HYPERSENSITIVITY (CSH)

- CSH is a syndrome with manifestations very similar to NMS (Table 10.2).
- Carotid sinus stimulation by triggers (washing of the face, shaving, head and neck movements) sends afferent neural signals, mainly from the cervical area (including the ipsilateral sternocleidomastoid) causing cardioinhibitory and vasodepressor responses.
- It is usually seen in men at 40 years.[5,30] Prodromal symptoms are usually absent. Two large studies of HUT testing in NMS patients showed a 6%–14% incidence of CSH.[4]
- A diagnosis is made by performing carotid sinus massage (CSM), both supine and dur-ing a HUT. A fall in systolic blood pressure (SBP) 50 mmHg or a pause (asystole) $ 3 s along with symptom reproduction is considered diagnostic of CSH.
- During HUT, even though the predominant response is cardioinhibitory, identifying an underlying vasodepressor component can significantly affect management. This can be iden-tified by repeating the HUT after correction of bradycardia (atropine or temporary pacing).

Table 10.3 Clinical features of situational syncopal syndromes

Situational syncope	Clinical features and comments
Cough syncope	Follows a vigorous coughing spell. Increase in CSF pressure causes increased cerebrovascular resistance, reducing CBF.[25] Cessation of smoking and bronchodilators are useful.
Deglutition syncope	Dysphagia induces vagal stimulation, especially in the setting of esophageal disorders (tumors, diverticulum, achalasia, stricture, and diffuse spasm), and with instrumentation (EGD, bronchoscopy). Syncope is due to cardioinhibition.
Postprandial syncope	Presyncope/syncope due to hypotension during the postprandial period is common in the elderly. Unclear mechanism, most likely explanations are meal-induced splanchnic pooling with an inadequate sympathetic compensation, inadequate postprandial increase in cardiac output, and release of gastrointestinal peptides. In a study of 113 elderly nursing home residents, 36% (41/113) showed a 1-h postprandial SBP decrease of 20 mmHg.[26] Octreotide infusion has been shown to be effective in reducing postprandial syncope.[27]
Defecation syncope	It is commonly seen among elderly people with bowel movements during the night or during manual fecal disimpaction.[28] Many such patients have underlying gastrointestinal malignancy.
Valsalva syncope	Forced exhalation against a closed glottis (Valsalva maneuver) can cause peripheral venous pooling and syncope.[2] Valsalva syncope can be a harbinger of syncope due to SND or cerebrovascular occlusive disease. Avoiding sustained Valsalva maneuvers can prevent recurrences.
Micturition syncope	LOC following urination is commonly seen in patients with nocturia, with consumption of large quantities of beverages, also following drainage of a distended urinary bladder and abdominal paracentesis.[29]

ORTHOSTATIC HYPOTENSION (OH)[40]

- Classical orthostatic hypotension is defined as a decrease of ≥20/10 mmHg in blood pressure within 3 min of change in posture. Progressive orthostatic hypotension is a decrease of ≥20/10 mmHg seen after 3 min of upright position.
- Measurement of BP should be done after 5 min of lying supine, and after 3 min of standing (see Table 10.2).
- OH is usually seen in the early morning hours or following prolonged recumbency. Symptoms of presyncope are seen, while bradycardia, sweating, and pallor are usually absent.
- The most common causes of OH are intravascular volume depletion (transient or chronic) and/or autonomic failure (primary or secondary). Table 10.4 lists the various causes of OH and its salient features.

CARDIAC CAUSES

Cardiac causes include arrhythmias and structural heart disease. Tables 10.5 and 10.6 list the various conditions.

Table 10.4 Causes of POH

Syndrome	Causes	Clinical features/comments
Primary autonomic failure	Pure autonomic failure (Bradbury Eggleston syndrome), POH, widespread autonomic failure (fecal and urinary incontinence, defective sweating and sexual function) decreased supine norepinephrine levels Autonomic failure with multiple system atrophy (Shy–Drager syndrome), autonomic dysfunction, parkinsonism, ataxia Parkinson's with autonomic failure	Autonomic failure is defined as an inadequate vasomotor reflex adaptation to orthostatic challenge; can be primary or secondary.
[a] Secondary autonomic failure	Diabetes mellitus [a]Volume depletion (gastroenteritis, hemorrhage), third space losses (adrenal insufficiency, diabetes insipidus, or hyperglycemia), medications antihypertensives, diuretics, nitrates, beta-blockers Autoimmune (Guillain–Barre syndrome, myasthenia gravis) Malignancy-induced autonomic neuropathy Metabolic (porphyria, Fabry's disease) CNS infections (syphilis, chagas) Hypothalamic and midbrain tumors/lesions (craniopharyngioma) Spinal cord lesions/tumors Prolonged physical inactivity associated with lengthy hospitalization	Volume depletion (mostly due to medications) is a common cause of orthostatic syncope. Medications are the most common causes of POH, especially in the elderly due to (1) reduced baroreceptor sensitivity, (2) reduced CBF, (3) renal sodium wasting, and (4) an impaired thirst mechanism.[31]
Drug/toxin-induced autonomic failure	Alcohol Diuretics Sedative/tranquilizers: phenothiazines, barbiturates Vasodilators ACE inhibitors Tricyclic antidepressants	
Acute autonomic failure	Rare acute pan-autonomic failure with POH, fecal and urinary incontinence, chronotropic incompetence, and fixed dilated pupils[32]	
Postural orthostatic tachycardia syndrome (POTS)	Thought to be a chronic form of autonomic failure, probably due to lack of peripheral vasoconstriction during an orthostatic challenge or ineffective norepinephrine clearance in the synaptic cleft (norepinephrine re-uptake gene mutation is shown in POTS patients' family members[33])	Characterized by ≥28 beats/min increase above the resting heart rate within 5 min of upright posture[5]

[a] Most common types.

Table 10.5 Clinical features of arrhythmic causes of syncope

Class	Causes, clinical features	ECG and diagnosis	Comments
Cardiac arrhythmias Sinus node dysfunction (SND)	Medications chamber enlargement, ANS influences, fibrosis Chronotropic incompetence (inability to increase HR in response to physical or emotional stress)	Sinus bradycardia, sinus pauses, sinoatrial exit block, chronotropic incompetence Symptom arrhythmia correlation by Holter/ event monitoring	CBF reduction is more pronounced in the elderly. Differential diagnosis includes PE, myocardial ischemia, new onset seizures.
AV conduction disturbances	Acquired progressive idiopathic fibrosis, myocardial ischemia/infarction, medications (digoxin, beta blockers, calcium channel blockers) congenital	Symptom AV block correlation by ambulatory ECG monitoring	Usually seen in patients with structural heart disease
First-degree AV block	Worsened by negative inotropes (beta-blockers, calcium-channel blockers)	PR interval >210 ms	If seen in syncope without structural heart disease, suspect NMS.
Second-degree AV block, Mobitz I		With narrow QRS, is benign. With wide QRS, especially >70 years suggests infranodal block warranting pacemaker placement.	
Second degree AV block, Mobitz II	Can progress to high-degree AV block warranting pacemaker placement	Usually infra-nodal level with HIS region subsidiary pacemakers which are slow and unreliable warranting pacemaker placement	
Third-degree AV block, acquired	Acquired: Syncope is reported in 38%–61% of patients.[34]	Usually at the AV nodal level hence benign. However if syncope is induced with exercise, pacemaker is indicated.[35]	
Third-degree AV block, congenital	Rare		
Bifascicular block	Common finding with rare progression to complete AV block		If an HV interval >100 ms pacing indicated
Supraventricular arrhythmias, atrial fibrillation, atrial flutter, AVNRT	In susceptible individuals (elderly with vascular disease, young with dehydration, hot weather, gravitational stress), sudden onset tachycardia can cause dizziness/syncope.	Syncope usually occurs at arrhythmia onset or termination.	Even among patients with established arrhythmic cause of syncope, HUT can identify an underlying vasodepressor component, which has therapeutic implications.

(Continued)

Table 10.5 (Continued) Clinical features of arrhythmic causes of syncope

Class	Causes, clinical features	ECG and diagnosis	Comments
Ventricular tachyarrhythmias VT, VF, Torsades			Among patients referred for EPS VT (20%) is > likely than SVT (15%) to cause syncope.[36] In patients with a high index of suspicion for ventricular arrhythmias and a negative EPS, SAECG can identify VT risk VT-induced syncope increases SCD risk, warranting ICD placement.
Long QT syndrome acquired (secondary)	Medications (Table 10.6), subarachnoid hemorrhage, poisoning (organophosphorus, arsenic), extreme bradycardia, liquid protein diets[37] Exacerbated by hypokalemia/hypomagnesemia		Though rarely causes syncope, treatable with prompt recognition Torsades induces syncope, usually during sleep (bradycardia) or after PVCs.
Long QT syndrome congenital		Abnormal ventricular repolarization (QT prolongation, notched T waves/T wave alternans)	Affected individuals are at high risk of SCD and recurrent syncope secondary to Torsades de pointes.
Structural cardiac disease	LV outflow tract lesions, aortic stenosis, HOCM LV inflow tract lesions, mitral stenosis, left atrial myxoma RV outflow tract lesions, PE, pulmonary hypertension, pericardial tamponade	Echocardiography	Recognizing structural heart disease among patients with syncope is of pivotal importance because patients with a cardiac cause of syncope have a 24% incidence of SCD at 1 year.[1] In AS (fixed) or HOCM (dynamic) arrhythmias and exercise can precipitate syncope due to CBF reduction or mechanoreceptor-mediated bradycardia/vasodilation.[38] In acute PE, syncope is due to both mechanical flow limitation and neurally mediated reflex vasodilation.

Table 10.6   Medications causing QT prolongation

Class of medication	Medication
Class IA anti-arrhythmics	Quinidine Procainamide Disopyramide
Class III	Sotalol Ibutilide Amiodarone NAPA (N-acetyl procainamide)
Anti-anginal	Bepridil
Psychoactive agents	Phenothiazines Thioridazine
Tricyclic antidepressants	Amitryptiline Imipramine
Antibiotics	Erythromycin Pentamidine Fluconazole
Antihistamines	Terfenadine Astemizole

CARDIAC ARRHYTHMIAS AS A PRIMARY CAUSE

- Cardiac arrhythmias are among the most common and potentially hazardous causes of syncope.
- Though hypotension due to arrhythmia (tachycardia/bradycardia) can be obvious, other mechanisms (depressed ventricular function, altered volume status, and impaired vascular reactivity) can be present, which can be deciphered by HUT testing.

CEREBROVASCULAR DISEASE

- Cerebrovascular disease is an infrequent cause of syncope. Table 10.2 lists the various conditions with salient features.

NON-SYNCOPAL CONDITIONS (SYNCOPE MIMICS)

- Non-syncopal conditions are several disorders without true LOC (no cerebral hypoperfusion). Table 10.7 lists the syncope mimics and their salient features.

Table 10.7 Causes of non-syncopal attacks: syncope mimics

	Type of disorder	Clinical features
Disorders without any impairment of consciousness	Falls Cataplexy Drop attacks Psychogenic pseudosyncope (factitious disorder, malingering, conversion reaction) Transient ischemic attacks (TIAs) of carotid origin	Medications used in psychiatric disorders (phenothiazines, tricyclics) can increase the risk of syncope.[12] Cataplexy, which is a generalized abrupt loss of muscle tone, can be triggered by emotional reactions and thus can mimic syncope. However in cataplexy, there is no TLOC. Drop attacks refer to sudden loss of postural tone with no LOC. Though the cause is unknown, vertebrobasilar atherosclerosis has been shown to compromise blood supply to the corticospinal tracts causing sudden lower extremity atonia.[39]
Disorders with partial or complete loss of consciousness	Metabolic disorders, including hypoglycemia,[a] hypoxia (pneumonia, CHF, pulmonary embolism), panic disorder/hyperventilation[a] with hypocapnia Epilepsy Intoxications[a] Vertebrobasilar transient ischemic attack Neurologic disorders (aneurysms, tumors)	Metabolic and endocrine causes of syncope are rare. They usually result in confusional states, but unlike syncope they seldom resolve spontaneously. Syncope/dizziness associated with hyperventilation (anxiety) is relatively common. Metabolic states including hypoxemia, hypoglycemia/hyperglycemia, severe metabolic acidosis often cause behavioral disturbances and altered mental status, but seldom result in syncope. Akinetic/complex partial seizures are particularly difficult to differentiate from syncope.[39]

[a] Major common causes.

REFERENCES

1. Kapoor W. Evaluation and outcome of patients with syncope. *Medicine* 1990; 69: 169–75.

2. Savage DD, Corwin L, McGee DL et al. Epidemiologic features of isolated syncope: The Framingham Study. *Stroke* 1985; 16(4): 626–9.

3. Benditt DG, Ferguson DW, Grubb BP et al. Tilt table testing for assessing syncope. *J Am Coll Cardiol* 1996; 28(1): 263–75.

4. Alboni P, Brignole M, Menozzi C et al. The diagnostic value of history in patients with syncope with or without heart disease. *J Am Coll Cardiol* 2001; 37: 1921–8.

5. Brignole M, Alboni P, Benditt DG et al. Task force on syncope, European Society of Cardiology. Guidelines on management (diagnosis and treatment) of syncope–update 2004. *Europace* 2004; 6(6): 467–537.

6. Lipsitz LA, Wei JY, Rowe JW. Syncope in an elderly, institutionalised population: Prevalence, incidence, and associated risk. *Q J Med* 1985; 55(216): 45–54.

7. Nyman JA, Krahn AD, Bland PC et al. The costs of recurrent syncope of unknown origin in elderly patients. *Pacing Clin Electrophysiol* 1999; 22(9): 1386–94.

8. Wieling W, van Lieshout JJ. Maintenance of postural normotension in humans. In: Low P, ed. *Clinical Autonomic Disorders*. Little, Brown. Boston, MA. 1993; 69–75.

9. Abboud F. Neurocardiogenic syncope. *N Engl J Med* 1993; 328: 117–1120.

10. Shalev Y, Gal R, Tchou PJ et al. Echocardiographic demonstration of decreased left ventricular dimensions and vigorous myocardial contraction during syncope induced by head-up tilt. *J Am Coll Cardiol* 1991; 18(3): 746–51.

11. Thoren P. Role of cardiac vagal C-fibers in cardiovascular control. *Rev Physiol Biochem Pharmacol* 1979; 86: 1–94.

12. Hoefnagels WAJ, Padberg GW, Overweg J et al. Transient loss of consciousness: The value of the history for distinguishing seizure from syncope. *J Neurol* 1991; 238: 39–43.

13. Cook P, James I. Drug therapy: Cerebral vasodilators (first of two parts). *N Engl J Med* 1981; 305(25): 1508–13.

14. Moya A, Brignole M, Menozzi C et al. Mechanism of syncope in patients with isolated syncope and in patients with tilt-positive syncope. *Circulation* 2001; 104: 1261–7.

15. Calkins H, Shyr Y, Frumin H et al. The value of clinical history in the differentiation of syncope due to ventricular tachycardia, atrioventricular block and neurocardiogenic syncope. *Am J Med* 1995; 98: 365–73.

16. Sheldon R, Rose S, Ritchie D et al. Historical criteria that distinguish syncope from seizures. *J Am Coll Cardiol* 2002; 40: 142–148.

17. Oberg B, Thoren P. Increased activity in left ventricular receptors during hemorrhage or occlusion of caval veins in the cat. A possible cause of the vaso-vagal reaction. *Acta Physiol Scand* 1972; 85: 164–73.

18. Kosinki D, Grubb BP, Temesy-Armos P. Pathophysiological aspects of neurocardiogenic syncope: Current concepts and new perspectives. *PACE Pacing Clin Electrophysiol* 1995; 18: 716–24.

19. Kuhn DM, Wolf WA, Lovenberg W. Review of the role of the central serotonergic neuronal system in blood pressure regulation. *Hypertension* 1980; 2: 243–55.

20. Saadjian AY, Levy S, Franceschi F et al. Role of endogenous adenosine as a modular of syncope induced during tilt testing. *Circulation* 2002; 106: 569.

21. Magerkurth C, Riedel A, Braune S. Permanent increase in endothelin serum levels in vasovagal syncope. *Clin Auton Res* 2005; 15(4): 299–301.

22. Ellenbogen KA, Morillo CA, Wood MA et al. Neural monitoring of vasovagal syncope. *Pacing Clin Electrophysiol* 1997; 20(3 Pt 2): 788–94.

23. Mattle HP, Nirkko AC, Baumgartner RW, Sturzenegger M. Transient cerebral circulatory arrest coincides with fainting in cough syncope. *Neurology* 1995; 45(3 Pt 1): 498–501.

24. Vaitkevicius PV, Esserwein DM, Maynard AK et al. Frequency and importance of postprandial blood pressure reduction in elderly nursing-home patients. *Ann Intern Med* 1991; 115(11): 865–70.

25. Jansen RW, Lipsitz LA. Postprandial hypotension: Epidemiology, pathophysiology, and clinical management. *Ann Intern Med* 1995; 122(4): 286–95.

26. Kapoor WN, Peterson J, Karpf M. Defecation syncope. A symptom with multiple etiologies. *Arch Intern Med* 1986; 146(12): 2377–9.

27. Godec CJ, Cass AS. Micturition syncope. *J Urol* 1981; 126(4): 551–2.

28. Kenny RA, Richardson DA, Steen N et al. Carotid sinus syndrome: A modifiable risk factor for nonaccidental falls in older adults (SAFE PACE). *J Am Coll Cardiol* 2001; 1: 1491–6.

29. Kapoor WN. Syncope in older persons. *J Am Geriatr Soc* 1994; 42(4): 426–36.

30. Low P, Mcleod J. The autonomic neuropathies. In: Low P, ed. *Clinical Autonomic Disorders*. Little, Brown. Boston, MA. 1993; 395–421.

31. Shannon JR, Flattem NL, Jordan J et al. Orthostatic intolerance and tachycardia associated with norepinephrine-transporter deficiency. *N Engl J Med* 2000; 342: 541–9.

32. Rowe JC, White PD. Complete heart block: A follow-up study. *Ann Intern Med* 1958; 49(2): 260–70.

33. Pordon CM, Moodie DJ. Adults with congenital complete heart block: 25-year follow-up. *Clev Clinic J Med* 1992; 59: 587–90.

34. Camm AJ, Lau CP. Syncope of undetermined origin: Diagnosis and management. *Prog in Cardiol* 1988; 1: 139–56.

35. Moss AJ, Schwartz PJ, Crampton RS et al. The long QT syndrome: Prospective longitudinal study of 328 families. *Circulation* 1991; 84: 1136–44.

36. Johnson AM. Aortic stenosis, sudden death, and the left ventricular baroreceptors. *Br Heart J* 1971; 33: 1–5.

37. Sulg IA. Differential diagnosis in syncope and epilepsy. Clinical neurophysiological and cardiological aspects. In: Refsum H, Sulg IA, Rasmussen K, eds. *Heart and Brain, Brain and Heart*. Springer-Verlag. Berlin, Germany. 1989; 202–21.

38. Moya A, Sutton R, Ammirati F et al. Guidelines for the diagnosis and management of syncope (version 2009): The task force for the diagnosis and management of syncope of the European Society of Cardiology (ESC). *Eur Heart J.* 2009; 30(21): 2631–71.

39. Sheldon RS, Grubb BP, Olshansky B et al. 2015 Heart rhythm society expert consensus statement on the diagnosis and treatment of postural tachycardia syndrome, inappropriate sinus tachycardia, and vasovagal syncope. *Heart Rhythm.* 2015; 12(6): e41–63.

40. Task Force for the Diagnosis and Management of Syncope; European Society of Cardiology (ESC); European Heart Rhythm Association (EHRA); Heart Failure Association (HFA); Heart Rhythm Society (HRS); Moya A, Sutton R, Ammirati F et al. Guidelines for the diagnosis and management of syncope (version 2009). The Task Force for the Diagnosis and Management of Syncope of the European Society of Cardiology (ESC). *Eur Heart J.* 2009; 30: 2631–2671.

41. Fedrowski A, Hamrefors V, Sutton R et al. Do we need to evaluate diastolic blood pressure in patients with suspected orthostatic hypotension? *Clin Auton Res.* 2017; 27(3): 167–173.

SYNCOPE MANAGEMENT FACILITIES

Subramanya Prasad, Robert Schweikert, Mina K. Chung,
Kenneth Mayuga, and Oussama M. Wazni

CONTENTS

BACKGROUND

- Syncope is a commonly encountered symptom representing the sixth commonest reason for hospitalization in adults, 65 years, with an average length of stay of 5–17 days.[1] The cost of an unstructured syncope evaluation can be high, with hospital admission alone accounting for 74% of the evaluation costs of syncope.[2]
- Currently, a wide variation exists among physicians and management facilities in the evaluation strategy for syncope. This has led to unnecessary diagnostic tests and a higher proportion of patients with unexplained syncope.[3–6]
- Establishment of syncope facilities, which maximize implementation of the guidelines and establish mechanisms for effective communication with the patient and other involved personnel can reduce costs.
- A coordinated syncope evaluation is vital for appropriate health-care delivery to patients with syncope. Studies have shown that 20% of cardiac syncope in patients, 70 years present as non-accidental falls. Studies of "falls" suggest that a multi-factorial intervention significantly reduces subsequent events among these patients.[7,8]

GUIDELINES FOR ESTABLISHING A SYNCOPAL FACILITY

- The complex nature of symptoms of syncope and presyncope requires a systematic approach to facilitate a cost-effective approach for management of syncope.
- Facilities caring for patients with syncope vary from primary care providers to tertiary care facilities with multiple specialist care. Thus a common management strategy that ensures implementation of the published practice guidelines should be agreed upon among all the personnel involved (patients, referring physicians, Emergency department, nurses, and other professionals) and practiced.

Table 11.1 Indications for hospitalization in syncopal patients

Diagnostic	• Suspected or known structural heart disease
	• Abnormal ECG
	• Exertional/exercise syncope
	• Significant injury
	• Family history of SCD
	• Occasionally
	  • No structural heart disease, but sudden onset of palpitations shortly before syncope, syncope in supine position, and frequent recurrence
	  • No structural heart disease, with high index of suspicion of cardiac syncope

Therapeutic	• Syncope due to cardiac arrhythmia, myocardial ischemia • Syncope due to structural cardiac or pulmonary disease • Cardioinhibitory NMS requiring pacemaker implantation

- Syncope is a common presenting symptom both in the outpatient and inpatient setting. The source of referral (Outpatient office vs Emergency department, vs specialists like neurologists) determines the amount of work-up necessary for further evaluation.
- Most patients with syncope can be investigated on an outpatient basis. Table 11.1 lists the criteria for hospitalization in syncope.
- A local integrated syncope clinic should set standards regarding:
  - The diagnostic criteria for the causes of syncope.
  - The preferred approach to the diagnostic work-up among selected groups of syncope patients.
  - Risk stratification of the patient with syncope.
  - Treatment to prevent recurrent episodes.
- An important goal of a syncope facility is to reduce frequent hospitalizations by providing a structured, quick, alternative evaluation pathway.
- Careful audit of the activity and performance of the syncope unit effectively maintains quality assurance.

PROFESSIONALS INVOLVED AT A SYNCOPE MANAGEMENT FACILITY

- Though specialized training in management of patients with syncope is desirable, it is not a requirement for a dedicated syncope facility.
- The requirements depend on criteria established by the local professional bodies, level of screening prior to referral, and the nature of the patient population encountered. In general, training and experience in key components of cardiology, neurology, emergency medicine, and geriatrics, with access to specialties including psychiatry, physiotherapy, occupational therapy, ENT, and clinical psychology, are desirable.
- Core medical and support personnel should be involved in managing the unit on a full time basis.

EQUIPMENT

- Core equipment includes: Surface ECG recording, phasic blood pressure monitoring, tilt table testing equipment, external and internal (implantable) ECG loop recorder systems, 24 h ambulatory blood pressure monitoring, 24 h ambulatory ECG monitoring, and autonomic function testing. The syncope clinic at our institution has a blood volume analysis facility as an integral part.
- Access to echocardiography, invasive electrophysiologic studies, stress testing, cardiac imaging, CT and MRI head scans, and EEG, should be present in the facility.
- Preferential access to hospitalization and therapeutic procedures, including pacemaker and defibrillator implantation, and catheter ablation of arrhythmias, should be present. Table 11.2 lists the ESC recommendations for a syncope facility.

Table 11.2 List of recommendations for a syncope facility

• A cohesive, structured core pathway—either delivered within a single syncope facility or as a more multi-faceted service—is recommended for the global assessment of the patient with syncope.
• Experience and training in key components of cardiology, neurology, emergency, and geriatric medicine are pertinent.
• Core equipment for the facility includes: Surface ECG recording, phasic blood pressure monitoring, tilt table testing equipment, external and internal (implantable) ECG loop recorder systems, 24 h ambulatory blood pressure monitoring, 24 h ambulatory ECG monitoring, and autonomic function testing.
• Preferential access to other tests or therapy for syncope should be guaranteed and standardized.
• The majority of syncope patients should be investigated as outpatients.

Source: Brignole, M. et al., *Europace*, 6, 467–537, 2004.

EXISTING SYNCOPE MODELS

- Facilities that are involved in the care of syncope patients range from general physicians to geriatricians/neurologists to cardiologists with an interest in cardiac pacing and electrophysiology. No evidence of superiority of any model exists.
- The Newcastle model involves a multi-disciplinary approach, where patients referred with falls or syncope are evaluated by a geriatrician or cardiologist. With this approach a significant reduction in expenditure towards evaluation of syncope has been seen (reduced rehospitalization rates, effective targeted treatment strategies).[2]
- The Italian model (similar to our institution) is a functional unit of cardiologists, with dedicated medical and support personnel. These patients have access to other investigations and specialist referral (neurologists) if deemed appropriate. This model was reported to substantially reduce the number of unnecessary investigations (2 tests in 66% of patients were enough to make a diagnosis).[9] Table 11.3 lists the common tests done in our syncope facility with their protocols.
- The Hamdan model[10,11] uses a standardized algorithm in evaluating patients presenting to the emergency department with syncope. Using an algorithm developed from contemporary guidelines and a proprietary software based decision-making tool, they report a decrease in admission rates, a decrease in test utilization and consultations, and an increased rate of diagnosis at 45 days.

Table 11.3 List of common tests with equipment and protocols

Test	Equipment	Protocol or procedure
HUT	ECG defibrillator Automatic BP monitor Tilt table Emergency equipment Oxygen source Medications (atropine) ECG leads	Patient rests for 20 min before starting the test. Support stockings of patient are removed. Venous access obtained, preferably in the antecubital vein. After 3 baseline readings, a graded HUT is done at 30 and 45 degrees for 2 min, followed by 70 degrees for 45 min or appearance of symptoms. Recovery for 5 min.
Isuprel tilt	ECG defibrillator Automatic BP monitor Tilt table Emergency equipment Oxygen source Medications (atropine) ECG leads Isuprel infusion bag at 1 μg/cc	Patient rests for 20 min. Venous access is obtained. Baseline BP and HR obtained for 3 min. Graded infusion of isoproterenol (at 0.01, 0.03, and 0.05 μg/kg) is done. The patient is tilted at 70 degrees with each dose of isoproterenol, with patient returning to baseline for 5 min in between, as tolerated by the patient and occurrence of symptoms.
Supine isuprel provocation test	ECG defibrillator Automatic BP monitor Tilt table Emergency equipment Oxygen source Medications (atropine) ECG leads Isuprel infusion bag at 1 μg/cc	Patient rests for 20 min. Venous access is obtained. Baseline BP and HR obtained for 3 min. Graded infusion of isoproterenol (from 0.01 μg/kg to 0.05 μg/kg) is done with the patient in supine position, as tolerated by the patient and occurrence of symptoms.

(Continued)

Table 11.3 (*Continued*) List of common tests with equipment and protocols

Test	Equipment	Protocol or procedure
Blood volume testing Exclude pregnancy, allergy to eggs, shellfish, IVP dye, or iodine	EDTA-coated 6 mL tubes for blood collection Multiple sample adapter 1-131 RISA syringe STAT-60 Centrifuge Dose calibrator	Plasma volume is measured using less than 50 µCi of 1-131 radioiodinated human serum albumin (iv), waiting for an 11 min equilibrium period. Total blood volume is calculated from the plasma volume and a simultaneously drawn venous hematocrit. Venous access established. After 20 min in supine position, baseline samples are obtained. Measure hematocrit by centrifuging method. RISA injected over 30 s. Post injection samples x5 are collected at 11,15,19, 23, and 27 min (with CHF, 6th sample is collected). After centrifugation and serum separation, serum samples are placed in vials in the BVA-100 analyzer (DAXOR). Quality control checked to exclude very high or low radioisotope background counts.
Hemodynamics	ECG defibrillator Dinamap BP monitor Technicare 420/450 Gamma camera and computer ADAC 3300 microprocessor Emergency equipment and medications Pyrophospate 1.0 mL injection 99mTcO4 at 0.5 mL, 4 mCi, 8 mCi, and 12 mCi (8 and 12 used with routine hemodynamics)	Venous access preferably in the antecubital vein (right basilic vein preferred) 1 mL of pyrophosphate is injected, waiting for 40 min to tag. *First cardiac output:* Patient is positioned at 45 degrees LAO. Patient lies still with normal breaths and no activity for 12 min. Simultaneously 4 mCi of 99mTc pertechnetate is injected and the camera is started (90 frame acquisition at 0.5 s intervals). 4 minute recovery. *Second cardiac output:* With the same position 8 mCi 99mTc pertechnetate is injected and frame acquisition is started, followed by 4 min recovery. *Third cardiac output:* After checking patient's HR and BP, with the patient at 45 degree tilt, the legs are dropped down, making sure the patient's chest and rest of the body remain still. 12 mCi 99mTc pertechnetate is injected and similar frame acquisition is done. *Ejection fraction:* Frame acquisition (24 frames for 20 min) is started during second output with HR and BP during that time frame recorded.

(*Continued*)

Table 11.3 (*Continued*) List of common tests with equipment and protocols

Test	Equipment	Protocol or procedure
Autonomic function testing	Has 4 components	
Valsalva:	ECG recorder Automatic beat-by-beat BP monitor (Finapres) Gould recorder[a] Respirometer Access to emergency equipment and medications Computer	After taking a deep breath, patient blows against the manometer, raising it to 40 mmHg and holding pressure for 15 s, while the gould recorder records breathing and BP.
Cold pressor test:		The patient's hand is completely dipped in ice cold water for 2 min Somatic pain generates efferent sympathetic input to the heart and peripheral arterioles, resulting in tachycardia and increased BP and peripheral resistance.
Phenylephrine:		Injection of 25 µg with 25 µg increments until a 20 mmHg rise in SBP with slowing of HR or maximum dose is reached.
Amyl nitrite inhalation:		A vial of amylnitrite is broken under the nose while the patient takes a deep sniff SBP decrease of 20 mmHg from baseline with increasing HR is seen.
HRV: (30:15 R-R ratio test)		HR recordings are done during the Valsalva test. Analysis of the R-R intervals at the 15th and 30th beats and obtaining the 30th to 15th beat ratio is done by HRV analysis in the software.

[a] Gould recorder also records BP and HR and RR while doing Valsalva for autonomic reflex testing.

REFERENCES

1. Brignole M, Alboni P, Benditt DG et al. Task Force on Syncope, European Society of Cardiology. Guidelines on management (diagnosis and treatment) of syncope—update 2004. *Europace* 2004; 6(6): 467–537.

2. Kenny RA, O'Shea D, Walker HF. Impact of a dedicated syncope and falls facility for older adults on emergency beds. *Age Ageing* 2002; 31(4): 272–275.

3. Ammirati F, Colivicchi F, Santini M. Diagnosing syncope in clinical practice. Implementation of a simplified diagnostic algorithm in a multicentre prospective trial—the OESIL 2 study (Osservatorio Epidemiologico della Sincope nel Lazio). *Eur Heart J* 2000; 21(11): 935–940.

4. Disertori M, Brignole M, Menozzi C et al. Evaluation of Guidelines in Syncope Study. Management of patients with syncope referred urgently to general hospitals. *Europace* 2003; 5(3): 283–291.

5. Ammirati F, Colivicchi F, Minardi G et al. [The management of syncope in the hospital: The OESIL Study (Osservatorio Epidemiologico della Sincope nel Lazio)]. *G Ital Cardiol* 1999; 29(5): 533–539 (in Italian).

6. Farwell DJ, Sulke AN. Does the use of a syncope diagnostic protocol improve the investigation and management of syncope? *Heart* 2004; 90(1): 52–58.

7. Kenny RA, Richardson DA, Steen N et al. Carotid sinus syndrome: A modifiable risk factor for nonaccidental falls in older adults (SAFE PACE). *J Am Coll Cardiol* 2001; 38(5): 1491–1496.

8. Shaw FE, Bond J, Richardson DA et al. Multifactorial intervention after a fall in older people with cognitive impairment and dementia presenting to the accident and emergency department: Randomised controlled trial. *BMJ* 2003; 326(7380): 73. *Erratum in BMJ* 2003; 326(7391): 699.

9. Croci F, Brignole M, Alboni P et al. The application of a standardized strategy of evaluation in patients with syncope referred to three syncope units. *Europace* 2002; 4(4): 351–355.

10. Daccarett M, Jetter TL, Wasmund SL et al. Syncope in the emergency department: Comparison of standardized admission criteria with clinical practice. *Europace* 2011; 13(11): 1632–1638.

11. Sanders NA, Jetter TL, Brignole M, Hamdan MH. Standardized care pathway versus conventional approach in the management of patients presenting with faint at the University of Utah. *Pacing Clin Electrophysiol* 2013; 36(2): 152–162.

SYNCOPE MANAGEMENT AND DIAGNOSTIC TESTING

Subramanya Prasad, Oussama M. Wazni, Robert Schweikert, Kenneth Mayuga, and Mina K. Chung

CONTENTS

MANAGEMENT

Throughout this chapter * denotes a class I recommendation, # denotes a class II recommendation and ^ denotes a class III recommendation from the 2018 ESC Guidelines for the diagnosis and management of syncope[1] or the 2017 ACC/AHA/HRS guideline for the evaluation and management of patients with syncope.[2]

Table 12.1 explains the strength of recommendations and levels of evidence.

INITIAL EVALUATION

- The sporadic and infrequent occurrence of syncopal episodes makes it highly impractical to evaluate the syncopal patient during an episode. Hence the primary goal during the initial evaluation of syncope is to arrive at a presumptive diagnosis.
- An initial evaluation (thorough history including bystander observations, a well-focused physical examination including orthostatic blood pressure measurements, and a standard ECG) can identify the probable cause of syncope in 75% of patients.[3,4]

Table 12.1 Strength of recommendations and levels of evidence

Class I*	When there is evidence for and/or general agreement
Class II#	Evidence is less well established or divergence of opinion exists
Class III^	Not useful and harmful in some cases
Level of evidence A	Data from multiple randomized clinical trials or meta-analyses
Level of evidence B	Data from one randomized clinical trial or multiple non-randomized studies
Level of evidence C	Expert consensus opinion

HISTORY AND PHYSICAL EXAMINATION

HISTORY

* A detailed history and physical examination is recommended in patients with syncope.[2]

- History and physical examination can lead to a suspected diagnosis in 40% of patients.
- A careful history should include bystander observations, circumstances surrounding the event, prodromal symptoms, rapidity of LOC, duration of event, and speed of recovery. A list of the historical features and their importance in syncope is given in Table 12.2.
- The history should focus on
    - Differentiating true syncope from "non-syncopal" conditions.
    - Identifying the presence of structural heart disease.
- Medication history including anti-arrhythmic and antihypertensive agents (diuretics, sympathetic blockers), which can predispose individuals to POH.

DIFFERENTIATING SEIZURES FROM SYNCOPAL EPISODES

- Although typical seizures are easy to diagnose (aura, generalized tonic/clonic movements, tongue biting) differentiating atypical/complex partial seizures from syncope can be challenging.
- Some syncopal patients have convulsive movements similar to seizures attributable to hypoxia due to a paradoxical cerebral vasoconstriction.[5]
- In a recent study of 74 patients with a diagnosis of epilepsy, with persistent episodes in spite of anticonvulsant therapy, HUT testing provided an alternative diagnosis in 31/74 (42%).[5] Table 12.3 lists the differentiating features of seizures from syncope.

PHYSICAL EXAMINATION AND MANEUVERS

- A well-focused physical examination, particularly cardiovascular and nervous (central and peripheral) systems, based on the historical clues can aid in diagnosis. A list of such physical findings can be seen in Table 12.4.

Table 12.2 Historical clues and interpretation

Historical feature	Interpretation
Age[3]	*Children, adolescents, young adults*: [a]NMS, POTS, SVT, VT, idiopathic LQTS, cardiomyopathy, ARVD, congenital heart disease, AV block, seizure disorder *Middle aged*: [a]NMS, POH, cardiac arrhythmias and obstructive lesions, seizure disorder, medications *Elderly*: [a]NMS, cardiac arrhythmias and obstructive lesions, POH, medications, cerebrovascular, CSH, seizure disorders, combined causes
Pre-existing medical conditions/medications	History of cardiac disease is a strong predictor of a cardiac cause of syncope.[4] Hyperventilation/anxiety with psychiatric illness. Autonomic neuropathy with diabetes, parkinsonism. Orthostatic hypotension due to antihypertensive/anti-arrhythmic medications.
Presyncopal features	
Position of the patient during syncopal occurrence	Standing suggests NCS. Supine suggests arrhythmia.
Activity (rest, during or after exercise) and events preceding syncopal onset (coughing, eating, drinking, micturition, defecation)	Situational syncope (NMS) Shaving, tight collars, head rotation suggests CSH
Exertional syncope	Usually seen in syncope associated with AS or HOCM (reduced flow due to outflow tract obstruction or vagally mediated hypotension) Can be rarely seen in NCS in young patients with structurally normal hearts
Predisposing factors	Crowded or warm places, prolonged standing, postprandial state, fear, pain s/o WS Neck movements s/o VBI, CSH
Onset of syncopal episode	
Prodromal symptoms (nausea, abdominal discomfort, pallor, warmth, lightheadedness, dizziness, blurred vision, diaphoresis)	Usually present in NCS Absent in elderly individuals and CSH
Auras (visual)	Associated with seizures
During syncopal episode	
Onset of symptoms, way of falling, skin color, duration of LOC, breathing pattern, movements with duration, tongue biting	With H/O structural heart disease sudden supine LOC suggests arrhythmia, while exertional LOC suggests AS, HOCM Presyncope s/o WS/benign causes Prolonged LOC with postictal weakness, tongue biting, and fecal/urinary soiling s/o epilepsy

(Continued)

Table 12.2 (*Continued*)   Historical clues and interpretation

Historical feature	Interpretation
Associated symptoms/signs	Nausea/vomiting/pallor after an episode suggest WS. Dyspnea suggests PE. Angina suggests ischemia. Focal neurologic deficits suggest CVA/TIA. Presence of urination/defecation after episode suggests seizure. Injury suggests higher mortality. Vertigo, dysarthria, diplopia suggests Vertebrobasilar TIA.
Duration of symptoms	Prolonged LOC suggests seizure or aortic stenosis. Brief LOC suggests arrhythmia or NCS (CBF is restored in supine position).
Number of episodes and time from first episode to subsequent episodes	<1 in lifetime or multiple episodes in many years have benign causes, and longer syncope-free intervals. Multiple episodes over a short time have a serious underlying disorder; >50% patients have recurrent episodes.
Recovery	Quick with persistence of nausea, pallor, and diaphoresis suggests NMS. Delayed with persistent neurologic changes and confusion suggests CVA/seizure.

[a]   Major common causes

Abbreviations: NMS, neurally mediated syncope; POTS, postural orthostatic tachycardia syndrome; SVT, supraventricular tachycardia; VT, ventricular tachycardia; LQTS, long QT syndrome; ARVD, arrhythmogenic right ventricular dysplasia; POH, postural orthostatic hypotension; CSH, carotid sinus hypersensitivity; AS, aortic stenosis; HOCM, hypertrophic obstructive cardiomyopathy; VBI, vertebro-basilar insufficiency; LOC, loss of consciousness; WS, vasovagal syndrome; PE, pulmonary embolism; CVA, cerebrovascular accident; TIA, transient ischemic attack; CBF, cerebral blood flow.

Table 12.3 Distinguishing seizures from syncope

Clinical findings	Seizure likely	Syncope likely	Arrhythmia likely
Demographics/clinical setting	Young (45 years)	Female > male Younger (<55 years) More episodes (>2) Standing/warm room, emotional upset	Male > female Older (>55 years) Fewer episodes (<3)
Findings during LOC (eyewitness account)	Prolonged syncope (>5 min). Tonic-clonic movements are usually prolonged coinciding with LOC onset Hemilateral clonic movement. Clear automatisms (chewing or lip smacking, or frothing at the mouth). Tongue biting. Blue face. Bowel and bladder incontinence. Elevated HR and blood pressure.	Tonic-clonic movements are always of short duration (15 s), starting after LOC onset, dilated pupils, bradycardia, hypotension.	Blue, not pale Incontinence can occur. Brief clonic movements can occur.
Symptoms preceding the event	Sudden onset Aura (déjà vu, olfactory, gustatory, visual)	Longer duration (>5 s) Nausea/vomiting, abdominal discomfort, cold sweating (neurally mediated), palpitations Lightheadedness, blurring of vision	Shorter duration (<6 s)
Symptoms after the event	Residual symptoms common, prolonged confusion. Aching muscles. Disoriented. Slow recovery. The presence of a slow and complete recovery with evidence of soft-tissue injury at multiple sites usually favors epilepsy.	Residual symptoms common, usually short duration Prolonged fatigue common (>90%) Nausea, vomiting, pallor (neurally mediated) Oriented	Residual symptoms uncommon (unless prolonged LOC) Oriented
Findings of low specificity	Family history Timing of the event (night) Paresthesias before the event Incontinence, injury, headache, drowsiness after the event		

Table 12.4   Physical findings in the diagnosis of syncope

Physical findings	Implications
Blood pressure	Postural change from supine to sitting or standing for 2–5 min: an SBP decrease of 20 mmHg, DBP decrease of 10 mmHg, *and/or* signs of cerebral hypoperfusion is diagnostic of POH
Heart rate	An increase in 28 beats above resting HR with postural change (supine to standing) is diagnostic of POTS.
Heart rhythm and respiratory rate	Marked sinus arrhythmia is indicative of high vagal tone, s/o VVS. Hyperventilation is s/o anxiety.
Cardiac auscultation findings	Ejection systolic murmur s/o AS, HOCM, PS Diastolic murmur s/o left atrial myxoma Sustained parasternal lift with loud P2 s/o pulmonary hypertension Sustained PMI with S3, S4 gallop s/o dilated cardiomyopathy (VT)
Physiologic maneuvers	Change in intensity of systolic murmur with Valsalva maneuver s/o HOCM
Localizing neurologic findings	s/o CVA
Fecal occult blood test	Positive s/o GI bleed
Carotid sinus massage	Positive response s/o CSH

Abbreviations: SBP, systolic blood pressure; DBP, diastolic blood pressure; HR, heart rate; POTS, postural orthostatic tachycardia syndrome; VVS, vasovagal syndrome; AS, aortic stenosis; HOCM, hypertrophic obstructive cardiomyopathy; PS, pulmonic stenosis; VT, ventricular tachycardia; s/o, suggestive of; CVA, cerebrovascular accident; GI, gastrointestinal; CSH, carotid sinus hypersensitivity.

ROLE OF ECG IN DIAGNOSIS OF SYNCOPE

* A 12-lead ECG is useful in the initial evaluation of syncope.[2]
● The presence of a normal ECG makes the diagnosis of a cardiac cause unlikely, thus making it an important part of the initial evaluation.
● The initial ECG can establish a diagnosis in 5% and suggests a diagnosis in 5% of cases.[3] ECG findings that contribute to syncopal diagnosis are listed in Table 12.5.

Table 12.5   ECG abnormalities suggesting an arrhythmic cause of syncope

ECG findings with a high likelihood of making a probable diagnosis	Less specific findings
• QT prolongation • A short PR interval and delta wave with pre-excited QRS complexes • Findings of acute myocardial infarction (MI) • High degree AVB • ARVD (negative T-waves in right precordial leads, epsilon waves, and ventricular late potentials) • Brugada syndrome (right bundle branch block pattern with ST-elevation in leads V1–V3)	• Asymptomatic sinus bradycardia (<50 bpm). • Sinoatrial block or sinus pause >3 s in the absence of negatively chronotropic medications. • Evidence of prior MI (Q waves). • BBB, bifascicular block. • Ventricular or septal hypertrophy and PVCs. • A prolonged QT interval may indicate Torsades de Pointes as the cause of syncope. Patients with LQTS may have a normal QT interval at rest. However, a diagnosis of LQTS can be made if the QT interval increases or fails to shorten during exercise.

Source: Brignole, M. et al., *Europace*, 6, 467–537, 2004.

- Since syncopal episodes are intermittent and unpredictable, documenting symptom–arrhythmia correlation is the gold-standard in syncope evaluation. A 30–60 s rhythm strip may aid such documentation in the symptomatic patient.

DIAGNOSTIC TESTING IN SYNCOPE

- An initial evaluation usually provides a probable diagnosis in 75% of syncopal patients. However, appropriate risk stratification, therapy, and prognostic estimates are possible once a reasonably accurate diagnosis has been established.
- Based on the initial evaluation, further testing may be necessary. Diagnostic testing should focus on establishing a strong correlation between symptoms and identified abnormalities, choosing appropriate therapy, and giving prognostic estimates.
- Routine hematologic and biochemical screens and brain CT or MRI, in the absence of focal findings, have a very low yield.[6]
- Though the treatment of a patient with syncope should be individualized, a systematic approach that ensures adherence to guidelines is most cost-effective. The evaluation of a patient with presyncope is the same as that for a patient with syncope.

Note: See Chapter 19 regarding Head Up Tilt Table Testing and Carotid Sinus Massage.

AMBULATORY ELECTROCARDIOGRAPHIC MONITORING (NON-INVASIVE AND INVASIVE)

- Due to the unpredictable nature of syncopal episodes, arrhythmic causes of syncope often require long-term ECG monitoring for successful symptom–arrhythmia documentation.
- * If initial evaluation suggests cardiovascular abnormalities, cardiac monitoring based on the frequency and nature of the syncope is recommended.[2]
- \# Long-term ambulatory ECG monitoring can be non-invasive (Holter monitor, event monitors/recorders, external loop recorders) or invasive (implantable loop recorder).[1,2]

ACTIVE STANDING
The ESC 2009 guidelines[1] recommend the following:

- * Manual intermittent determination with sphygmomanometer of BP supine and during active standing for 3 min is indicated as initial evaluation when orthostatic hypotension is suspected.
- \# Continuous beat-to-beat non-invasive pressure measurement may be helpful in cases of doubt.

INPATIENT VS. OUTPATIENT ECG MONITORING
The ACC/AHA/HRS 2017 guidelines[2] recommend:

- * Hospital evaluation and treatment for patients with syncope who have a serious medical condition potentially relevant to the syncope.
- \# Outpatient management is reasonable in patients with presumptive reflex-mediated syncope without serious medical conditions.

\# A structured emergency department observation protocol may reduce hospital admission in intermediate-risk patients with syncope of unclear cause.

\# Outpatient management may be reasonable in select patients with suspected cardiac syncope but without serious medical conditions.

The ESC 2018 guidelines[1] recommend:

* Immediate in-hospital monitoring is indicated in high-risk patients.

HOLTER RECORDERS

● Holter monitors are low-cost external recorder devices used over 24–48 h periods.
● Holter monitors or event recorders are more useful in excluding an arrhythmic cause than establishing a diagnosis.[7] Many studies of ambulatory monitoring showed symptom–arrhythmia correlation of 1%–2% among unselected patients.

The ESC 2018 guidelines[1] recommend:

\# Holter monitoring should be considered in patients who have very frequent syncope or pre-syncope (≥1 per week).

LONG-TERM NON-INVASIVE EVENT MONITORS

● Event monitors are patient-activated, portable ECG recording devices that can be used for longer periods of time.
● Event recorders can be prospective, retrospective, or both.
● Retrospective external loop recorders have a higher yield.[8]
● Studies regarding the use of event monitors are mixed. While Linzer et al., using retrospective external loop recorders, showed a higher yield (25% of patients recorded in a 1-month period),[8] a recent study of syncopal patients (3 6 4 episodes in 6 months), with a negative HUT test and no structural heart disease, showed event recorders as not useful.[9]
● A study showed that, despite patient education, 23% failed to activate the recorder at the appropriate time.[7]

The ESC 2018 guidelines[1] recommend:

\# External loop recorders should be considered in patients who have an inter-symptom interval ≤4 weeks.

IMPLANTABLE LOOP RECORDER

● The implantable loop recorder (ILR) is a small subcutaneous device with 2 electrodes, an 18–24 month battery life, and is usually implanted in the left prepectoral chest wall.
● It is most useful in patients with unexplained syncope after a negative or inconclusive conventional work-up.[10] A study of 60 patients with unexplained syncope that randomized patients to conventional testing (external loop recorder, HUT, and EPS) vs ILR monitoring showed that ILR use in the initial phase of work-up was more likely to provide a diagnosis (52% vs 20%).[11]
● Pooled data of 287 patients from four studies showed a symptom–arrhythmia correlation in 34% (52% asystole/bradycardia, 11% tachycardia, 37% no rhythm variation).[10,12,13]

The 2017 ACC/AHA/HRS syncope guidelines[2] recommend:

\# For selected ambulatory patients with suspected arrhythmic syncope, an ILR can be useful.[2]

The 2018 ESC syncope guidelines[1] recommend:

* ILR is indicated in patients an early phase of evaluation in patients with recurrent syncope of uncertain origin, absence of high-risk criteria, and a high likelihood of recurrence within battery longevity.

* ILR is indicated in high-risk patients in whom a comprehensive evaluation did not demonstrate a cause of syncope or lead to a specific treatment.
# ILR should be considered in patients with suspected or certain reflex syncope with frequent or severe syncope episodes and may be considered in patients with suspected epilepsy but ineffective therapy, or in patients with unexplained falls.

ADVANCED CARDIAC TESTING

ECHOCARDIOGRAPHY
The ESC 2018 guidelines[12] recommend the following:

* Echocardiography is indicated for diagnosis and risk stratification in patients who are suspected of having structural heart disease.

The ACC/AHA/HRS 2017 guidelines[2] recommend:

Transthoracic echocardiography can be useful in selected patients if structural heart disease is suspected.

EXERCISE TESTING
* Exercise testing can be useful in patients who experience syncope or presyncope during[1,2] or shortly after exertion.[1]

CARDIAC CATHETERIZATION
Cardiac catheterization techniques should be carried out in suspected myocardial ischemia or infarction and to rule out ischemia-driven arrhythmias.[1]

COMPUTED TOMOGRAPHY (CT) OR MAGNETIC RESONANCE IMAGING (MRI)
CT or MRI may be useful in selected patients with syncope of suspected cardiac etiology, especially if other noninvasive studies are inconclusive.[2]

ELECTROPHYSIOLOGIC TESTING (EPS)
The ACC/AHA/HRS 2017 guidelines recommend:

EPS can be useful for selected patients with suspected arrhythmic cause for syncope.[2]
^ EPS is not recommended for syncope patients with a normal ECG and normal cardiac structure and function, unless an arrhythmic cause is suspected.[2]

The ESC 2018 guidelines[1] recommend:

* In patients with prior myocardial infarction or other scar-related conditions, EPS is indicated syncope remains unexplained after initial non-invasive evaluation suggests an arrhythmic cause of syncope unless there is already an established indication for ICD.
# In patients with bifascicular BBB, EPS should be considered when non-invasive tests have failed to make the diagnosis.[1]
# In patients with syncope preceded by sudden and brief palpitations, EPS may be considered when other non-invasive tests have failed to make the diagnosis.[1]
# In patients with asymptomatic sinus bradycardia, EPS may be considered in selective cases when non-invasive tests have failed to correlate syncope and bradycardia.[1]
^ EPS is generally not useful in patients with normal ECG, no heart disease, and no palpitations.

- Electrophysiological studies can be non-invasive (transesophageal) or invasive. Invasive EPS tests are considered in patients with recurrent syncopal symptoms due to an unexplained cause.
- The role of transesophageal EPS, which is similar to performing a TEE, is limited to:
  - Screening for rapid AtrioVentricular Nodal Reentrant Tachycardia (AVNRT)
  - AtrioVentricular Reentrant Tachycardia (AVRT) in patients with palpitations and a normal ECG
  - Evaluation of SND in syncope due to bradycardia
  - Risk evaluation in accessory pathways
- Similar to other diagnostic tests, the yield of an EPS depends on the pretest likelihood of an arrhythmic cause. Demonstration of an inducible arrhythmia during an EPS does not prove an arrhythmic cause of syncope, unless there is symptom correlation.
- EPS is considered in patients with recurrent syncope due to an unexplained cause. EPS is used to diagnose sinus node dysfunction, atrioventricular block (AVB), and supraventricular/ventricular tachyarrhythmias.
- In patients with a high likelihood of an arrhythmic cause, a negative EPS does not exclude arrhythmia; further studies (ILR) are recommended.
- Identification of abnormal EP findings is not always diagnostic of an arrhythmic cause.
- Though EPS can easily induce supraventricular tachyarrhythmias and ventricular tachycardia, induction of polymorphic ventricular tachycardia (PVT)/Torsades de pointes is difficult despite isuprel provocation, or using long–short sequence stimulation.
- The minimum testing required during an EPS for syncope diagnosis per ESC guidelines is:
  - Measurement of sinus node recovery time and corrected sinus node recovery time by repeated sequences of atrial pacing for 30–60 s with at least one low (10–20 beats/min higher than sinus rate) and two higher pacing rates.
  - Assessment of the His Purkinje system includes measurement of the HV interval at baseline and His Purkinje conduction with stress by incremental atrial pacing. If the baseline study is inconclusive, pharmacologic provocation with slow infusion of ajmaline (1 mg/kg iv), procainamide (10 mg/kg iv), or disopyramide (2 mg/kg iv) is added unless contraindicated.
  - Assessment of ventricular arrhythmia inducibility by ventricular program-med stimulation at two right ventricular sites (apex and outflow tract), at two basic drive cycle lengths (100 or 120 beats/min), with up to 2 extra stimuli. Use of a third extra stimulus can increase sensitivity but decreases specificity.
  - Assessment of supraventricular arrhythmia inducibility by any atrial stimulation protocol.
- The diagnostic yield of EPS is high among patients with structural heart disease, especially when an SVT with hypotension or sustained monomorphic VT is induced, and low with induction of NSVT, PVT (torsades), or VF. In a study of patients with unexplained syncope, EPS provided a diagnosis in 56% (71% with structural heart disease vs 36% with none).[14] Other predictors of a positive EPS include impaired ventricular function, male sex, prior myocardial infarction, BBB, and non-sustained VT.[15]

EPS IN SND

- Though EPS is frequently used to document sinus node dysfunction, it is seen as a cause of syncope in 5% of patients undergoing EP testing.[16]
- The sinus node recovery time (SNRT) is defined as the interval between the last paced atrial depolarization and the first spontaneous atrial depolarization resulting from the activation of the sinus node.

- A prolonged SNRT or corrected SNRT (CSNRT), sino-atrial conduction time (SACT), or chronotropic incompetence with exercise stress testing indicates SND.
- An SNRT of 1.6 s to 2 s or a CSNRT (SNRT–sinus cycle length) greater than 525 ms is indicative of abnormal sinus node automaticity, sino-atrial conduction, or both (sensitivity 50%–80%; specificity 95%).[17] A study by Menozzi et al showed an 8-fold increase in the risk of syncope in patients with a CSNRT $800 ms.[18]
- When the baseline EPS is inconclusive, pharmacologic challenge with atropine (0.04 mg/kg) or propranolol (0.2 mg/kg) can cause complete autonomic blockade of the sinus node, differentiating intrinsic and extrinsic SND.[19] Although the intrinsic heart rate (IHRp) in relation to age can be calculated using a linear regression equation (IHRp 5 118.1 2 [0.57 3 age]), its sensitivity is low.[20]

EPS IN AV BLOCK

- Patients with varying degrees of AV block can present with syncope.
- AV conduction is measured by the HV interval (His bundle to ventricular conduction time) and/or the response of AV conduction to incremental atrial pacing.
- The presence of alternating bifascicular or trifascicular block is an ominous sign due to the possibility of impending or intermittent high-grade AV block. Documenting transient/intermittent bifascicular block requires extended ambulatory ECG monitoring.
- A history of syncope and a prolonged HV interval increase the risk of AV block.
- Ventricular arrhythmias are more common in patients with AV block. Pacemaker implantation reduces recurrent syncope in patients with AV block.[21]
- Studies have shown that although there is a 12% SCD incidence in patients with AV block, it is not associated with syncope or a prolonged HV interval, suggesting that the increased SCD incidence is probably related to the underlying structural heart disease and not syncope.
- The diagnostic yield of EPS in evaluating AV block can be increased by pharmacologic provocation (procainamide: 10 mg/kg; disopyramide: 2 mg/kg, ajmaline: 1 mg/kg) and/or incremental atrial pacing/short sequence ventricular pacing.[22]

EPS IN SUPRAVENTRICULAR ARRHYTHMIAS

- Among syncopal patients of unknown cause undergoing EPS, SVT causing syncope is seen in 5%.[23] The hemodynamic effects of the SVT causing syncope can be studied by EPS (transesophageal or invasive), with or without isoproterenol/atropine provocation.

EPS IN VENTRICULAR ARRHYTHMIAS

- VT is the most common abnormality seen during EPS for syncope (20% of patients undergoing EPS).[15] Ventricular tachycardia can present as syncope with or without palpitations. A study by Moasez et al showed that identification of MMVT on Holter was a strong predictor of inducing MMVT during EPS.[16]
- While induction of MMVT during EPS indicates a high risk of SCD, a negative EPS predicts a low risk of SCD among CAD patients with preserved LV function.[24,25]
- The value of inducing polymorphic ventricular tachycardia (torsades) or VF during EPS depends on the clinical scenario:
    - In the setting of syncope with CAD, the induction of PVT or VF during EPS does not predict syncopal events.[26]
    - However, induction of PVT during EPS predicts survival in patients with (i) Brugada syndrome,[27] (ii) cardiac arrest survivors undergoing coronary bypass surgery, and (iii) idiopathic ventricular fibrillation.[28]

REFERENCES

1. Brignole M, Moya A, de Lange FJ et al. 2018 ESC Guidelines for the diagnosis and management of syncope. *Eur Heart J* 2018 1; 39: 1883–1948.

2. Shen WK, Sheldon RS, Benditt DG et al. 2017 ACC/AHA/HRS Guideline for the Evaluation and Management of Patients with Syncope. *J Amer Coll* Cardiol 2017; 70: e39–110.

3. Kapoor W. Evaluation and outcome of patients with syncope. *Medicine* 1990; 69: 169–175.

4. Alboni P, Brignole M, Menozzi C et al. The diagnostic value of history in patients with syncope with or without heart disease. *J Am Coll Cardiol* 2001; 37: 1921–1928.

5. Sheldon R, Rose S, Ritchie D et al. Historical criteria that distinguish syncope from seizures. *J Am Coll Cardiol* 2002; 40: 142–148.

6. Sarasin FP, Louis-Simonet M, Carballo D et al. Prospective evaluation of patients with syncope: A population-based study. *Am J Med* 2001; 111: 177.

7. Sivakumaran S, Krahn AD, Klein GJ et al. A prospective randomized comparison of loop recorders versus Holter monitors in patients with syncope or presyncope. *Am J Med* 2003; 115: 1.

8. Linzer M, Pritchett EL, Pontinen M et al. Incremental diagnostic yield of loop electrocardiographic recorders in unexplained syncope. *Am J Cardiol* 1990; 66(2): 214–219.

9. Smit AA, Halliwill JR, Low PA, Wieling W. Pathophysiological basis of orthostatic hypotension in autonomic failure. *J Physiol* 1999; 519 (Pt 1) 1–10.

10. Krahn A, Klein GJ, Yee R et al. Use of an extended monitoring strategy in patients with problematic syncope. *Circulation* 1999; 99: 406–410.

11. Alboni P, Menozzi C, Brignole M et al. An abnormal neural reflex plays a role in causing syncope in sinus bradycardia. *J Am Coll Cardiol* 1993; 22: 1130–1134.

12. Moya A, Brignole M, Menozzi C et al. Mechanism of syncope in patients with isolated syncope and in patients with tilt-positive syncope. *Circulation* 2001; 104: 1261–1267.

13. Nierop P, Van Mechelen R, Elsacker A et al. Heart rhythm during syncope and presyncope. *Pacing Clin Electrophysiol* 2000; 23: 1532–1538.

14. Kapoor WN, Hammil SC, Gersh BJ. Diagnosis and natural history of syncope and the role of invasive electrophysiologic testing. *Am J Cardiol* 1989; 63: 730.

15. Morady F, Shen F, Schwartz A et al. Long term follow-up of patients with recurrent unexplained syncope evaluated by electrophysiologic testing. *J Am Coll Cardiol* 1983; 2: 1053.

16. Moasez F, Peter T, Simonson J et al. Syncope of unknown origin: clinical, noninvasive, and electrophysiologic determinants of arrhythmia induction and symptom recurrence during long-term follow-up. *Am Heart J* 1991; 121(1 Pt 1): 81–88.

17. Narula OS, Samet P, Javier RP. Significance of the sinus-node recovery time. *Circulation* 1972; 45(1): 140–158.

18. Menozzi C, Brignole M, Alboni P et al. The natural course of untreated sick sinus syndrome and identification of the variables predictive of unfavorable outcome. *Am J Cardiol* 1998; 82(10): 1205–1209.

19. Benditt DG, Gornick CC, Dunbar D et al. Indications for electrophysiologic testing in the diagnosis and assessment of sinus node dysfunction. *Circulation* 1987; 75(4 Pt 2): III93–III102.

20. Jose AD, Collison D. The normal range and determinants of the intrinsic heart rate in man. *Cardiovasc Res* 1970; 4(2): 160–167.

21. Kaul U, Dev V, Narula J et al. Evaluation of patients with bundle branch block and 'unexplained' syncope: A study based on comprehensive electro-physiologic testing and ajmaline stress. *Pacing Clin Electrophysiol* 1988; 11(3): 289–297.

22. Englund A, Bergfeldt L, Rosenqvist M. Pharmacological stress testing of the His-Purkinje system in patients with bifascicular block. *Pacing Clin Electrophysiol* 1998; 21(10): 1979–1987.

23. Bachinsky WB, Linzer M, Weld L, Estes NA III. Usefulness of clinical characteristics in predicting the outcome of electrophysiologic studies in unexplained syncope. *Am J Cardiol* 1992; 69(12): 1044–1049.

24. Link MS, Kim KM, Homoud MK et al. Long-term outcome of patients with syncope associated with coronary artery disease and a nondiagnostic electrophysiologic evaluation. *Am J Cardiol* 1999; 83(9): 1334–1337.

25. Olshansky B, Hahn EA, Hartz VL et al. Clinical significance of syncope in the electrophysiologic study versus electrocardiographic monitoring (ESVEM) trial. The ESVEM Investigators. *Am Heart J* 1999; 137(5): 878–886.

26. Menozzi C, Brignole M, Garcia-Civera R et al. International Study on Syncope of Uncertain Etiology (ISSUE) Investigators. Mechanism of syncope in patients with heart disease and negative electrophysiologic test. *Circulation* 2002; 105(23): 2741–2745.

27. Brugada P, Brugada R, Mont L et al. Natural history of Brugada syndrome: The prognostic value of programmed electrical stimulation of the heart. *J Cardiovasc Electrophysiol* 2003; 14(5): 455–457.

28. Viskin S, Lesh MD, Eldar M et al. Mode of onset of malignant ventricular arrhythmias in idiopathic ventricular fibrillation. *J Cardiovasc Electrophysiol* 1997; 8(10): 1115–1120.

DEVICE PROCEDURES

IMPLANTATION OF PACEMAKERS AND ICDs

Kushwin Rajamani, Michael P. Brunner, Oussama M. Wazni, and Bruce L. Wilkoff

CONTENTS

PATIENT SELECTION AND PREPARATION

- Patients must have an indication for pacemaker or implantable cardioverter-defibrillator (ICD) according to ACC/AHA guidelines as discussed elsewhere.[1,2] The informed consent should include discussion of the indication, the potential risks associated with the procedure, and alternatives to the procedure. The incidence of any type of complication with the initial implantation of leads and the pulse generator is about 1.0%.[3] However the major complication rate for generator change alone is about 4% and if lead replacement or upgrade performed the risk increases to 15%.[4] Major risks include pneumothorax, venous laceration, cardiac perforation, pericardial effusion, infection, and pulseless electrical activity associated with defibrillation testing. Minor risks include pocket hematoma, device migration, and diaphragmatic stimulation. Patients should be aware of lifelong maintenance of the device and the need for generator replacements in the future.
- Before the procedure, screening labs should include coagulation parameters, electrolytes, and complete blood count. In a metanalysis including 2321 patients, uninterrupted warfarin therapy throughout pacemaker or ICD implantation was associated with decreased risk of bleeding without increasing the risk of thromboembolic events compared to heparin bridging.[5] We generally proceed with implantation as long as the international normalized ratio (INR) is less than 3. Heparin should be delayed as long as possible after the procedure, but should not be restarted before 24 h.
- Once patients are in the EP lab, there should be meticulous attention paid to sterility. The implantation site should be clear of any superficial wounds, be clipped and not shaven, and be prepped with either betadine or chlorohexidine and a head-to-toe drape. All personnel involved in the procedure should undergo a surgical scrub. Moderate sedation in the form opiates and anxiolytics (e.g., fentanyl and versed) is most often used. Local analgesia is achieved using agents such as lidocaine.

POCKET FORMATION

- Most devices are placed in a left prepectoral pocket since most patients are right-handed and implantation of the leads is easier from the left versus the right side. Further, since a significant part of the left ventricular mass is not along the shock vector in right-sided implants, higher defibrillation thresholds may be encountered. Other implantation sites include infra-mammary, sub-pectoralis major muscle, sub-xiphoid, and iliac fossa. The former two positions may be considered for cosmetic reasons. The pocket should not be created in the fat layer but just above the pectoral fascia with sharp and blunt dissection and sized to the implanted device. Hemostasis may be achieved with either electrocautery, manual pressure, and with sutures applied during closure of the pocket.[6]
- There are variations in the location of the incision line. However, most implanters use the clavicle and deltopectoral groove as landmarks. If the subclavian or axillary vein is used for venous access then an incision line is extended 2–3 cm below the clavicle for a total length of 3–5 cm (dependent on the size of the device), which brings the lateral extension of the incision line just medial to the deltopectoral groove. If the cephalic vein is accessed then the incision extends over the deltopectoral groove.

VEIN ACCESS

- Veins may be accessed by either direct visualization, anatomic landmarks, or fluoroscopy. The "first-rib" approach involves the use of fluoroscopy to access the axillary vein ("extrathoracic" subclavian vein) lateral to the medial edge of the first rib (see Figure 13.1). The vein is accessed using a percutaneous introducer needle and a guidewire is inserted through the needle (see Figure 13.2). The guidewire should be advanced to the inferior vena cava to assure that the vein and not the artery has been entered. The process is repeated for the number of leads to be inserted. Another technique involving retained guidewires requires only one venous access with guidewires left in place to allow for more than one lead to pass through a single venotomy site. The length of the guidewire (often 45 cm) can be used as a guide to determine the required lead length.

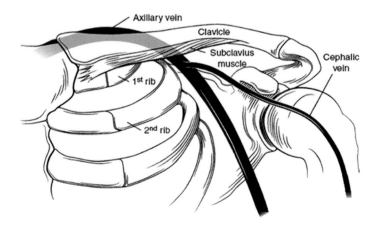

Figure 13.1 The "first rib" approach.

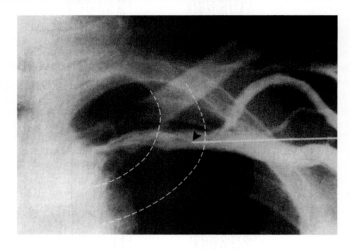

Figure 13.2 Guidewire is inserted through a percutaneous introducer needle.

- Of note, in patients who have prior leads, central catheters or radiation therapy that included the subclavian veins, there may be stenosis that prevents vein access. In such patients, the use of venograms through a peripheral intravenous line placed in the ipsilateral arm can delineate stenosis and guide therapy.

LEAD PLACEMENT

- Sheaths are placed over the guidewires, typically 7 French size for pacemaker leads and 9 French size for ICD leads. The sheaths are either slittable or usually splittable, which allows removal of sheaths once the leads are placed in the endocardium. Leads come in two basic types: those with plastic projections called tines (passive fixation) or those with retractable helical screws (active fixation) at the lead tip. Leads are introduced through the sheath with a metal stylet inserted into the hollow center of the lead to provide shape and stiffness to the distal aspect of the lead.
- For the ventricular lead, a curved stylet is inserted which allows passage of the lead into the right ventricular outflow tract (RVOT). The presence of ventricular ectopy and placement in the RVOT ensures that the lead is in the right ventricle and not the coronary sinus. From this position, either a "gentle" curved or straight stylet is inserted to place the lead along the septum or at the apex respectively. The current of injury and the signal amplitude is assessed at the site prior to the lead being screwed into place with confirmation by fluoroscopy in multiple views. Passive fixation leads are usually only stable in the apex but they can be also trapped in the right ventricular trabeculations above the apex.
- The lead is then tested for sensing, capture threshold, impedance, and injury pattern. Acceptable sensing for the R-wave is usually greater than 5 mV and acceptable capture threshold is less than 1 V with a pulse duration of 0.5 ms. Impedance varies with the type of lead and the amount of scar in the myocardium, but should be between 200 and 1200 ohms. Acutely, especially after a lead is "screwed in," an injury pattern (ST-segment-like elevation of the electrogram) is indicative of good contact with myocardium.

- For atrial leads, a straight stylet is used to advance the lead into the right atrium. A preformed J-shaped stylet is used to place the atrial lead into the right atrial appendage (RAA), lateral wall, or septum. This involves ensuring free movement of the lead in the atrial body and then pulling it back slowly until it is "hooked" firmly onto atrial tissue with adequate electrical signal and injury. The active fixation is then screwed with fluoroscopic confirmation. Passive fixation leads are usually only placed in the RAA. The acceptable sensing of the P-wave is typically greater than 2 mV with a capture threshold less than 1 V. Stimulation impedance should also be between 200 and 1200 ohms.
- Once the leads are positioned properly, suture sleeves are tied down with non-absorbable sutures to secure the leads. It is important to allow for adequate slack in both leads to accommodate the movement of the heart and diaphragm when the patient stands and for growth (pediatric patients). It is crucial, to prevent dislodgement, that the leads are tied down to the muscle surface which moves little with muscular efforts and that the leads and pulse generator are not in the adipose or breast that is mobile with gravity and physical activity. The ventricular lead usually takes the shape of a boot with the curve of the boot just proximal to the tricuspid valve in the right atrium. The atrial lead should have sufficient slack in its distal loop and should not be intertwined with the ventricular lead.
- Once the leads are secured, the pocket should be re-inspected for hemostasis. The leads are then inserted into the connector block (header) of the pacemaker or ICD and the set-screws tightened. It is important to ensure correct placement of leads into the header both in terms of alignment and matching the right lead to the port. The pocket is then copiously irrigated with antibiotic solution (e.g., vancomycin) and the device is then placed in the pocket with the leads neatly curled behind it. At this point it is vital to perform a "system check" fluoroscopy from the lead tip to the can to identify any issues prior to closure of the pocket and also serve as a reference image. Two subcutaneous layers of absorbable suture and one subcuticular layer of suture are used to close the pocket.

DEFIBRILLATION THRESHOLD TESTING

- For ICDs, defibrillation efficacy testing (DFT) can be performed to assure that the ICD can detect and terminate ventricular fibrillation with an adequate safety margin for defibrillation. DFT is based on probabilistic calculations. If defibrillation is successful, then there is a high probability of successful shocks in the future, but this is not guaranteed. However, if defibrillation is unsuccessful, additional measures need to taken to rectify this.
- What defines a successful defibrillation efficacy test? It varies from center to center, but a fairly common definition is defibrillation, often twice, with a 10 J safety margin in reference to the maximum delivered output of the device. If this is not achieved, then polarity of the shocking coils may be reversed, shock properties can be altered (pulse width, tilt, etc.) or additional coils implanted, either subcutaneously or in the azygous vein.
- Defibrillation efficacy testing had historically been performed routinely but is now considered controversial because studies have shown that patients who do not undergo testing at the time of implant have similar survival using the current generation of devices. In a single-blind, non-inferiority study of 2500 patients receiving an initial ICD in the left pectoral region for standard primary or secondary prevention indications, followed-up for 3 years, no DFT testing was non-inferior to DFT testing.[7] Right-sided implants, replacement devices, and subcutaneous ICDs were not studied in this trial.

- After the device is implanted and the pocket closed, the device is usually interrogated through the device, for atrial and ventricular sensing, capture thresholds, and impedance. This can help identify problems such as early lead dislodgement or a loose set-screw prior to the patient leaving the lab.

- In addition, initial programming of the device is often performed at this stage. Although programming options have grown significantly over the years, the fundamental parameters remain unchanged. The low pacing rate, high pacing rate (if applicable), rate responsiveness, and the atrioventricular (AV) interval are some of the basic options that are programmed. The AV interval has become more important in recent years with the realization that high degree of ventricular pacing may result in left ventricular dysfunction and heart failure symptoms. The AV interval is usually set slightly longer than the native AV interval to allow for AV conduction. Most devices now have a feature which searches for native AV conduction by extending the paced AV interval. For ICDs, the various tachycardia detection zones are programmable along with tailored delivery of ATP and shocks. Empiric use of ATP in the ventricular tachycardia zone has been shown to decrease shocks without compromising patient safety. Further, in primary prevention ICD programming high rate therapy and delayed ICD therapy reduces the incidence of inappropriate shocks and mortality.

- Patients usually require an overnight stay in hospital with inpatient Holter monitoring, follow-up chest X-ray to check lead position and exclude a pneumothorax, and a device interrogation to re-assess lead function. Figure 13.3 shows a chest X-ray with typical location and appearance of a dual chamber ICD. If these tests and the pocket site is satisfactory, then the patient is usually seen at 6–8-week follow-up for a device interrogation.

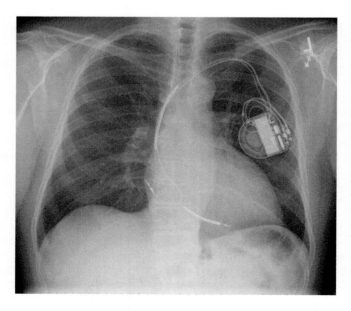

Figure 13.3 Chest X-ray showing the typical location and appearance of a dual chamber ICD.

- When a lead is screwed into atrial or ventricular tissue, there is an initial current of injury. Over the subsequent 6–8 weeks, the lead matures as the injured myocardium surrounding the lead fibroses. This can cause an increase in the capture threshold from the time of implantation to time of lead maturation at 6–8 weeks. Thus, at the time of device implantation, pacing output is set to a high output (usually 5 V). Thresholds checked at 6–8 weeks post-implantation are usually stable and pacing outputs are then set to 1.7 to 2 times the capture thresholds.

NOVEL DEVICES

- Leadless pacemakers (Figure 13.4) are totally self-contained devices which are smaller than a AAA battery placed endovascularly within the right ventricle.[8] They eliminate the weakest link in a device—the lead. They are implanted in patients who would be eligible for a VVIR pacemaker (i.e., permanent atrial fibrillation with AV block, sinus rhythm with 2nd or 3rd degree AV block or sinus bradycardia with infrequent pauses). Safety and efficacy results of postmarket studies are awaited prior to FDA approval.
- The subcutaneous ICD (Figure 13.5) was introduced in 2009 and avoids the vascular space completely.[9] It is ideal for patients with challenging vascular access, prior infections, and younger patients. The sensing/defibrillation coil lead is tunneled subcutaneously along the left sternal edge and connected to a pulse generator located in the left mid-axillary line for rhythm identification and defibrillation. The device provides limited post-defibrillation pacing and is therefore contraindicated among patients with a pacing indication or need for antitachycardia pacing.

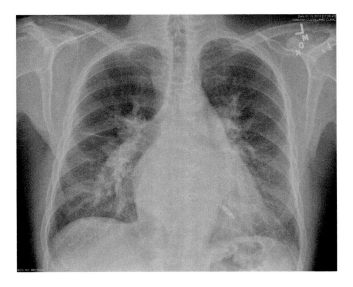

Figure 13.4 Leadless pacemaker.

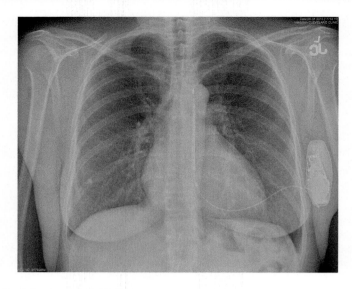

Figure 13.5 Subcutaneous defibrillator.

ACKNOWLEDGMENT

The authors would like to thank Mohammed Khan and Jennifer Cummings for their contributions to the prior edition of this chapter.

REFERENCES

1. Epstein, A. E. et al. ACC/AHA/HRS 2008 Guidelines for Device-Based Therapy of Cardiac Rhythm Abnormalities: A report of the American College of Cardiology/American Heart Association Task Force on Practice Guidelines (Writing Committee to Revise the ACC/AHA/NASPE 2002 Guideline Update for Implantation of Cardiac Pacemakers and Antiarrhythmia Devices) developed in collaboration with the American Association for Thoracic Surgery and Society of Thoracic Surgeons. *J Am Coll Cardiol.* 2008; 51(21): e1–e62.

2. Tracy, C. M. et al. 2012 ACCF/AHA/HRS focused update of the 2008 guidelines for device-based therapy of cardiac rhythm abnormalities: A report of the American College of Cardiology Foundation/American Heart Association Task Force on Practice Guidelines. *J Am Coll Cardiol.* 2012; 60(14): 1297–1313.

3. Aggarwal, R. K. et al. Early complications of permanent pacemaker implantation: No difference between dual and single chamber systems. *Br Heart J.* 1995; 73(6): 571–575.

4. Poole, J. E. et al. Complication rates associated with pacemaker or implantable cardioverter-defibrillator generator replacements and upgrade procedures: Results from the REPLACE registry. *Circulation.* 2010; 122(16): 1553–1561.

5. Ghanbari H. et al. Meta-analysis of safety and efficacy of uninterrupted warfarin compared to heparin-based bridging therapy during implantation of cardiac rhythm devices. *Am J Cardiol.* 2012; 110(10): 1482–1488.

6. Bellot, P. H. and Reynolds, D. W. Permanent pacemaker and implantable cardioverter-defibrillator implantation in adults. In: Ellenbogen, K. A., Wilkoff, B. L., Kay, G. N., Lau, C. P., Auricchio, A. (eds.) *Clinical Cardiac Pacing, Defibrillation and Resynchronization Therapy*, 5th ed. WB Saunders, Philadelphia, PA; 2017. pp. 631–691.

7. Healey, J. S. et al. Cardioverter defibrillator implantation without induction of ventricular fibrillation: A single-blind, non-inferiority, randomized controlled trial (SIMPLE). *Lancet.* 2015; 385(9970): 785–791.

8. Reddy, V. Y. et al. Permanent leadless cardiac pacing: Results of the LEADLESS trial. *Circulation.* 2014; 129(14): 1466–1471.

9. Bardy, G. H. et al. An entirely subcutaneous implantable cardioverter-defibrillator. *N Engl J Med.* 2010; 363(1): 36–44.

LEFT VENTRICULAR LEAD IMPLANTATION FOR CARDIAC RESYNCHRONIZATION THERAPY

Kushwin Rajamani, Michael P. Brunner, Oussama M. Wazni, and Bruce L. Wilkoff

CONTENTS

BACKGROUND

Cardiac resynchronization therapy (CRT) has proven to be an invaluable tool in improving both the quality of life and survival in patients with left ventricular dysfunction, congestive heart failure, and interventricular conduction delay.[1] Patients who receive CRT have improved functional capacity estimated by 6 min walk, New York Heart Association classification, and quality of life based on Minnesota Living with Heart Failure questionnaires, and they are protected from the associated increased risk of sudden cardiac death when combined with an implantable cardioverter-defibrillator (ICD) system.[2]

CRT implantation has been rising exponentially coupled with increasing number of operators comfortable with placing leads in coronary sinus (CS) tributaries. Despite the improvements in technology specifically designed to assist with the CS lead implantation, this step remains the main obstacle in delivering optimal CRT. One of the most important factors in delivering CRT is the placement of the CS lead in the appropriate location. The posterior and lateral locations should theoretically offer the most benefit. These locations are directly opposite the anterior and apically located right ventricular or ICD lead. Although the anterior branches of the CS tend to be easier to cannulate, it appears that shorter distances and conduction times between the right and left ventricular stimulation sites may be responsible for some of the CRT non-response.[3] The MADIT-CRT study recommended that a favorable CRT response could be seen at all non-apical sites of LV pacing.[4] This appears to be in part due to an increased separation from the RV pace/sense lead encompassing a greater ventricular mass. The two major anatomical obstacles to delivering optimal CRT are coronary sinus ostium cannulation and delivering a lead to the appropriate branch in a posterior and lateral location. Although most implantations of CRT systems are relatively uncomplicated, this chapter outlines an approach to recognize and overcome potential challenges and continue moving forward with the procedure. Benefit of cardiac resynchronization has been best demonstrated in patients with significantly delayed ventricular depolarization and left bundle branch block morphology and likely these particular techniques, including the targeting of the posterior and lateral branches of the cardiac venous system are dependent on appropriate patient selection. We discuss some of the major techniques employed to achieve appropriate LV lead implantation, but the implanter should assess each patient individually and adapt the available techniques and tools available to leverage the opportunities the patient's anatomy provides.

CANNULATION OF THE CORONARY SINUS

The first step in CS lead delivery is cannulation of the coronary sinus. After cannulation, the system in place must be stable and provide a support structure or "backbone" to allow controlled force to be transmitted to the lead tip without dislodging the system. Several methods to engage the CS ostium exist and the choice is operator dependent. These include dedicated sheaths and guide-wire systems, sheaths with steerable and telescoping inner catheters, and steerable electrophysiologic catheters that provide electrical clues to the location of the CS ostium, with the typical larger atrial electrogram and smaller ventricular electrogram. Fluoroscopy, which is frequently performed in the left anterior oblique (LAO) position, also provides guidance to the location.

CS cannulation can be performed with either contrast-based or electrogram-based techniques. Although electrophysiologists are generally very comfortable with CS cannulation guided fluoroscopically with electrograms, contrast is required for optimal final lead placement and allows the opportunity to take advantage of the anatomical variations invisible to the electrogram-guided techniques.

Anatomically, there are two potential impediments to entering the CS ostium. Laterally, the Eustachian ridge may prevent the advancement of a catheter to the ostium. Inferiorly, the thebesian valve may prevent entry to the ostium from an approach below (Figure 14.1). The optimal method of avoiding these impediments is approaching the ostium from a superior and medial approach. Regardless of the equipment used or the fluoroscopic approach, to avoid the Eustachian ridge and the thebesian valve, advance the system initially into the right ventricle and withdraw the system, while applying counterclockwise torque. When the catheter or sheath appears to be freed from the tricuspid valve, it should then be advanced while continuing counterclockwise torque. This technique avoids both impediments in most cases, and as long as counterclockwise torque is applied, this will also tend to avoid the atrial sulcus inferior and anterior to the CS os, below the tricuspid valve. Using a sheath or catheter with a proximal curve allows direction over the Eustachian ridge with ease.

Even if electrogram guidance is initially attempted, when difficulty persists after performing this maneuver, "puffing" contrast dye through the sheath or catheter is frequently revealing. It may show the atrial sulcus, in which case the approach should be more posterior and superior. Contrast may also reveal either an early or separate take-off of a middle cardiac vein that is preferentially cannulated by the system. Slight manipulation of the system while using contrast may allow the main CS lumen to be selected. Other possibilities include an acutely angled ostium, vertical or tortuous initial segments, or narrowing in the CS from a mid-CS valve or stenosis resulting from prior surgery. In these situations, contrast is invaluable to determine the cause of difficulty and aid in determining the optimal remedy. In cases such as these, an inner guide-wire or diagnostic electrophysiology catheter may facilitate manipulation and provide support to allow passage of the outer sheath.

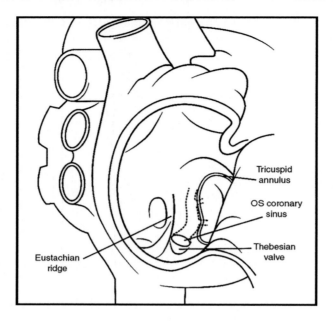

Figure 14.1 The Eustachian ridge and the thebesian valve may prevent advancement of a catheter to the ostium.

Several fluoroscopic clues may disclose the location of the CS. If an ICD lead has been placed in the RV apex, the ostium is generally in the vicinity of the proximal end of the distal coil in most usual projections. The "fat stripe" or radio-lucency of the atrioventricular groove can be seen best in the right anterior oblique (RAO) view. In the LAO oblique view, the coronary sinus will appear to course more toward the left side of the chest, while the right ventricle is *en face*. This orientation may more clearly reveal the posterior position of the sheath or catheter, especially if the operator's difficulty is repeatedly advancing into the right ventricle, indicating that the position is not posterior enough.

LV LEAD DELIVERY INTO THE APPROPRIATE CORONARY SINUS TRIBUTARY

After intubation of the CS ostium, the second major obstacle is cannulation of the appropriate branch so that the pacing electrodes are positioned at a stable non-LV apical location. The most important tool to accomplish this is the use of an appropriate support structure or "backbone" that will allow force to be transmitted to the tip of the lead when advancing it without dislodging or pushing the system back. The sheath that is used to deliver the lead needs to be designed so that it rests firmly against the lower lateral right atrium and superior vena cava. These sites provide the best support, and the sheath should be stiff enough to allow pressure at these sites without changing the conformation of the sheath. Available sheaths used for this purpose generally have a long straight segment followed by an extended curve, with the proximal curve intended to rest against the lower lateral right atrium. The next straight segment lies anterior to the Eustachian ridge and the secondary curve enters the coronary sinus. The size of the primary curve and length of the segment between the curves may need to be larger if the right atrium is significantly dilated, as is the case in some patients with tricuspid regurgitation. This "backbone" or workstation provides the support necessary for the force required to advance the lead into the appropriate branch.

At this point, it is frequently helpful to assess the available options in the venous anatomy with coronary venography. Several balloon-tipped catheters are available for this purpose. Of note, one may wish to use a guidewire to advance the balloon-tipped catheter because this catheter alone may cause coronary vein dissection. In order to obtain an optimal image, the coronary sinus should be occluded during contrast injection. After the distal tributaries are well visualized, the balloon should be released to view contrast enhancement of the proximal branches. It is vital to perform fluoroscopy in 2 planes (RAO and LAO) to determine the better inform branch orientation of the branches. Pay careful attention to vessel collateralization since it is principally about the pacing site and not how you get there. Often the main CS is too large to occlude and direct intubation of one of the branches allows direct injection or sometimes balloon-occluded injection with retrograde filling of the rest of the venous drainage. The images should ideally be saved on a separate monitor, and special attention should be paid to the initial segments of the appropriately located branches and the caliber of the branches.

CORONARY SINUS ANATOMY

After performing coronary venography the operator must then select the coronary vein tributary that will deliver the lead to a posterolateral location. Due to discrepancies between physicians in naming the branches of the coronary sinus and tributaries we rely on academic sources and journal reports for the correct nomenclature.[5-13] The coronary veins are described to commence with the anterior interventricular vein (AIV), which is located at the lower or middle third of the anterior interventricular groove. It connects with diagonal veins (DVs) supplying the lateral and anterolateral portion of the left ventricle. It continues to run vertically turning posterior at the AV groove and as it courses horizontally it becomes the great cardiac vein (GV). The GV courses medially over the summit of the left ventricle (Figure 14.2).

The great cardiac vein becomes the CS at the left atrial oblique vein of Marshall (LAOV). In cases where the LAOV is not present the CS begins at the valve of Vieussens.

The tributaries of the CS that originate off the lateral wall are referred to as marginal veins. These marginal veins are further defined by the location where they empty into the CS in

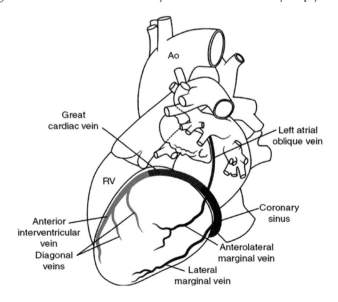

Figure 14.2   The coronary veins.

the LAO projection, such as the anterolateral marginal (AM), lateral marginal (LM), and inferolateral marginal (IM) (Figure 14.3). Since posterior is not an accepted terminology in echocardiographic standards, inferolateral is used in naming the CS tributary here for consistency, but posterolateral marginal may be used.

The posterior ventricular vein (PVV) drains the inferior (posterior) aspect of the left ventricle. The PVV is often confused with the posterolateral marginal vein due to the similar location. The PVV is usually larger in caliber than the posterolateral marginal and sometimes drains into the middle cardiac vein (MCV). The MCV originates near the apex, runs in the posterior interventricular groove, and drains either directly into the right atrium or into the CS just before it opens into the right atrium (Figure 14.4).

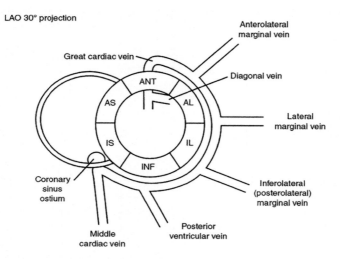

Figure 14.3   LAO 30° projection.

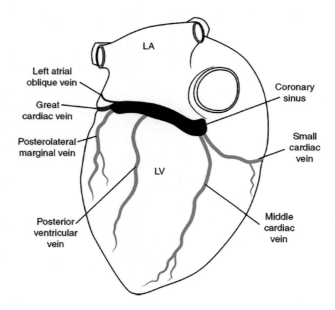

Figure 14.4   Vein drainage.

We also prefer to use fluoroscopy for the identification of the location of the left ventricular lead tip after completion of the procedure. Since implantation of a left ventricular lead occurs in the electrophysiology lab with fluoroscopy, we therefore use fluoroscopic views to correspond with the short axis and long axis views of the heart. Using this method, an accurate and consistent description of the location of the LV lead tip can be made at the time of implant and entered into the operative report, rather than relying on the CXR for documentation of lead position.

The RAO 30 projection is used to define the location of the left ventricle along the vertical axis of the heart, dividing it into a basal, mid, and apical third (Figure 14.5). The LAO 30 projection is used for the short axis views to define the circumferential location of the lead.

Based on the anatomy, the operator may make several decisions at this point, including the size of the lead used and the approach to the cannulate the branches. In the case of an uncomplicated branch cannulation, a hydrophilic wire is introduced into the central lumen of the lead and lead advanced (without wire protruding) until the tip of the sheath is reached. A torquing tool can then be threaded over the wire and used to steer the wire into the desired branch and wedged distally. This is then used as a rail to advance the lead. Manufacturers now produce leads that are of different sizes and shapes, such as a distal coil or sigmoid shape, that facilitates lead stability in larger branches.

The common impediments to cannulating branches of the CS include an angulated take-off of the branch, a tortuous initial segment, or a small or stenosed branch. Once again, proceeding from this point requires adequate support from the outer sheath. If the initial segment of the selected branch is slightly angulated, then using an over-the-wire lead system may be the only tool necessary. The wire is used to navigate the branch, and the lead is inserted over the wire.

Occasionally, it is difficult to even get the wire into the selected branch. For this problem, inner catheters may be used to intubate the selected branches, and the wire is advanced through this catheter into the branch. The catheter is removed, and the lead is advanced over the wire. Newer generation inner catheters permit introduction of the lead over the wire without the need to remove the catheter, providing added support. At points where it becomes difficult to advance the lead, simultaneously advancing the lead and withdrawing the wire (push–pull technique) is sometimes helpful. The optimal set-up for this is similar to an angioplasty system. On the exteriorized end of the catheter, a system with an adjustable valve and side port should be attached. The wire goes through the valve, and the side port allows contrast to opacify the vein and branch, when the valve is closed.

For selected branches that have a very angulated or tortuous initial segment, a range of inner catheters with variable curves at the tip facilitates intubation of the selected branch. The hydrophilic wire could then be advanced through this and then depending on the subselection

RAO 30° projection

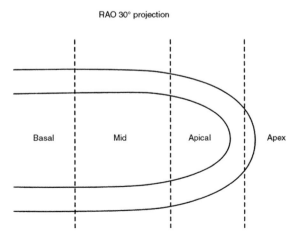

Figure 14.5 RAO 30° projection.

catheter used the lead may be advanced over the wire through the catheter or the catheter exchanged out and then the lead advanced over the wire. The advantage of having the lead introduced while the subselection catheter is still in place is that extra support is provided to advance the lead or else you will need to be confident that sufficient force can be transmitted to the lead tip to overcome the tortuosity. The characteristics of these inner sheaths must be similar to the outer sheath. It must be stiff enough to allow pressure to be transmitted to the tip of the lead without buckling. The design feature should be in a fashion that uses the wall of the CS opposite the selected branch as well as the outer sheath for support (Figure 14.6). Currently, there are three available shapes. The multi-purpose shape will provide support for most mild angulations. The renal and hockey stick shapes are appropriate for more severe angulations or very tortuous initial segments. In fact, these inner catheters by virtue of their shape and stiffness will straighten branches and allow deeper intubations of these branches (Figure 14.7). They can be used like angioplasty catheters with contrast and manipulated to locate the ostium

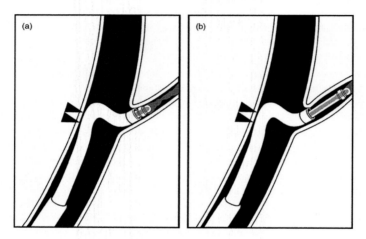

Figure 14.6 Intubation of catheter into selected branch a) Support of the opposing wall of the vein allows engagement into the branch vessel (b) Back support of the back wall of the vein allows advancement of the lead to the distal branch vessel.

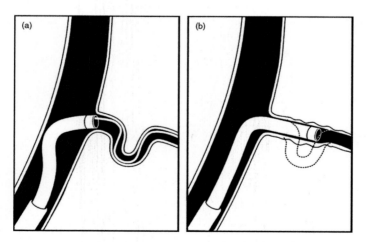

Figure 14.7 Straightening of branch segment (a) Flexible guide wire is advanced through tortuous proximal segment of the branch vein. (b) Catheter is advanced over the guide wire to straighten the tortuosity.

of the selected branch. Another way to straighten tortuous branch segments is the use of a buddy wire. In this case, a relatively stiff wire is used to cannulate the branch, and another wire is used to cannulate the branch and deliver the lead.

VENOPLASTY TECHNIQUES

Another obstacle to delivering the lead may be due to limitations in the size or a stenosed segment of the appropriately located vein. The solution to this problem is venoplasty. The outer sheath and inner catheter system should be used to intubate the ostium of the branch. A guidewire should be passed to the most distal portion of this vein. A non-compliant balloon of appropriate length for the stenosed or small segment should be used. In general, the sizes necessary for accepting coronary venous pacing leads are 3–3.5 mm in diameter. The segment is dilated using a long slow inflation. The balloon is deflated, removed, and replaced with the over-the-wire pacing lead. The dilated vein tends to return to its original size and serves to aid in keeping the lead in place.[14]

ASSESSMENT OF LEAD FUNCTION

Once the lead is in place, it is tested for impedance and capture threshold. A capture threshold of <2 V is usually acceptable. The impedance can vary between 400 and 2000 ohms with unipolar pacing having lower impedance values. Assessment of phrenic nerve capture at high voltage output is also made. With the advent of quadpolar leads, the operator is provided with several pacing options, which combines the goals of avoiding phrenic nerve capture, low pacing threshold, and narrower biventricular paced QRS width (Figure 14.8).[15]

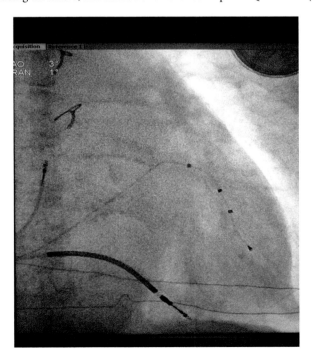

Figure 14.8   Fluoroscopic image of a quadpolar lead.

Since on many occasions, the number of suitable branches are limited, the major advantage of the quadpolar lead is that it rarely needs to be repositioned if you encounter one of the aforementioned problems, but instead use a different bipolar or unipolar pacing vector.

SUMMARY

Anatomical variations can make delivery of a left ventricular lead extremely challenging. However, a thorough understanding of the anatomic structure and its variations along with the tools available to overcome this is key. The method of approaching the CS ostium from the right ventricle avoids the pitfalls of the Eustachian ridge and the overriding thebesian valve. The use of an outer sheath serves as a strong, supportive workstation, and the philosophy of always moving forward with the available tools is a useful strategy. Familiarity with inner sheaths that allow selective branch intubation and delivery of the pacing lead plus venoplasty techniques, permits an operator to confidently manage many of the barriers for a successful CS lead implantation.

ACKNOWLEDGMENTS

The authors would like to thank Kenneth Civello, Mohammed Khan, and Jennifer Cummings for their contribution to the prior edition of this chapter.

REFERENCES

1. Cleland JG, Daubert JC, Erdmann E et al. The effect of cardiac resynchronization on morbidity and mortality in heart failure. *N Engl J Med* 2005; 352(15): 1539–1549.
2. Abraham WT, Fisher WG, Smith AL et al. Cardiac resynchronization in chronic heart failure. *N Engl J Med* 2002; 346(24): 1845–1853.
3. Butter C, Auricchio A, Stellbrink C et al. Effect of resynchronization therapy stimulation site on the systolic function of heart failure patients. *Circulation* 2001; 104(25): 3026–3029.
4. Kandala J, Upadhyay GA, Altman RK et al. QRS morphology, left ventricular lead location, and clinical outcome in patients receiving cardiac resynchronization therapy. *Eur Heart J* 2013; 34(29): 2252–2262.
5. Gensini G, Digorgi S, Coskun D et al. Anatomy of the coronary circulation in living man: Coronary venography. *Circulation* 1965; 31: 778–784.
6. McAlpine WA, Coskun D et al. *Heart and The Coronary Arteries: An Anatomical Atlas for Clinical Diagnosis, Radiological Investigation, and Surgical Treatment.* Springer-Verlag, New York, NY, 1978.
7. Schumacher B, Tebbenjohanns J, Pfeiffer D et al. Prospective study of retrograde coronary venography in patients with posteroseptal and left-sided accessory atrioventricular pathways. *Am Heart J* 1995; 130(5): 1031–1039.
8. Maric I, Bodinac D, Ostojc L et al. Tributaries of the human and canine coronary sinus. *Acta Anat (Basel)* 1996; 156(1): 61–69.
9. Gilard M, Mansourati J, Etienne Y et al. Angiographic anatomy of the coronary sinus and its tributaries. *Pacing Clin Electrophysiol* 1998; 21(11 Pt 2): 2280–2284.
10. Ortale JR, Sabriel CA, Lost C et al. The anatomy of the coronary sinus and its tributaries. *Surg Radiol Anat* 2001; 23(1): 15–21.

11. Meisel E, Pfeiffer D, Engelman L et al. Investigation of coronary venous anatomy by retrograde venography in patients with malignant ventricular tachycardia. *Circulation* 2001; 104(4): 442–447.

12. Kawashima T, Sato K, Sato F et al. An anatomical study of the human cardiac veins with special reference to the drainage of the great cardiac vein. *Ann Anat* 2003; 185(6): 535–542.

13. Bales GS. Great cardiac vein variations. *Clin Anat* 2004; 17(5): 436–443.

14. Ellenbogen KA, Kay Neal G, Wilkoff Bruce L. *Device Therapy for Congestive Heart Failure*. Saunders, Philadelphia, PA, 2004.

15. Forleo GB, Mantica M, Di Biase L et al. Clinical and procedural outcome of patients implanted with a quadripolar left ventricular lead: Early results of a prospective multi-center study. *Heart Rhythm* 2012; 9(11): 1822–1828.

EXTRACTION OF DEVICES

Oussama M. Wazni and Bruce L. Wilkoff

CONTENTS

Percutaneous intravascular lead extraction has evolved from simple traction through a weight-and-pulley system to a more advanced modern day technique utilizing telescoping and powered sheaths. As the number of new and replacement devices increase due to expanding indications and an ageing population so too has the need for extraction. This chapter will address indications and general techniques of percutaneous lead extraction.

INDICATIONS

Infection remains the main indication for extraction. It is important to note here that both endovascular and pocket infections are class I indications. Antibiotic therapy without extraction is ineffective with very high rates of relapse in infection.[1,2]

The most recent guidelines published in 2009[3] divide indications into those for infection and other non-infection related indications.

In summary, extraction is a class I indication when infection is clearly present as in cases of endocarditis, gram positive bacteremia or pocket infection. Extraction is also indicated in cases of significant thrombosis and symptomatic vein stenosis and in cases when a lead poses risks to the patient. Other indications include extraction for lead recall, access retention in upgrade situations, and chronic pain.

EXTRACTION TOOLS

The tools used for extractions are shown in Tables 15.1 and 15.2.

LOCKING STYLETS

Locking stylets provide tensile strength to the lead all the way to the tip electrode. This permits the advancement of the telescoping sheaths and withdrawal of the entire lead, without leaving fragments behind.

TELESCOPING SHEATHS

The inner and outer telescoping sheaths provide for flexibility and strength as they are passed over the lead to the endocardial surface. Balanced traction on the locking stylet allows first

Table 15.1 Extraction tools

Locking stylets	Liberator (Cook-Vandergrift, PA) Lead Locking Device (Spectranetics, Colorado Springs, CO) VascoMED (Weil am Rhein, Germany)[7]	3rd generation locking stylet, locks at the distal end of the conductor coil. One size fits all leads. Locking mechanism locks along the entire length of the conductor coil, 4 sizes are used depending on the coil inner diameter. T-shaped end screws down the conductor coil to the tip. Available in Europe only.
Telescoping sheaths	Stainless steel sheaths Plastic sheaths (Teflon or polypropylene)	Used to break through the tissue at the vein entry site. Once access to the vein is obtained, replacement with flexible sheaths that adapt better to the vein's shape is recommended.[7] Used to maneuver around curves and forcing through circumferential bands of fibrous tissue in the vein tracts.
Laser ablation	Excimer laser light (Spectranetics, Colorado Springs, CO)	Light dissolves the fibrotic tissue along the entire circumference as it advances over the lead. The sheaths are provided in 12, 14, and 16 French.
Electrosurgical ablation	Electrosurgical energy, modified from a standard surgical Bovie unit	The spark is produced between two tungsten wires and cuts the fibrosis along about 15% of the arc of the Teflon sheath.
Byrd femoral workstation and femoral snares	Teflon sheaths used to snare the snare in the heart or veins (Cook-Vandergrift, PA)	Several snares (needle's eye snare, Dotter basket with tip deflecting guidewire, Amplatz gooseneck snare) are used to grasp the lead and the Teflon sheath is advanced over the lead to the heart to provide countertraction.[10,11]

Table 15.2 Specific procedures

Conventional mechanical extraction	Conventional tools including the blunt but angled Teflon or steel telescoping sheaths with appropriate locking stylets using the principles of counterpressure and countertraction
Excimer laser extraction	Conventional technique plus Excimer laser inner telescoping sheaths for dissolution of the fibrotic tissue
Electrosurgical extraction	Conventional technique plus e electrosurgical sheath for cutting the fibrotic tissue
Rotating Cutting Tip	Conventional sheath with rotating cutting tip (Evolution and Tight Rail)

the inner and then the outer sheath to break through the scar tissue and down over the lead to the endocardium. Their use is based on the two important concepts of *counterpressure* and *countertraction*.[8] Telescoping sheaths may be powered or non-powered.

BYRD FEMORAL WORKSTATION AND FEMORAL SNARES

Some leads that have been cut or fractured are not accessible from the venous entry site. In these cases, the femoral approach for lead extraction may be favored. Femoral extraction requires the use of a large 16 French sheath (Byrd workstation), which is carefully inserted via the femoral vein. The sheath has many functions, including protection of the vein or heart from damage during femoral snare insertion, and it acts as the outer telescoping sheath for counter-traction. A snare can then be inserted through the sheath to grasp the lead and pull it down from the superior veins and from the heart with countertraction.[4]

Femoral venous and arterial access must be obtained before the extraction starts. The anesthesia method would depend on the team preferences, general status of the patient, and the quality and quantity of leads to be extracted. Measures must be taken to provide appropriate temporary pacing in pacer-dependent patients. Extraction should only be performed with available surgical backup that is able to rescue the patient in case of catastrophic complications such as SVC-RA perforation.[3]

The following are the basic *principles* for a successful lead extraction:

1   Control of the lead body and tip, which is achieved by binding of all its separate components with the application of uniform force on the entire length of the lead, to remove it in one piece with minimal disruption. The locking stylets previously described are the appropriate tool to use.

2   Controlled disruption of the fibrous tissue using counterpressure and if needed powered lysis using laser, electrocautery, or rotational cutting.

3   Bracing the cardiac wall using countertraction, which involves opposing the traction placed on the lead by bracing the myocardium with the overlying blunt sheath. This focuses the traction force perpendicular to the heart wall and limits the counterpressure to the scar tissue immediately surrounding the lead tip (Figure 15.1).

GENERAL TECHNICAL PRINCIPLES

1   A linear incision is made to obtain better access to the vein of insertion and the generator is explanted.

2   The terminal pin of each lead is cut, leaving sufficient length of the proximal end outside the venous insertion. The cut end is prepared by circumferentially incising the insulation.

3   A standard pacemaker stylet is passed through the electrode to its distal tip to ascertain the distance through which the locking stylet has to travel and to clear the debris.

4   A locking stylet is advanced to the farthest reach of the lead and then deployed. A 0 gauge suture is tied around the insulation tightly with a square knot. The long end of the suture is then tied to the looped end of the locking stylet, providing for parallel and simultaneous traction on the outer insulation and on the conductor coil. A One Tie may be used when preparing an ICD lead. The One Tie binds all the components of the ICD lead to each other and to the locking stylet (Figure 15.2).

5   Sheaths:
    (a)   With the use of the locking stylet the lead is pulled through the extraction sheath and used as a rail for sheath advancement. As binding sites are encountered these are broken using the blunt end of the sheaths or by activating a powered mechanism.
    (b)   The sheaths should always be advanced under direct fluoroscopic guidance.
    (c)   Sheaths should not be advanced directly against the vessel wall but rather the leads should be peeled away from the wall of the vessel, bringing the lead into the center of the vascular lumen.

6   With infected devices, the generator pocket should be completely excised to prevent microbial reseeding, and closed with mattress sutures. In a non-infected extraction new hardware can be implanted during the same procedure.

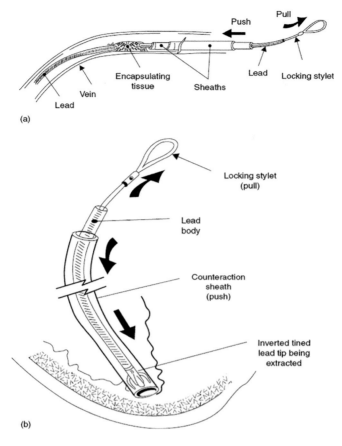

(a)

Push

Pull

Encapsulating
tissue

Sheaths

Lead

Locking stylet

Vein

Lead

(b)

Locking stylet
(pull)

Lead
body

Counteraction
sheath
(push)

Inverted tined
lead tip being
extracted

Figure 15.1 Panel (a): Counter-Pressure involves the controlled disruption of the fibrosis along the lead by concentrating the forces at the tip of the extraction sheath as the sheath is advanced over the lead without allowing the lead to be pushed in but also not retracting the lead from the vessel. Thus the lead is kept steady, the sheath is advanced, and the fibrosis is broken up. Panel (b): Counter-Traction involves the release of the lead from the myocardium after the extraction sheath has been advanced to a few mm from the endocardial surface. The lead is held so it is neither advanced or removed and the lead is pulled into the sheath. This prevents myocardial laceration.

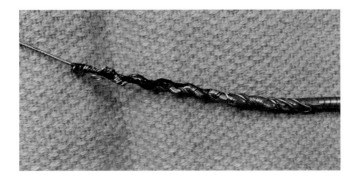

Figure 15.2 One Tie is applied over the insulation and binds the insulation and all of the conductors (inner, outer, and cables) together.

SPECIFIC POWERED TOOLS (TABLE 15.2)

EXCIMER LASER EXTRACTION

The laser sheath is one of the most effective extraction tools and has been prospectively studied in the randomized PLEXES trial in comparison to traditional extraction with locking stylets and telescoping sheaths. Laser resulted in a higher percentage of complete lead removal (94% versus 64%, $p = 0.001$) and also reduced the time required for removal (10.1 +/− 11.5 min compared with 12.9 +/− 19.2 min, $p < 0.04$). Life-threatening complications (including one death) occurred in the laser group, while none occurred in the traditional group, but this difference was not statistically different given the small numbers overall.[5] The LeXiCon study, in 2010, reported on 2405 lead extractions in 13 centers. Major complications related to the procedure were seen in 1.4% of patients and death in 0.4%.[6] Multiple other studies from experienced centers worldwide have reported similar results (Figure 15.3).

ELECTROSURGICAL DISSECTION EXTRACTION

The electrosurgical dissection sheath is less expensive than a laser system. It uses electrocautery at the tip of the sheath instead of laser. In general it has achieved similar results as laser extraction.[7]

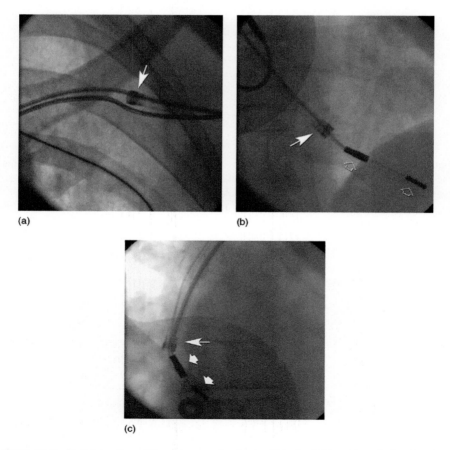

(a)

(b)

(c)

Figure 15.3 (a–c) Extraction of the old pacemaker leads within the left brachiocephalic vein using excimer laser sheath (long arrow). (Atrial lead, short solid arrow; ventricular lead, short open arrow.)

ROTATIONAL CUTTING SHEATHS

There are two such sheaths with distal rotating cutting tips. The earlier one is the Evolution R/L from Cook medical and the other is the Tight Rail from Spectranetics. Both are helpful in managing calcified binding sites.[8,9]

SPECIAL CONSIDERATIONS

Defibrillator Lead Extraction

The extraction of ICD leads can be more difficult due to exuberant fibrotic tissue surrounding the defibrillator coils, especially the proximal one located at the superior vena cava. Extraction of defibrillator leads more commonly requires the use of powered sheaths and is associated with more major complications. Given that the most dreaded complication is perforation at the SVC-RA junction, whenever possible, single-coil defibrillator leads should be used to minimize the extent of fibrosis and binding at that site. Newly designed defibrillator leads with coated and backfilled defibrillation coils may reduce tissue ingrowth and fibrosis.[10]

Coronary Sinus Lead Extraction

Given their smaller profiles, CS leads can be removed by simple traction explantation in most instances. In cases with significant binding can be extracted by powered or non-powered extraction. Sheaths can be advanced into the coronary sinus and even its venous branches but it is best to avoid the use of the powered mechanisms in this area as any complications could be very difficult to manage in this location. Although the Attain Starfix® (Medtronic, Minneapolis, MN, USA) has an active fixation mechanism that consists of lobes at the tip, it has extracted with use of traction and counter traction once the distal end of the lead is reached, in most cases without incident.[11-13]

DEFINING CLINICAL OUTCOMES

Clinical success is one in which the clinical goal is achieved whether it is elimination of infection, creation of venous access, or elimination of risk attributed to an extracted lead. Complete procedural success is when all targeted lead material is removed without complications.[3]

SURGICAL APPROACH

A more invasive open-heart surgical technique through a midline sternotomy or a limited atriotomy technique was developed, and continues to be a last resort answer to difficult lead extractions that are not suitable for percutaneous techniques. Such cases include very large vegetations or situations when concomitant surgical repair or replacement of infected valves is anticipated.

REFERENCES

1. Chua, J.D. et al. Diagnosis and management of infections involving implantable electrophysiologic cardiac devices. *Ann Intern Med* 2000; **133**(8): 604–608.

2. Klug, D. et al. Systemic infection related to endocarditis on pacemaker leads: Clinical presentation and management. *Circulation* 1997; **95**(8): 2098–2107.

3. Wilkoff, B.L. et al. Transvenous lead extraction: Heart Rhythm Society expert consensus on facilities, training, indications, and patient management: This document was endorsed by the American Heart Association (AHA). *Heart Rhythm* 2009; **6**(7): 1085–1104.

4. Byrd, C.L. Advances in device lead extraction. *Curr Cardiol Rep* 2001; **3**(4): 324.

5. Wilkoff, B.L. et al. Pacemaker lead extraction with the laser sheath: results of the pacing lead extraction with the excimer sheath (PLEXES) trial. *J Am Coll Cardiol* 1999; **33**(6): 1671–1676.

6. Wazni, O. et al. Lead extraction in the contemporary setting: The LExICon study: An observational retrospective study of consecutive laser lead extractions. *J Am Coll Cardiol* 2010; **55**(6): 579–586.

7. Neuzil, P. et al. Pacemaker and ICD lead extraction with electrosurgical dissection sheaths and standard transvenous extraction systems: Results of a randomized trial. *Europace* 2007; **9**(2): 98–104.

8. Hussein, A.A. et al. Initial experience with the Evolution mechanical dilator sheath for lead extraction: Safety and efficacy. *Heart Rhythm* 2010; **7**(7): 870–873.

9. Aytemir, K. et al. Initial experience with the TightRail Rotating Mechanical Dilator Sheath for transvenous lead extraction. *Europace*, 2015; **18**(7): 1043–1048.

10. Epstein, L.M. et al. Superior vena cava defibrillator coils make transvenous lead extraction more challenging and riskier. *J Am Coll Cardiol* 2013; **61**(9): 987–989.

11. Cronin, E.M. et al. Active fixation mechanism complicates coronary sinus lead extraction and limits subsequent reimplantation targets. *J Interv Card Electrophysiol* 2013; **36**(1): 81–86; discussion 86.

12. di Cori, A. et al. Large, single-center experience in transvenous coronary sinus lead extraction: Procedural outcomes and predictors for mechanical dilatation. *Pacing Clin Electrophysiol* 2012; **35**(2): 215–222.

13. Zucchelli, G. et al. Cardiac resynchronization therapy after coronary sinus lead extraction: Feasibility and mid-term outcome of transvenous reimplantation in a tertiary referral centre. *Europace* 2012; **14**(4): 515–521.

PERFORMING BASIC EP STUDIES

VENOUS AND ARTERIAL ACCESS, EP CATHETERS, POSITIONING OF CATHETERS

Ching Chi Keong, J. David Burkhardt, Thomas Dresing, and Andrea Natale

CONTENTS

FEMORAL ARTERY AND VEIN PUNCTURES

These vessels are common sites of entry for catheterization of right and left heart chambers for electrophysiologic recordings. The femoral artery typically begins in the midpoint of the inguinal ligament and ends at the junction of the middle and lower third of the thigh to become the popliteal artery. Its proximal course of about 4 cm lies within the femoral sheath and the arterial pulse can be felt at the inguinal skin crease. The femoral vein lies medial to the femoral artery, approximately one finger-breadth medial to the femoral artery. Adequate local anesthesia is given before vessel puncture to ensure patient comfort and cooperation.

FEMORAL VEIN PUNCTURE

The arterial course is outlined with three fingers while skin incisions are made medial to the arterial pulsation over the intended sites of entry. This small skin incision can be further enlarged by the use of a curved hemostat to prevent potential crimping of the intravascular sheath, though the sheath can almost always be advanced over the guide-wire safely and easily without having to first enlarge the skin defect. A Cook needle is then introduced through the skin incision and advanced along the anesthetized track at a 30–45 degree angle to the skin surface. Gentle suction is applied to the syringe as the needle is advanced until a clear flashback of non-pulsatile venous blood occurs. The syringe and the needle are depressed to be more parallel to the skin surface. The syringe is then detached and a

J-tipped guide-wire is advanced into the hub of the needle and forward into the vessel without any resistance. If resistance is encountered, a downward depression of the needle hub to secure an intravascular position of the needle can be attempted. Otherwise the guide-wire should be removed and a syringe re-attached and the whole assembly advanced or withdrawn slightly until a free flow of blood is encountered. If there is no free flow, the whole assembly is removed and pressure is held and landmarks rechecked before further venous punctures.

When the guide-wire is successfully advanced intravascularly, the needle is removed and an intravascular sheath is then inserted over the guide-wire until it protrudes from its proximal end. The whole assembly is then advanced with firm forward pressure and slight rotation. Once the sheath is intravascular and completely advanced, the guide-wire and introducer can be removed and the side port flushed with heparinized saline. As illustrated in Figure 16.1, the intended site of entry should be within the femoral sheath. A lower site of entry may inadvertently puncture one of several branches of the femoral vein that traverse medially. The procedure can be repeated to accommodate up to three venous sheaths.

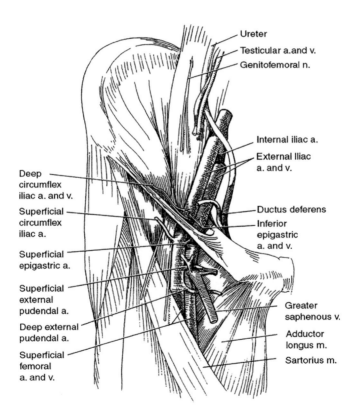

Figure 16.1 Relationship of the femoral vessels. Note the medial course of superficial and deep pudendal branches of the femoral artery. (From Valentine, R.J., *Anatomic Exposures in Vascular Surgery*, Lippincott Williams and Wilkins, Philadelphia, PA, 2003. With permission.)

FEMORAL ARTERY PUNCTURE

Femoral artery puncture is performed lateral to the femoral vein puncture sites just below the inguinal ligament. With three fingers outlining the course of the femoral artery, the tip of an open lumen Cook needle is inserted at the site of maximal pulsation and carefully advanced. A pulsatile jet of flashback occurs when the needle enters the arterial lumen. With the left hand holding the hub steadily, a J-tipped guide-wire is then introduced through the needle into the arterial lumen and advanced into the lumen. Under fluoroscopy, the guide-wire should to the left of the vertebrae. If resistance is encountered or if the patient complains of discomfort, the guide-wire may be within the subintimal wall of the artery. Other causes may be due to a kink in the intra-vascular sheath or tortuous vasculature. Alternatively, a subintimal dissection may occur, in which case the needle is removed, a 5 French dilator is introduced over the wire, and a small bolus of contrast agent is injected to verify the cause of obstruction. If arterial dissection is the cause, the whole assembly is removed and digital pressure is maintained for 5–10 min. If there is no dissection, other guide-wires may be tried. If resistance is encountered just beyond the tip of the needle, a downward depression of the needle hub should move the tip more intravascular and facilitate passage of the guide-wire. At all times, the backflow of blood must be pulsatile. When the guide-wire is adequately advanced without further resistance, the needle is withdrawn and the guide-wire wiped with wet gauze. The desired intravascular sheath is then advanced over the guide-wire. The guide-wire is then removed and the side port of the sheath flushed with heparinized saline.

SUBCLAVIAN VEIN PUNCTURE

The left subclavian vein is the continuation of the axillary vein and extends from the outer border of the first rib to the sternal end of the clavicle. It lies posterior to the clavicle and often rests in a depression on the first rib and upon the pleura. The subclavian artery lies posterosuperior to the vein and is separated medially by the scalenus anterior. The site of puncture is immediately lateral to the ligament that joins the clavicle to the first rib, at the junction of the proximal two-thirds and distal one-third of the clavicle. Adequate anesthesia is given along the track of intended puncture. A Cook needle attached to a syringe is directed to the sternal notch, parallel to the clavicle. Gentle aspiration is performed as the needle is advanced slowly. Return of dark venous blood without pulsatile flow indicates entry in the subclavian vein. The syringe is detached, the needle stabilized, and a guide-wire is advanced into the lumen without resistance. If resistance is encountered, the guide-wire is likely to be extravascular. The guide-wire should be visualized under fluoroscopy to ascertain its position and adjusted accordingly to direct it into the superior vena cava. If the guide-wire fails to advance, it should be withdrawn, the needle slightly pulled back or advanced to obtain a free flow of venous blood, and the wire re-advanced. With fluoroscopic guidance, the guide-wire should be advanced into the inferior vena cava, which lies to the right of the vertebrae, to ensure that the guide-wire has not inadvertently been introduced into the subclavian artery. The needle is then removed and a desired intravascular sheath advanced over the guide-wire and the side port flushed with heparinized saline.

If pulsatile blood is aspirated, the needle has punctured the subclavian artery. The needle should be removed and digital pressure maintained for 5–10 min to allow proper hemostasis.

If air is aspirated, the pleural space is entered and the puncture is too deep or too lateral. Other complications include hemothorax and subclavian arteriovenous fistula.

INTERNAL JUGULAR VEIN PUNCTURE

The internal jugular vein is located anterior and lateral to the carotid artery. It lies behind the clavicular head of the sternocleidomastoid muscle. The site of puncture is approximately at the level of the apex formed by both heads of the sterno-cleidomastoid muscle and medial to the lateral border of the clavicular head. The Trendelenberg position is helpful in distending the vein. The syringe and needle are directed lateral to the carotid artery. When a free flow of venous blood is encountered, the syringe is detached, the needle held firmly, and a guide-wire advanced. At all times the guide-wire should be advanced without any perceived resistance. The needle is then removed and an intravascular sheath advanced as described previously. The potential complications of internal jugular vein access include carotid artery puncture with resultant hematoma, potential air embolism, and pneumothorax. Digital pressure should be maintained for 5–10 min in the event of inadvertent carotid artery puncture. Air embolism can be prevented by keeping the patient in the Trendelenberg position until the sheath is advanced. The risk of pneumothorax can be minimized by obtaining access in the neck at a higher level.

VENOUS ACCESS DURING A PROCEDURE WITH AGGRESSIVE ANTICOAGULATION OR THERAPEUTIC INR

Many centers perform catheter ablation in patients on warfarin with therapeutic international normalized ratio (INR). Additionally, intravenous infusion of heparin is given to maintain an activated clotting time (ACT) of over 300 s for procedures that necessitate left atrial instrumentation. There is little margin for error in obtaining venous access in these patients. An inadvertent arterial puncture may result in a large hematoma requiring early termination of the procedure. Therefore, venous access of the femoral veins is obtained with a modified Seldinger technique to avoid possible venous hematoma. An ultrasound-guided internal jugular vein puncture is performed to avoid inadvertent arterial puncture or through and through venous punctures. Standing at the head of the patient, an ultrasound probe is placed over the right side of the neck bordered by the two heads of the sterno-cleidomastoid (Figure 16.2). Two vascular structures are seen deep to it. Identification of the internal jugular vein can be easily made by noting flattening of the vessel with gentle compression (Figure 16.3). Thereafter the venous access to the internal jugular vein is performed using a modified Seldinger technique (Figure 16.4). Care is taken to avoid intramuscular route of venous access. Often an intramuscular hematoma ensues in these patients who are adequately anticoagulated. Alternatively, a guide-wire can be advanced from the femoral vein to the right internal jugular vein. With fluoroscopic guidance, venous access to the right internal jugular can then be performed, targeting the intravascular guide-wire. With these measures, the complication rate of vascular access is comparable to patients who are not on anticoagulation.

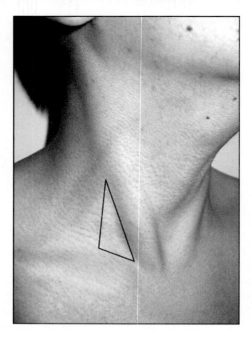

Figure 16.2 Surface anatomy of the neck. The two heads of the sternocleidomastoid muscle are depicted. Venous puncture is attempted between these two heads to avoid intramuscular anesthesia or an intramuscular route.

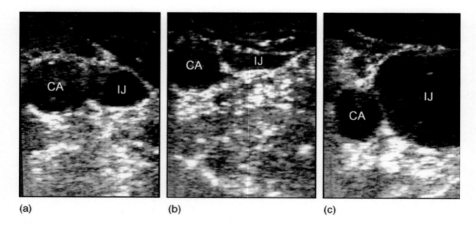

(a)   (b)   (c)

Figure 16.3 Ultrasound-guided internal jugular vein puncture. (a) The carotid artery is seen medial to the vein. (b) Gentle compression distinguishes the vein. (c) A Valsalva maneuver from the same patient distends the vein. IJ: internal jugular vein; CA: carotid artery.

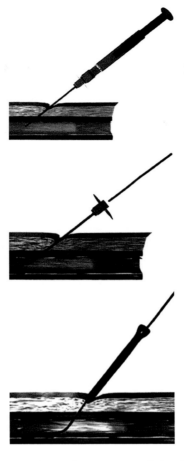

Figure 16.4 Modified Seldinger technique for venous cannulation. (From Singer, I., *Interventional Electrophysiology*, Lippincott Williams and Wilkins, Philadelphia, PA, 2001. With permission.)

STANDARD CATHETER POSITIONS

HIGH RIGHT ATRIUM
A fixed curve quadripolar catheter is advanced from the femoral vein and placed in contact with the right atrial wall. It should be at the lateral wall near the superior vena cava/right atrial junction.

RIGHT VENTRICULAR APEX
A fixed curve quadripolar catheter is advanced from the femoral vein and placed with the tip at the apical right ventricular septum. For many ablation procedures, a more basal site on the RV septum is preferred.

CORONARY SINUS
The coronary sinus allows recording of left atrial and ventricular electrograms. The availability of wide range of multi-polar catheters including steerable catheters makes venous access flexible. The catheter is advanced from the femoral vein or right internal jugular vein into

the coronary sinus until the proximal electrode overlies the lateral border of the vertebrae in the anteroposterior projection.

HIS BUNDLE

A quadripolar steerable or fixed-curve catheter is used for His bundle recording. This is advanced from the femoral vein to the superior tricuspid annulus, around 1 to 2 o'clock in the left anterior oblique fluoroscopic view.

OTHER CATHETERS

More specialized catheters are mentioned in the relevant sections of this book. The standard left anterior oblique and right anterior oblique views of these catheters are depicted in Figures 16.5 and 16.6.

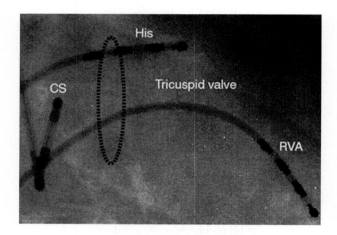

Figure 16.5 Right anterior oblique view of the His bundle catheter in relation to the tricuspid annulus. Right ventricular and coronary sinus catheters are shown. CS: coronary sinus; RVA: right ventricular apex.

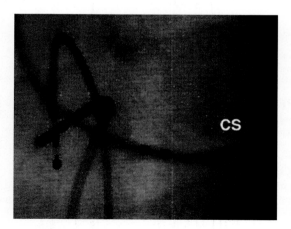

Figure 16.6 Left anterior oblique view of the coronary sinus catheter. *Abbreviation*: CS: coronary sinus.

BIBLIOGRAPHY

1. Singer I. *Interventional Electrophysiology*, 2nd ed. Philadelphia, PA: Lippincott Williams and Wilkins, 2001.
2. Valentine RJ. *Anatomic Exposures in Vascular Surgery*, 2nd ed. Philadelphia, PA: Lippincott Williams and Wilkins, 2003.

BASIC INTRACARDIAC INTERVALS

Duc H. Do and Noel G. Boyle

CONTENTS

The electrophysiologic study is performed by inserting electrode-tipped catheters into the body and positioning them within the heart (Figure 17.1). Intracardiac electrograms (EGMs) are recordings from these electrodes. In contrast to surface electrocardiogram (ECG), which records the summation of cardiac electrical activity, intracardiac EGMs record localized cardiac activity between two electrodes on the catheter, called a bipolar electrode recording. EGMs contain several rapid deflections, representing depolarization of myocardial tissue between the two recording electrodes (Figure 17.2). Remote (far field) cardiac electrical activity can also be seen, characterized by less rapid deflections (Figure 17.3). Less commonly used are unipolar lead configurations, which measure cardiac electrical activity directly beneath the electrode. High-pass and low-pass filters are applied to EGMs for display to reduce noise and interference. The usual filter range for bipolar EGM recording is 30–500 Hz.

EGMs are displayed on the recording screen by the position of the catheter (e.g., HRA for high right atrial, CS for coronary sinus, HIS for His bundle, and RV for right ventricular) or by the name of the catheter (e.g., DD for duodecapolar or Abl. for ablation catheter) and the pair of electrodes from which the recording is originating. In a basic diagnostic study, quadripolar catheters inserted in the HRA, HIS, and RV, with 2 or 3 EGMs displayed for each catheter. Other catheters are multipolar catheters with multiple pairs of recording electrodes. Pairs of electrodes can be distinguished by a subscript p for proximal, m for middle, and d for distal (e.g., HIS_p, HIS_m, HIS_d) or by number pair, where by convention, electrode 1 is the most distal, electrode 2 is next sequentially (e.g., CS 1,2 representing the most distal bipolar recording pair of electrodes, CS 3,4 representing the second most distal pair, etc.) (Figure 17.3).

The amplitude of the EGMs depends on multiple factors: electrode contact to the myocardial tissue, the proximity of an electrode to the tissue from where the EGM originates, and the health of the myocardial tissue. Catheters placed on the annulus will record atrial and ventricular EGMs with approximately the same amplitude. As the catheter moves away from the annulus and towards the atrium, the atrial EGM will progressively become higher amplitude than the ventricular EGM, and vice versa for a catheter moving away from the annulus from the ventricular side. Areas of myocardium with a significant amount of fibrosis will have relatively lower amplitudes than normal myocardial tissue. On the display screen, the gain can be adjusted to improve visualization of low amplitude signals.

In a typical diagnostic study, baseline intracardiac intervals: RR, AH, and HV are measured, and the responses to pacing from different sites in the atria and ventricles are analyzed. The interval between two consecutive instances of the same recurring EGM is called the cycle length, and is measured in milliseconds (msec). In order to convert cycle length to beats per minute (bpm), which is used more routinely in surface ECG terminology, the conversion formula is: heart rate (bpm) = 60,000/cycle length (msec).

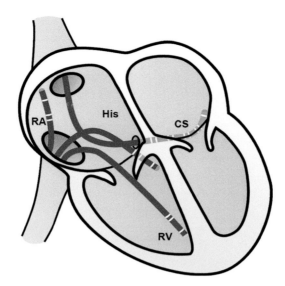

Figure 17.1 Basic positioning of intracardiac electrode catheters for diagnostic electrophysiology study. Three of the basic catheters used in electrophysiologic studies are quadripolar catheters including the RA (right atrium), His bundle, and RV (right ventricle), all of which are generally inserted through femoral venous access. The CS (coronary sinus) catheter is usually a decapolar electrode catheter, which is commonly inserted via the right internal jugular vein.

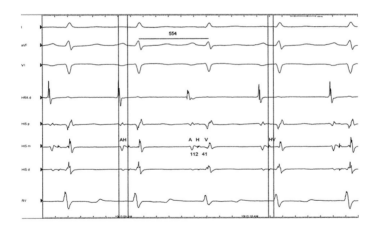

Figure 17.2 Basic intervals: RR, AH, and HV. All measurements are in milliseconds (msec). Three surface electrocardiographic (ECG) leads are shown along with high right atrium (HRA), His bundle, and right ventricle (RV) electrogram (EGM) recordings. Subscripts denote recording pair of electrodes on each quadripolar catheter: p: proximal, m: middle, d: distal. The RR interval (554 msec) is measured between two R waves and can be measured on any lead from surface ECG or from ventricular EGMs on intracardiac recordings. The AH and HV intervals are measured on the mid-His bundle catheter in this case, where the onset of the His bundle EGM, denoted by H is most clearly seen as a small sharp deflection. The AH interval (114 msec, normal 50–120 msec) is measured from the beginning of the atrial EGM (A) on the HISm lead to the His bundle EGM (H). The HV interval (41 msec, normal 35–55 msec) is measured from the His bundle EGM (H) to the first ventricular activation (V) on any surface ECG lead or intracardiac lead.

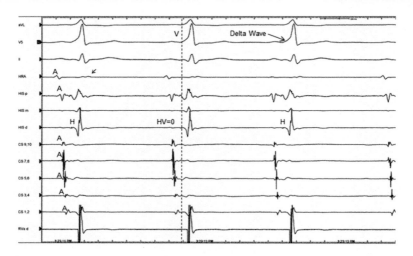

Figure 17.3 Intracardiac recording in sinus rhythm in a patient with a posteroseptal bypass tract. This shows 3 surface electrocardiographic leads with a standard array of intracardiac electrogram (EGM) recordings obtained from 4 catheters: HRA: High Right Atrium, HIS: His bundle, CS: coronary Sinus, RVa: Right Ventricular Apex. Subscripts denote recording pair of electrodes on each quadripolar catheter: p: proximal, m: middle, d: distal. Number pairs denote recording pair of electrodes on a multipolar catheter where 9,10 is the most proximal pair and 1,2 is the most distal pair. The atrial EGM is labeled "A" in the figure, and activation moves from HRA to His to CS (proximal to distal). The dotted vertical line shows the time of first ventricular activation, labeled V, which coincide on the surface leads and the intracardiac His tracings resulting in a short HV interval of 0 msec (normal 35–55 msec), indicative of a bypass tract. A far field ventricular EGM, denoted by the arrow, is seen in the atrial electrode.

BASIC INTERVALS

Precise measurements of AV conduction can be performed with intracardiac recording. In addition to the basic surface ECG measurements of the PR, QRS, QT, PP, and RR intervals, in an electrophysiologic study, atrioventricular conduction can be further analyzed by quantifying the AH and HV intervals. These are measured at the His bundle catheter, which due to its location on the superior tricuspid annulus between atrial and ventricular tissue can simultaneously record atrial, His bundle, and ventricular depolarization (Figure 17.2).

The AH interval is the time measured between the initial atrial depolarization and the His bundle depolarization as measured on by the His bundle catheter. Normal values are 50–120 msec. This measures conduction across the atrioventricular (AV) node and is highly dependent on vagal, sympathetic tone, as well as medications such as beta blockers or calcium channel blockers, which slow conduction (negative dromotropy), or isoproterenol, which speeds up conduction (positive dromotropy). Significantly prolonged AH intervals in the lack of reversible factors may represent high vagal tone, intrinsic AV nodal disease, or conduction down the slow pathway of the AV node (Figure 17.4).

The HV interval is the time measured between His bundle depolarization and the earliest ventricular depolarization either on surface ECG or on EGM. Normal values are 35–55 msec. Shorter values may represent pre-excitation via bypass, tracts, which depolarize ventricular tissue independent of the AV node and the His Purkinje system (Figure 17.3). Longer values usually represent Purkinje system disease though in rare cases, this may be the manifestation of conduction delay within the His bundle itself (Figure 17.5).

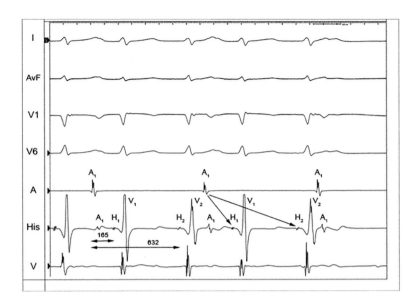

Figure 17.4 Sinus rhythm with 1:2 atrioventricular (AV) response. Sinus rhythm is seen on intra-cardiac atrial (A_1) recording. Following each atrial electrogram (EGM), there are two His bundle and ventricular EGMs, one conducting with a normal AH interval (representing fast AV pathway conduction), and one with a very prolonged AH interval (slow pathway conduction). There is prolongation of AH intervals prior to AV block, indicating 2nd degree Type I (Mobitz I) AV block in both pathways. (Modified from Bradfield, J. et al., *J. Cardiovasc. Electrophys.*, 21, 1062–1063, 2010. With permission.)

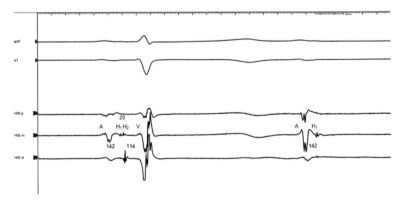

Figure 17.5 Intra-Hisian block. All measurements are in milliseconds (msec). His bundle catheter recordings are shown in addition to surface electrocardiogram (ECG). AV block is seen on surface ECG. On the first beat, intracardiac recording shows an AH interval of 140 msec (normal 50–120 msec), two His electrograms (EGMs) denoted by H_1 and H_2, with a prolonged HV interval of 114 msec (normal 35–55 msec) as measured from H_1 to the first ventricular depolarization (V), with an H1H2 interval of 20 msec. On the second beat, the AH interval remains constant with an H_1 EGM present, but loss of H_2 and V, indicating that AV block occurs within the His bundle.

Distinguishing the site of conduction delay or block by recording the AH and HV intervals during electrophysiologic study can assist with determining whether a pacemaker should be implanted in cases where the etiology of atrioventricular block is uncertain.

Retrograde conduction, measured by the VA interval, the time between ventricular depolarization to the earliest atrial depolarization is also helpful in the study of supraventricular tachycardias. The manner by which the atrium is depolarized in the retrograde direction can also indicate whether a bypass tract is present. Retrograde conduction through the AV node depolarizes the atrium in a midline (or concentric) fashion where atrial EGMs propagate from CS 9,10, which is the most midline electrode pair in the CS catheter, towards CS 1,2, which is the most lateral electrode pair. Other patterns of depolarization are consistent with bypass tracts, though midline depolarization may also be seen with a septal bypass tract, which can insert into the atrium at a similar location to the AV node.

BIBLIOGRAPHY

Bradfield, J., Buch, E., Tung, R., and Shivkumar, K. Recurrent Irregular Tachycardia that Consistently Terminates on a P Wave: What is that Mechanism? *J Cardiovasc Electrophys* 2010, 21, 1062–1063.

Fogoros, Richard N. *Electrophysiologic Testing.* John Wiley & Sons, Chichester, UK, 2012.

Josephson, Mark E. *Josephson's Clinical Cardiac Electrophysiology*, 5th ed. Lippincott Williams & Wilkins, Philadelphia, PA, 2015.

Prystowsky, Eric N., and George J. Klein. *Cardiac Arrhythmias: An Integrated Approach for the Clinician.* McGraw-Hill, New York, 1994.

BASICS OF ELECTROPHYSIOLOGY STUDY

Jonathan R. Hoffman and Marmar Vaseghi

CONTENTS

OVERVIEW

The clinical electrophysiology (EP) study plays an important role in the evaluation and diagnosis of both tachy- and brady-arrhythmias as well as in assessing the heart's atrial and ventricular conduction system. During the standard EP study, multipolar catheters are placed in various locations within the heart. The particular locations can vary depending on the purpose of the study, but typical locations include the high right atrium, the right ventricular apex or base, the His bundle, and the coronary sinus (Figure 18.1). These catheters are used to record electrograms, which can be measured as difference between electromyographic signals from two different electrodes (bipolar recording), or in relation to a single electrode (unipolar recording). Using these catheters, the electrophysiologic properties of the heart's conduction system, including the sinus node, the atrioventricular node, the His Purkinje system, and the atrial and ventricular myocardium can be assessed both at baseline and in response to pharmacologic agents such as isoproterenol, adenosine, atropine, procainamide, and epinephrine, among others. In addition, multiple pacing maneuvers are performed using these catheters, both to assess the response of the heart's conduction system to stress, as well as to attempt to induce various arrhythmias.

BASELINE MEASUREMENTS

CONDUCTION INTERVALS

During a standard EP study, there are several baseline conduction times or intervals that are measured. These include the cardiac cycle length, commonly measured as the duration between two consecutive R waves and recorded as the "RR" interval; the PR interval, measured from the onset of the P wave to the onset of the following QRS complex; the QRS duration; the QT interval, measured from the onset of the QRS complex to the point where the most negative slope of the terminal portion of the T wave intersects with the baseline;

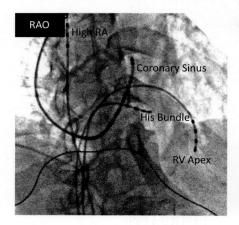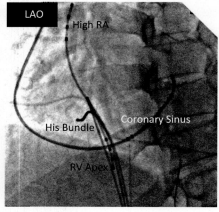

Figure 18.1 Fluoroscopic positions of the catheters for a standard EP study are shown in the right anterior oblique (RAO), left panel, and left anterior oblique (LAO), right panel, views. A quadripolar catheter is placed in the high right atrium (High RA), a decapolar catheter is placed in the coronary sinus, a quadripolar catheter is used for His bundle recordings, and a quadripolar catheter is placed in the right ventricular apex (RV apex).

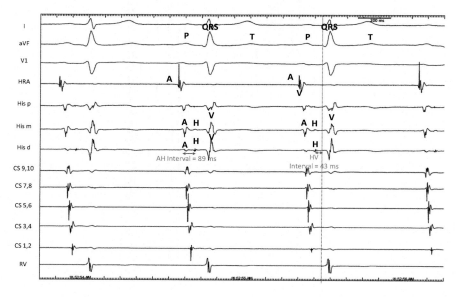

Figure 18.2 Measurements of basic intracardiac intervals are shown. These including the A–H interval, measured from the beginning of the atrial electrogram to the His potential recording, the HV interval, measured from the His potential recording to the earliest ventricular activation on the surface electrocardiogram. CS 9,10 is the proximal coronary sinus electrode and CS 1,2 is the most distal coronary sinus electrode. His p = proximal, His m = middle, His d = distal His bundle electrodes. HRA = high right atrium. RV = right ventricle.

the A–H interval, measured from the earliest intracardiac atrial activity to the His potential; and the HV interval, measured from the His potential to the earliest ventricular activity on the surface ECG (Figure 18.2). These conduction times are typically recorded in milliseconds, and are often repeated following administration of pharmacologic agents such as isoproterenol.

BASIC PACING CONCEPTS

Intracardiac pacing is generally performed in a bipolar fashion. An electrical impulse is applied through a catheter with the current flowing from the most distal electrode, stimulating the heart, and returning to a second, typically adjacent electrode, with the goal of depolarizing the local myocardium. This often results in a stimulation artifact on the pacing catheter recordings. When the stimulation current successfully depolarizes the myocardium, the impulse is said to have captured the myocardium. If the impulse does not depolarize the myocardium, the impulse is said to have failed to capture. In order to capture the myocardium, both the amplitude and duration of the impulse can be adjusted, controlling the amount of current delivered.

There are several common terms used to describe certain pacing maneuvers. Most maneuvers are initiated with a series of consecutive paced beats with a constant pacing interval, called a drive train. The delivered stimulus comprising the drive train is called the S1 stimulus. Frequently, one or more stimulus is/are delivered at the end of the drive train with a shortened coupling interval. These stimuli are called extrastimuli, and are demarcated as S2, S3, S4, and so forth to represent the first, second, third, and any additional extrastimuli. Intracardiac electrograms associated with myocardial capture of these stimuli are named based on the initiating stimulus and the structure activated; for example, atrial, ventricular, or His bundle electrograms associated with the drive train (S1) are named A1, V1, or H1, respectively. An atrial electrogram associated with the first, second, or third extrastimulus (S2, S3, or S4) is named A2, A3, A4, respectively. Nomenclature for ventricular or His bundle electrograms associated with extrastimuli follows the same pattern.

PACING MANEUVERS

There are multiple pacing maneuvers that can be performed during an EP study. The most common maneuvers will be covered below. These include extrastimulus testing, decremental pacing, burst pacing, differential pacing, and pacing with variable output.

EXTRASTIMULUS PACING

During extrastimulus pacing, a drive train of 6–10 beats (typically at intervals between 400 and 600 ms) is followed by one or more extrastimuli (premature beat) that is placed at a coupling interval less than the drive train (generally starting between 300 and 500 ms, Figure 18.3). Initially, the drive train is followed by a single extrastimulus beat. This is repeated multiple times with progressive shortening of the coupling interval between the drive train and extrastimulus beat (S1S2 interval), usually by 10–20 ms, until the extrastimulus fails to capture the myocardium. The interval at which the extrastimulus fails to capture is called the effective refractory period. Additional extrastimuli can then be added, with the S1S2 coupling interval increased and generally set at 10–20 ms above the S2 refractory period. Progressive shortening of the coupling interval between the additional extrastimuli (S_xS_{x+1}), again by 10–20 ms is performed, until these also fail to capture. The coupling intervals are typically not decreased below 200 ms due to the risk of inducing non-specific arrhythmias. Extrastimulus pacing has multiple roles during the standard EP study. It is used to define atrial, ventricular, and AV nodal effective refractory periods, investigating dual AV nodal physiology, and induce arrhythmias (described in more detail below).

DECREMENTAL PACING

During decremental pacing, a cardiac chamber is initially paced at a cycle length slightly shorter than the sinus rate. The cycle length is then gradually shortened every few beats, usually by 10–20 ms. This maneuver is used to define the Wenckebach cycle length, or the cycle length at which conduction from the paced chamber to the opposing chamber begins to prolong until conducted beats are intermittently blocked (Figure 18.4). For example, while performing decremental pacing in the atrium, the rate at which conduction from the atrium to the ventricle changes from 1:1 to intermittent conduction to the ventricle (3:1, 4:1, etc.)

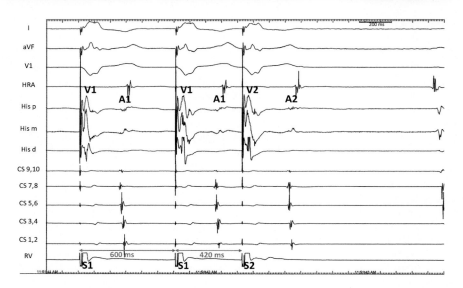

Figure 18.3 During extrastimulus pacing, a drive train (S1) of 6–10 beats (typically at intervals between 400 and 600 ms) is followed by one or more extrastimuli (premature beat) that is placed at a coupling interval less than the drive train (generally starting between 300 and 500 ms). In this case the drive train (S1 train) is at 600 ms with an extra-stimulus (S2) placed at an interval of 420 ms. CS 9,10 is the proximal coronary sinus electrode and CS 1,2 is the most distal coronary sinus electrode. His p = proximal, His m = middle, His d = distal His bundle electrodes. HRA = high right atrium. RV = right ventricle. S = stimulus.

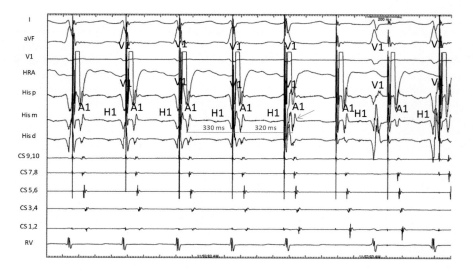

Figure 18.4 Decremental pacing in the high right atrium is performed to determine the antegrade AV node Wenckebach cycle length, the rate at which conduction from the atrium to the ventricle changes from 1:1 to intermittent conduction (3:1, 4:1, etc.). In this case the antegrade AV node Wenckebach cycle length occurs at 320 ms. Arrow points to the atrial beat that fails to conduct to the ventricle. CS 9,10 is the proximal coronary sinus electrode was CS 1,2 is the most distal coronary sinus electrode. His p = proximal, His m = middle, His d = distal His bundle electrodes. HRA = high right atrium. RV = right ventricle.

due to decremental properties of the AV nodal is the antegrade AV node Wenckebach cycle length. If retrograde AV nodal conduction is present, the cycle length at which paced beats fail to conduct from the ventricle to the atrium, assuming lack of accessory pathway presence, is called the retrograde AV nodal Wenckebach cycle length.

BURST PACING

During burst pacing, a group of beats is delivered at a fixed cycle length faster than the intrinsic cardiac rate. This can be done in sinus rhythm from either the atrium or ventricle to attempt to induce arrhythmias, or can be performed during tachycardia at a cycle length slightly shorter than the tachycardia cycle length to try to overdrive the arrhythmia's circuit in a maneuver called overdrive pacing.

DIFFERENTIAL PACING

Differential pacing consists of pacing at the same rate from different locations within a cardiac chamber and measuring conduction times to downstream cardiac structures. For example, differential pacing from the right ventricular apex versus the base and measuring the conduction time from the ventricle to the atrium, is often performed to differentiate between retrograde conduction through the AV node versus retrograde conduction utilizing a septal accessory pathway.

PACING AT VARIABLE OUTPUT

By pacing at different outputs, different cardiac structures can be captured. For example, during parahisian pacing, low-output pacing near the His bundle captures the local myocardium, while high-output pacing captures the His Purkinje system as well as the ventricular myocardium (Figure 18.5). This maneuver can also be useful in identifying presence of accessory pathway.

REFRACTORY PERIODS

As mentioned above, in addition to baseline conduction times, the refractory periods of important cardiac structures including the conduction system are also measured. The most commonly measured refractory period is the effective refractory period (ERP), or the longest coupling interval between captured beats, which fails to capture or conduct to a given cardiac structure. For example, when pacing the atrium at a drive train of 600 ms, if both the drive train and extrastimulus beat with an S1S2 coupling interval of 250 ms capture the atrium (eliciting both an A1 and A2), but when the coupling interval is decreased to 240 ms, the S2 fails to capture the atrium (only an A1 is observed), the atrial ERP is reported to be 240 ms at a drive cycle length of 600 ms.

Ventricular effective refractory period and AV node effective refractory period are two other parameters that are measured as part of a standard EP study. AV node effective refractory period is defined as the longest A1A2 interval, when pacing the atrium, that fails to conduct to the His bundle (no H2 is observed). Let's assume in the above example that while pacing at a drive train of 600 ms, an extrastimulus beat with an S1S2 coupling interval of 260 ms captures the atrium eliciting an A2, and the action potential then propagates through the AV node, His, and ventricle, eliciting an H2 and V2. However, when the S1S2 coupling interval is decreased to 250 ms, the extrastimulus elicits an A2, but does not propagate through the His bundle to the ventricle (H2 and V2 are absent) (Figure 18.6). Here, the AV node ERP is 250 ms at a drive train of 600 ms.

In addition to the ERP, the relative refractory period (RRP) and functional refractory period (FRP) can also be measured. The RRP is the longest coupling interval that results in a conduction delay. For example, while pacing in the atrium, the conduction time from the atrium to the His bundle will initially be constant, but as the A1A2 coupling interval is decreased, the AH conduction time will begin to prolong (i.e., the A2H2 time becomes longer than the A1H1 time). The AV node RRP occurs at the longest A1A2 coupling interval where A2H2 is longer than A1H1. The FRP is defined the shortest output interval that can be observed with any given input interval (i.e., when pacing the atrium, the shortest V1V2 that can be elicited with any A1A2).

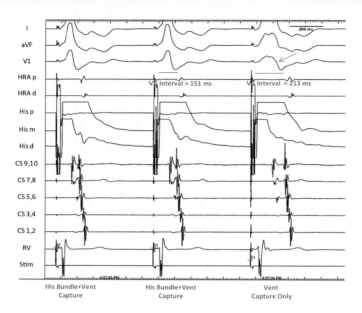

Figure 18.5 Example of parahisian pacing is shown. High-output pacing from the His bundle catheter initially shows His bundle and ventricular capture with ventricular surface QRS beats that are narrower than when the output is lowered slightly and the His bundle is no longer captured resulting in a wider QRS (arrow) and ventricular capture only. The ventricular to atrial activation time (VA time) during His bundle capture is shorter than during ventricular myocardial capture alone, consistent with AV nodal retrograde conduction. Note that the VA interval is measured from the earliest ventricular activation on the surface ECG to a designated atrial electrogram, in this case, the high right atrial electrogram, for each paced beat. Vent = ventricular. CS 9,10 is the proximal coronary sinus electrode and CS 1,2 is the most distal coronary sinus electrode. His p = proximal, His m = middle, His d = distal His bundle electrodes. HRA p = proximal and HRA d = distal high right atrial electrodes. RV = right ventricle. S = stimulus.

SINUS NODE TESTING

Sinus node function can be assessed during an EP study by the sinus node recovery time (SNRT). To test the sinus node, the atrium is paced at a rate greater than the sinus rate for at least 30 s. The SNRT is the time from the last paced atrial electrogram, from the high right atrium, to the first spontaneous atrial electrogram that is observed. This should be repeated with at least 3 different pacing cycle lengths with the longest SNRT noted. The corrected SNRT is the measured SNRT minus the spontaneous sinus cycle length prior to pacing. A normal value is less than 550 ms; longer values indicate abnormal sinus node function.

TYPICAL EP STUDY

The EP study will vary depending on the purpose of the study, but certain measurements are standard to most studies. In general, catheters are placed in the high RA, RV apex, and His bundle. In many cases, a coronary sinus catheter is also placed. A basic EP study will almost always involve baseline measurements, pacing in the atrium, and pacing in the ventricle.

BASELINE MEASUREMENTS

Baseline intervals should always be obtained, including the cardiac cycle length, PR, QT, AH, and HV intervals, as well as QRS duration.

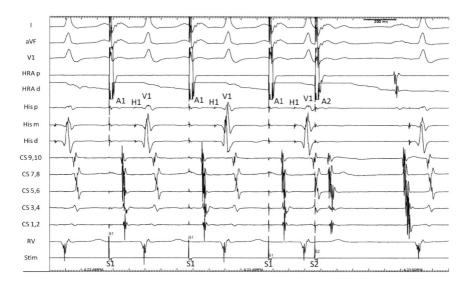

Figure 18.6 AV nodal effective refractory period is shown. The S2 extra-stimulus interval is shortened until the captured atrial beat (A2) fails to propagate through the AV node and does not reach the ventricle. CS 9,10 is the proximal coronary sinus electrode and CS 1,2 is the most distal coronary sinus electrode. His p = proximal, His m = middle, His d = distal His bundle electrodes. HRA p = proximal and HRA d = distal high right atrial electrodes. RV = right ventricle. S = stimulus.

ATRIAL PACING

During a basic EP study, the following maneuvers are typically performed during atrial pacing:

- Assessment of sinus node function by measurement of the SNRT at least 3 different cycle lengths.
- Decremental pacing to assess AV node antegrade Wenckebach cycle length and from the ventricle to assess presence of retrograde atrial conduction.
- Extrastimulus pacing from the atrium. This will evaluate for dual AV nodal physiology (demonstrated when conduction from the atrium to the His bundle increases by more than 50 ms with a 10 ms shortening of the A1A2 coupling interval; i.e., when A1A2 is decreased by 10 ms, A2H2 increases by >50 ms, signifying the transition from conduction over the fast pathway to conduction over the slow pathway and is referred to as a "jump" (Figure 18.7). Extrastimulus pacing is also used to determine the AV node ERP, atrial ERP, and to induce arrhythmias.
- Burst pacing to induce arrhythmias.

VENTRICULAR PACING

The following maneuvers are typically performed during ventricular pacing:

- *Assessment of presence and pattern of retrograde atrial activation*: Retrograde conduction from the ventricle to the atrium is present in 40%–60% of patients. If retrograde conduction is present, the pattern of atrial activation is examined to determine whether activation occurs in a concentric manner the atrial septum outwards (for example, by His bundle distal to proximal activation and by coronary sinus proximal to distal atrial activation, Figure 18.8). Eccentric atrial activation occurs when an accessory pathway is present or in the setting of atrial tachycardia. In this case, atrial activation is not earliest at the atrial septum and may be earlier in the lateral right atrium (in case of right-sided accessory pathway) or lateral left atrium (in case of left-sided accessory pathway).

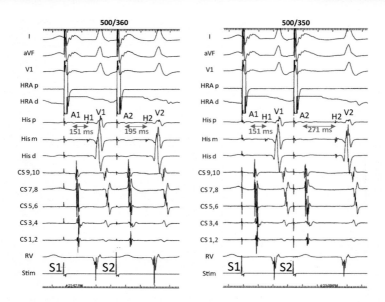

Figure 18.7 Extrastimulus pacing from the right atrium in this case show that when the A1A2 is decreased by 10 ms, A2H2 increases by >50 ms (from 195 to 271 ms), and an "AH jump", is therefore observed, signifying the transition from conduction over the fast AV nodal pathway to conduction over the slow pathway. CS 9,10 is the proximal coronary sinus electrode and CS 1,2 is the most distal coronary sinus electrode. His p = proximal, His m = middle, His d = distal His bundle electrodes. HRA p = proximal and HRA d = distal high right atrial electrodes. RV = right ventricle. S = stimulus.

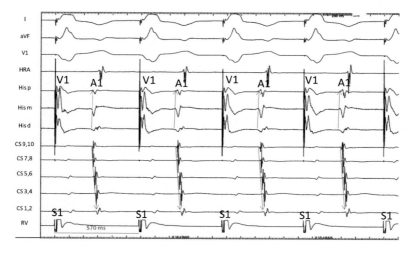

Figure 18.8 Concentric retrograde atrial activation is shown. The pattern of atrial activation shows His bundle distal to proximal activation and by coronary sinus proximal to distal atrial activation. CS 9,10 is the proximal coronary sinus electrode and CS 1,2 is the most distal coronary sinus electrode. His p = proximal, His m = middle, His d = distal His bundle electrodes. HRA = high right atrium. RV = right ventricle.

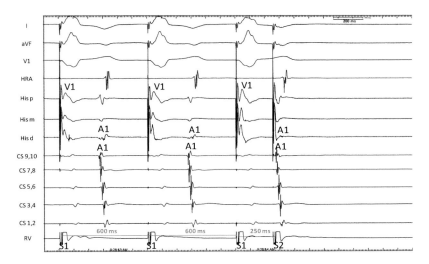

Figure 18.9 Ventricular extrastimulus pacing is used to determine ventricular effective refractory period, or the longest extra-stimulus interval where S2 no longer captures the ventricle, as observed on both surface ECG and intracardiac ventricular electrograms. CS 9,10 is the proximal coronary sinus electrode was CS 1,2 is the most distal coronary sinus electrode. His p = proximal, His m = middle, His d = distal His bundle electrodes. HRA = high right atrium. RV = right ventricle.

- *Decremental pacing*: Assuming that retrograde conduction is present, decremental pacing is used to determine the retrograde AV nodal Wenckebach cycle length.
- *Ventricular extrastimulus pacing*: Ventricular extrastimulus pacing is used to determine the ventriculo-atrial ERP, as well as the ventricular ERP (Figure 18.9). In addition, it is frequently used to risk stratify patients for ventricular arrhythmias, or for induction of ventricular tachycardias for mapping and/or ablation. Ventricular extrastimulus pacing is often performed with single, double, and triple extrastimuli, from two different locations (often apex and base of the right ventricle), and at two different drive cycle lengths.

In summary, although many laboratories follow different protocols during an EP study, the above represents many of the basic maneuvers commonly utilized during these studies. It's important to note that multiple other maneuvers, described elsewhere in this book, can be added depending on the goals of the study, such as the use of isoproterenol to facilitate arrhythmia induction; adenosine to block the AV node; and differential pacing and/or paraHisian pacing to assess for presence of septal accessory pathways. In addition, if the patient enters the study in a persistent arrhythmia, or an arrhythmia is induced during the study, maneuvers such as overdrive pacing are frequently performed to further characterize the arrhythmia. While the above protocol is by no means comprehensive, it provides a firm foundation for the basics of an EP study.

BIBLIOGRAPHY

1. Josephson ME. *Clinical Cardiac Electrophysiology: Techniques and Interpretations*, 4th ed. Lippincott Williams and Wilkins, Philadelphia, PA, 2008.
2. Zipes D, Jailfe J. *Cardiac Electrophysiology: From Cell to Bedside*, 5th ed. Saunders, Philadelphia, PA, 2009.

HEAD-UP TILT (HUT) TABLE TESTING

Subramanya Prasad, Amer Kadri, J. David Burkhardt,
Thomas Dresing, and Kenneth Mayuga

CONTENTS

INTRODUCTION/BACKGROUND

- HUT testing with or without adjunctive pharmacologic agents is the most commonly used test for syncope evaluation. Several studies have shown that the vasodepressor-cardioinhibitory response seen during a HUT test is comparable to spontaneous neurally mediated syncope (NMS).[1,2]
- In the young healthy individual or the elderly with syncope of unknown etiology, it is considered the gold standard test.[3,4]

  Throughout this chapter, * denotes a Class I recommendation; # denotes a Class II recommendation, and ^ denotes a Class III recommendation.
- The physiologic basis for HUT testing is discussed in detail under pathophysiology.
- Briefly, in healthy humans, orthostatic stress causes peripheral pooling of 500–1000 mL of blood, triggering arterial mechanoreceptors (major role) and thoracic wall and cardiac mechanoreceptors (minor role) to stimulate the vasomotor center (VMC) via afferent C fibers.
- The VMC sends efferent vagal signals (cardioinhibitory) and neuroendocrine modulators causing reflex vasoconstriction of the splanchnic, musculocutaneous, and renal vascular beds, thus maintaining systemic arterial blood pressure during standing.
- In patients with NMS, these responses are deficient, resulting in syncope.

HUT INDICATIONS

The European Society of Cardiology (ESC) guidelines in 2009[31] recommend the following Indications and Contraindications for HUT:

* HUT is indicated in the case of unexplained single syncopal episode in high-risk settings.
* HUT is indicated when it is of clinical value to demonstrate susceptibility to reflex syncope to the patient.
# HUT should be considered to discriminate between reflex and orthostatic hypotension syncope.

HUT may be considered to differentiate syncope with jerking movements from epilepsy.

HUT may be considered for evaluating patients with recurrent unexplained falls.

HUT may be considered for evaluating patients with frequent syncope and psychiatric disease.

^ HUT is **not recommended** for assessment of treatment.

^ Isoproterenol is **contraindicated** in patients with ischemic heart disease.

The Heart Rhythm Society 2015 Expert Consensus Document[39] recommends the following indications and contraindications for HUT:

HUT can be useful for assessing patients with suspected vasovagal syncope who lack a confident diagnosis after the initial assessment.

HUT is a reasonable option for differentiating between convulsive syncope and epilepsy, for establishing a diagnosis of pseudosyncope, and for testing patients with suspected vasovagal syncope but without clear diagnostic features.

HUT may be considered to identify patients with a hypotensive response who would be less likely to respond to permanent cardiac pacing for vasovagal syncope.

HUT may be considered for selected patients being assessed for Postural Tachycardia Syndrome (POTS).

^ HUT is **not recommended** for predicting the response to specific medical treatments for vasovagal syncope.

TEST PROCEDURE/TILT TESTING PROTOCOLS

PROCEDURE

- The HUT is usually performed in an EP lab using a specialized tilt table.
- HUT testing with pharmacologic provocation has been used to increase the sensitivity of HUT testing.
- The set-up of a HUT test is relatively straightforward. The HUT table is set up in a quiet room with minimal distractions.
- The table should have a footboard and safety restraints and be capable of passive swinging in a smooth yet rapid fashion, from 0 to 90 degrees within 10 s.
- Infusion pumps capable of giving IV fluids and medications should be kept close.
- The patient is usually advised to be in a fasting state (the rationale being to avoid postprandial splanchnic pooling, or vomiting during the procedure) for at least 2 h prior to the procedure.
- After excluding orthostatic BP changes at baseline, and obtaining peripheral venous access, the patient should rest in the supine position for 20–45 min to decrease the likelihood of a vasovagal response due to venous cannulation.
- After obtaining supine heart rate (HR) and BP measurements for 3–5 min, HUT testing is performed between 60 and 90 degrees for 30–45 min.[5]
- Tilting at an angle of 60 degrees may decrease the sensitivity but may increase the specificity.[38]
- Blood pressure, HR, and symptoms are recorded every minute along with continuous ECG monitoring, throughout the test. The possibility of profound asystole >10 s requires careful monitoring.
- Though continuous beat-to-beat arterial BP monitoring is the preferred method, most centers use intermittent sphygmomanometer measurements, especially in children. Another option is the use of beat-to-beat finger plethysmography, which allows for continuous non-invasive measurement of blood pressure.
- The patient is returned to baseline if the test becomes positive (loss of consciousness, unable to maintain posture with hypotension, or bradycardia) or upon completion of the protocol.

HUT TESTING PROTOCOLS

- HUT testing with or without pharmacologic provocation has proved to be a useful tool for diagnosis of syncope.
- Though the Westminster protocol (non-pharmacologic) is most preferred, other protocols utilizing pharmacologic provocation with isoproterenol, nitroglycerin (NTG), and clomipramine (less commonly edrophonium and adenosine) have been used due to higher positivity rates. Table 19.1 lists the features of the various HUT protocols.
- Since the Westminster protocol is the most commonly used protocol, it is discussed first in detail, followed by other specific protocols which are used less frequently.

METHOD

- The Westminster protocol (passive HUT at 60–70 degrees from 20 to 45 min) is the commonly preferred protocol in the initial evaluation of syncope.
- If the passive phase is negative, pharmacologic provocation using intravenous isoproterenol or sublingual NTG is performed.

ADVANTAGES AND PITFALLS

- HUT testing is a safe procedure with minimal complications. Most patients have symptoms ranging from nausea/vomiting to the effects of a syncopal episode reproduced by HUT testing.
- Symptoms reported during tilt (other than syncope) range widely and include dizziness, diaphoresis, nausea, paleness, general weakness, and parasthesia.[35,36]
- Asystole during VVS as long as 73 s has been reported.[7] A quick return of the table to the supine position and raising the legs is enough to restore consciousness in most patients.
- Rarely ventricular arrhythmias (especially with isoproterenol provocation) in patients with cardiac ischemia[8] and self-limited atrial fibrillation[9] have been reported. Hence isoproterenol provocation is contraindicated in patients with coronary artery disease.

HUT WITH CAROTID SINUS MASSAGE

- Carotid sinus massage (CSM), when performed carefully, can provide a clinical diagnosis of carotid sinus syndrome. Similar to NMS, stimulation of the mechanoreceptors of the carotid sinus results in VMC-mediated parasympathetic and sympathetic responses.
- CSM should be performed preferably in conjunction with HUT in syncope due to unexplained cause, especially among patients >40 years because, in addition to an increased rate of positive responses, an additional vasodepressor component (usually seen in carotid sinus hypersensitivity [CSH]) can be identified.
- A CSM is contraindicated if (i) carotid bruit is present, (ii) CVA/TIA has occurred in the last 3 months, (iii) myocardial infarction within the last 6 months, and (iv) there is a history of VT or VF.[10]

The ESC 2009 guidelines[31] recommend the following indication for CSM:

* CSM is indicated in patients >40 years old with syncope of unknown etiology after initial evaluation.

^ CSM should not be done in patients with previous TIA or stroke within the past 3 months and in patients with carotid bruits (except if Doppler studies excluded significant carotid stenosis).

- The CSM should be done as follows:
  - The carotid arteries should be palpated on both sides and auscultated for the presence of bruits (indicative of carotid disease).

Table 19.1 The various HUT protocols including methods, endpoints, response, and interpretation

HUT protocol	Method	Endpoints	Response and diagnosis	Comments
HUT testing	*Supine pretilt phase of at least 5 min (without iv) and at least 20 min (with iv). *Tilt angle of 60–70 degrees with a passive phase of 20 min (minimum) and 45 min (maximum) Westminster protocol is the commonly preferred protocol (90% specificity) in the initial evaluation of syncope. *Pharmacologic provocation using intravenous isoproterenol or sublingual nitroglycerin if passive phase is negative. *Drug challenge phase duration of 15–20 min.	*While most physicians consider steadily decreasing BP with symptoms as the endpoint, some prefer to terminate the test with occurrence of LOC.[20] *In patients with structural heart disease, spontaneous syncope during HUT is diagnostic and requires no further testing.	Three responses are seen 1. Cardioinhibitory (type 2) 2. Vasodepressor (type 3) 3. Mixed (type 1). A typical vasovagal response starts invariably with Prodromal symptoms which precede WR by 1 min.[21,22] The WS usually lasts for <3 min.[20] Marked hypotension is seen during the prodromal phase followed by bradycardia[20–22] While presyncope is seen with an SBP decrease of 90 mmHg, syncope is seen with an SBP decrease of 60 mmHg.[21]	The sensitivity of HUT testing can be as high as 80% with a specificity of 70%–86%, depending on the protocol and patient selection.[7,8,23,24] Studies of HUT testing in syncopal patients by Fitzpatrick et al[5] in 1991 reported low positive response rates with angles <60 degrees. By using >60 degree tilt for 45 min (based on a mean time to positive response of 24+/– 10 min plus 2 SD) they reported a positive response rate of 75% (specificity 93%). Even among patients with syncope and a negative EPS, a positive HUT was shown in 75% of patients.[5] The clinical response may be different from the response elicited during HUT,[25] which could explain the varied response to therapy. Thus a negative HUT does not rule out NMS.
Isoproterenol infusion	Single or escalating doses (1, 3, 5 μg/kg) of isoproterenol are infused at baseline to increase the HR (20%–30% > baseline), followed by tilting for 20–30 min during isoproterenol infusion. For isuprenaline, an incremental infusion rate from 1–3 μg/min in order to increase average heart rate by about 20%–25% over baseline, administered without returning the patient to supine position.	The patient is returned to baseline if the test becomes positive or upon completion of the protocol.	LOC with hypotension or loss of postural tone is considered a positive test. Modest BP decrease with symptoms is non-specific.	Studies by Almquist et al using single dose isoproterenol infusion during HUT increased the frequency of positive responses (56% vs 32%) and reduced the duration of HUT.[13] In 1995, Natale et al using incremental low dose isoproterenol infusion during HUT, showed a 61% positive response rate (92% specificity).[27]

(Continued)

Table 19.1 (*Continued*) The various HUT protocols including methods, endpoints, response, and interpretation

HUT protocol	Method	Endpoints	Response and diagnosis	Comments
Nitrates	*Nitroglycerin by intravenous or sublingual route can be used for provocation of hypotension/syncope. *For NTG, a fixed dose of 400 μg NTG administered sublingually, in the upright position.	The patient is returned to baseline if the test becomes positive or upon completion of the protocol.	LOC with hypotension or loss of postural tone is considered a positive test.	In 1994 Raviele et al. used iv nitroglycerin (NTG) infusion in unexplained syncopal patients showing a 53% positive response rate.[27] Later studies by Graham et al[28] and Raviele et al compared sublingual NTG to isoproterenol infusion showing similar positive response rates and specificity, with a better side-effect profile with NTG.
Clomipramine	*A dose of 5 mg (1 mg/min iv) is given during the first 5 min of tilting. HUT is done for the next 15 min, or until syncope occurs	The patient is returned to baseline if the test becomes positive or upon completion of the protocol	LOC with hypotension or loss of postural tone is considered a positive test	A study of 55 patients with WS showed more positive response rates (80% vs 53%) in the clomipramine group.[29]
HUT with CSM	The CSM should be done in conjunction with HUT for 5–10 s in both supine and erect positions. If asystole is seen, CSM is repeated after 1 mg atropine infusion.	The procedure is considered positive if syncope is reproduced during or immediately after massage in the presence of asystole longer than 3 s and/or a fall in systolic blood pressure ≥50 mmHg.	Three responses are seen 1. Cardioinhibitory (type 2) 2. Vasodepressor (type 3) 3. Mixed (type 1). A positive response is diagnostic in the absence of any other competing diagnosis.	Elderly patients undergoing CSM should be monitored for 2 h postprocedure for neurologic events.[10] A study of elderly patients found a 0.28% incidence of neurologic events after CSM, although the events were transient and full recovery was the rule.[10] In a study of 80 patients with unexplained syncope, a 9% positive response was seen during CSM during supine position, as opposed to 60% during a HUT, suggesting that 50% of patients with CSH are missed if CSM is done only in the supine position.[30]

(*Continued*)

Table 19.1 (Continued) The various HUT protocols including methods, endpoints, response, and interpretation

HUT protocol	Method	Endpoints	Response and diagnosis	Comments
ATP infusion[16,17]	# As proposed by Flammang,[18] 20 mg of ATP dissolved in 10 mL of saline is given as a rapid (<2 s) bolus, followed by a 20 mL dextrose solution flush during ECG monitoring.	The test is considered positive if a pause >10 s (even if interrupted by escape beats) is seen[19] Asystole lasting >6 s, or AV block lasting >10 s is considered positive.	ATP testing produces an abnormal response in some patients with unexplained syncope, but not in controls.	ATP infusion is rarely used in the United States. In a study of 316 patients with presyncope/syncope, using this protocol, 41% had a positive response. When they were followed for 50 months, patients with long pauses (>10 s) were more likely to have recurrent symptoms than those with <10 s pauses. The test was positive in 5% of controls.[18] In two studies of unexplained syncope, ATP testing was abnormal in 28% and 41%.[18,19] In a study of patients with syncope due to ECG documented pauses, ATP test reproduced AVB in 53% of patients with AV block but not sinus arrest.[19] These findings suggest that ATP testing may be useful in establishing intermittent AV block as the cause in patients with unexplained syncope.

Note: *Class 1, #Class II, ^Class III.

- Though the presence of a carotid bruit increases the likelihood of stenosis, the absence of bruit does not rule it out, especially in patients with risk factors of atherosclerosis.[32] In patients at increased risk, consideration should be made for imaging the carotids prior to CSM.
  - If no bruits are heard in patients with lower likelihood, a vigorous and circular pressure is applied on the carotid artery anterior to the sternocleidomastoid at the level of the cricoid cartilage (carotid sinus) for 5–10 s in both supine and erect positions, with simultaneous electrocardiographic monitoring.
  - If no response is seen on one side, CSM is repeated on the other side 1–2 min later.
  - If a cardioinhibitory (asystolic) response is seen, the test can be repeated after 1 mg atropine infusion, to look for an additional vasodepressor response.
- In the elderly, CSM should be done cautiously. Elderly patients undergoing CSM should be monitored for 2 h postprocedure for neurologic events.[10]

The ESC 2009 guidelines recommend the following regarding CSM interpretation:[31]

* CSM is considered diagnostic if syncope is reproduced in the presence of asystole >3 s and/or a fall in systolic blood pressure >50 mmHg.

ISOPROTERENOL INFUSION

- Most investigators will use isoproterenol (escalating doses) during a HUT, in patients with a negative HUT and a high index of suspicion of NMS. The use of pharmacologic provocation (isoproterenol) increases positive responses but reduces specificity.[26]
- Isoproterenol infusion is contraindicated in patients with coronary artery disease to avoid provocation of serious arrhythmias or angina.[11]
- HUT with isoproterenol provocation can falsely raise sensitivity.[12]

NTG INFUSION

- NTG is a potent venodilator, which causes venous pooling, but spares the sympathetic compensatory responses to syncope. Thus it is particularly useful in duplicating the vasodepressor response.
- This is known as the Italian protocol.
- Though NTG infusion was used initially, recently many authors have used 400 mg of NTG sublingual spray after a 20 min baseline phase.[13–15]
- It has a superior side-effect profile when compared to isoproterenol with comparable positivity rates.
- HUTT with NTG may have higher sensitivity and specificity than HUTT with Isoproterenol.[38]
- Head-up tilt testing with nitroglycerin has been studied in the elderly.[34]
- Presyncope induced by this protocol seems to be induced by drop in systemic vascular resistance rather than drop in cardiac output.[37]

CLOMIPRAMINE PROTOCOL

- Clomipramine is a central serotonin reuptake inhibitor, leading to sympathetic withdrawal.
- Clomipramine has a reported higher sensitivity and specificity than NTG.[33]

HUT INTERPRETATION AND DIAGNOSIS

HUT interpretation as suggested by Brignole et al.[6,40] includes the following classifications:

- *Type 1 mixed:* HR falls at the time of syncope, but not to <40 bpm, or falls to <40 bpm for <10 s with or without asystole of <3 s. Blood pressure falls before the heart rate falls.

- *Type 2A, cardioinhibition without asystole:* Heart rate falls to a ventricular rate <40 bpm for >10 s, but asystole of >3 s does not occur. Blood pressure falls before the heart rate falls.
- *Type 2B, cardioinhibition with asystole:* Asystole occurs for >3 s. Heart rate fall coincides with or precedes blood pressure fall.
- *Type 3 vasodepressor:* Heart rate does not fall more than 10%, from its peak, at the time of syncope.
- *Exception 1—chronotropic incompetence:* No significant heart rate rise during the tilt (<10% from the pre-tilt rate).
- *Exception 2—excessive heart rate rise:* Excessive heart rate rise both at the onset of the upright position and throughout its duration before syncope (>130 bpm).

The ESC 2009 guidelines[31] outline the following regarding Tilt test diagnosis:

* In patients without structural heart disease, reflex hypotension/bradycardia with reproduction of syncope is diagnostic of reflex syncope.
* In patients without structural heart disease, progressive orthostatic hypotension with reproduction of syncope is diagnostic of orthostatic hypotension.
# In patients without structural heart disease, reflex hypotension/bradycardia *without* reproduction of syncope may be diagnostic of reflex syncope.
# In patients with structural heart disease, arrhythmia, or other cardiovascular cause of syncope should be excluded prior to considering positive tilt test results as diagnostic.
# Induction of loss of consciousness in the absence of hypotension and/or bradycardia should be considered diagnostic of psychogenic pseudo-syncope.

REFERENCES

1. Fitzpatrick A, Williams T, Ahmed R et al. Echocardiographic and endocrine changes during vasovagal syncope induced by prolonged head-up tilt. *Eur J Cardiac Pacing Electrophysiol* 1992; 2: 121–128.
2. Benditt DG, Lurie KG, Adler SW et al. Rationale and methodology of head-up tilt table testing for evaluation of neurally mediated (cardioneurogenic) syncope. In: Zipes DP, Jalife J, eds. *Cardiac Electrophysiology. From Cell to Bedside,* 2nd ed. WB Saunders, Philadelphia, PA, 1995: 115–128.
3. Brignole M, Alboni P, Benditt DG et al. Task Force on Syncope, European Society of Cardiology. Guidelines on management (diagnosis and treatment) of syncope-update 2004. *Europace* 2004; 6(6): 467–537.
4. Oribe E, Caro S, Perera R et al. Syncope: The diagnostic value of head-up tilt testing. *Pacing Clin Electrophysiol* 1997; 20: 874.
5. Fitzpatrick A, Theodorakis G, Vardas P et al. Methodology of head-up tilt testing in patients with unexplained syncope. *J Am Coll Cardiol* 1991; 17: 125–130.
6. Sutton R, Petersen M, Brignole M et al. Proposed classification for tilt induced vasovagal syncope. *Eur J Cardiac Pacing Electrophysiol* 1992; 2; 180–183.
7. Maloney JD, Jaeger FJ, Fouad-Tarazi FM, Morris HH. Malignant vasovagal syncope: Prolonged asystole provoked by head-up tilt. Case report and review of diagnosis, patho-physiology, and therapy. *Cleve Clin J Med* 1988; 55(6): 542–548.
8. Leman RB, Clarke E, Gillette P. Significant complications can occur with ischemic heart disease and tilt table testing. *Pacing Clin Electrophysiol* 1999; 22(4 Pt 1): 675–677.
9. Kapoor WN, Karpf M, Maher Y et al. Syncope of unknown origin. The need for a more cost-effective approach to its diagnosis evaluation. *JAMA* 1982; 247(19): 2687–2691.

10. Davies AJ, Kenny RA. Frequency of neurologic complications following carotid sinus massage. *Am J Cardiol* 1998; 81: 1256.

11. Sheldon R, Rose R, Koshman ML. Isoproterenol tilt-table testing in patients with syncope and structural heart disease. *Am J Cardiol* 1996; 78: 700.

12. Almquist A, Goldenberg IF, Milstein S et al. Provocation of bradycardia and hypotension by isoproterenol and upright posture in patients with unexplained syncope. *N Engl J Med* 1989; 320(6): 346–351.

13. Del Rosso A, Bartoli P, Bartoletti A et al. Shortened head-up tilt testing potentiated with sublingual nitroglycerin in patients with unexplained syncope. *Am Heart J* 1998; 135(4): 564–570.

14. Natale A, Sra J, Akhtar M et al. Use of sublingual nitroglycerin during head-up tilt-table testing in patients >60 years of age. *Am J Cardiol* 1998; 82(10): 1210–1213.

15. Del Rosso A, Bartoletti A, Bartoli P et al. Methodology of head-up tilt testing potentiated with sublingual nitroglycerin in unexplained syncope. *Am J Cardiol* 2000; 85(8): 1007–1011.

16. Belardinelli L, Linden J, Berne RM. The cardiac effects of adenosine. *Prog Cardiovasc Dis* 1989; 32(1): 73–97.

17. Flammang D, Chassing A, Donal E et al. Reproducibility of the adenosine-5′-triphosphate test in vasovagal syndrome. *J Cardiovasc Electrophysiol* 1998; 9(11): 1161–1166.

18. Flammang D, Church T, Waynberger M et al. Can adenosine 5′-triphosphate be used to select treatment in severe vasovagal syndrome? *Circulation* 1997; 96(4): 1201–1208.

19. Brignole M, Gaggioli G, Menozzi C et al. Adenosine-induced atrioventricular block in patients with unexplained syncope: The diagnostic value of ATP testing. *Circulation* 1997; 96(11): 3921–3927.

20. Brignole M, Menozzi C, Del Rosso A et al. New classification of haemodynamics of vasovagal syncope: Beyond the VASIS classification. Analysis of the pre-syncopal phase of the tilt test without and with nitroglycerin challenge. Vasovagal Syncope International Study. *Europace* 2000; 2(1): 66–76.

21. Alboni P, Dinelli M, Gruppillo P et al. Haemodynamic changes early in prodromal symptoms of vasovagal syncope. *Europace* 2002; 4(3): 333–338.

22. Brignole M, Croci F, Menozzi C et al. Isometric arm counter-pressure maneuvers to abort impending vasovagal syncope. *J Am Coll Cardiol* 2002; 40(11): 2053–2059.

23. Sheldon R, Killam S. Methodology of isoproterenol–tilt table testing in patients with syncope. *J Am Coll Cardiol* 1992; 19: 773–779.

24. Fitzpatrick AP, Lee RJ, Epstein LM et al. Effect of patient characteristics on the yield of prolonged baseline head-up tilt testing and the additional yield of drug provocation. *Heart* 1996; 76: 406.

25. Moya A, Brignole M, Menozzi C et al. Mechanism of syncope in patients with isolated syncope and in patients with tilt-positive syncope. *Circulation* 2001; 104: 1261–1267.

26. Natale A, Akhtar M, Jazayeri M et al. Provocation of hypotension during head-up tilt testing in subjects with no history of syncope or presyncope. *Circulation* 1995; 92(1): 54–58.

27. Raviele A, Gasparini G, Di Pede F et al. Nitroglycerin infusion during upright tilt: A new test for the diagnosis of vasovagal syncope. *Am Heart J* 1994; 127(1): 103–111.

28. Graham LA, Gray JC, Kenny RA. Comparison of provocative tests for unexplained syncope: Isoprenaline and glyceryl trinitrate for diagnosing vasovagal syncope. *Eur Heart J* 2001; 22(6): 497–503.

29. Theodorakis GN, Livanis EG, Leftheriotis D et al. Head-up tilt test with clomipramine challenge in vasovagal syndrome—a new tilt testing protocol. *Eur Heart J* 2003; 24(7): 658–663.

30. Morillo CA, Camacho ME, Wood MA et al. Diagnostic utility of mechanical, pharmacological and orthostatic stimulation of the carotid sinus in patients with unexplained syncope. *J Am Coll Cardiol* 1999; 34: 1587.

31. Moya A, Sutton R, Ammirati F et al. Guidelines for the diagnosis and management of syncope (version 2009): The Task Force for the Diagnosis and Management of Syncope of the European Society of Cardiology (ESC). *Eur Heart J* 2009; 30(21): 2631–2671.

32. Sauvé J, Laupacis A, Østbye T et al. Does this patient have a clinically important carotid bruit? *JAMA* 1993; 270(23): 2843–2845. doi:10.1001/jama.1993.03510230081040.

33. Flevari P, Leftheriotis D, Komborozos C et al. Recurrent vasovagal syncope: Comparison between clomipramine and nitroglycerin as drug challenges during head-up tilt testing. *Eur Heart J* 2009; 30(18): 2249–2253.

34. Gieroba ZJ, Newton JL, Parry SW et al. Unprovoked and glyceryl trinitrate–provoked head-up tilt table test is safe in older people: A review of 10 years' experience. *J Am Geriatr Soc* 2004; 52(11): 1913–1915.

35. Naschitz JE, Hardoff D, Bystritzki I et al. The role of the capnography head-up tilt test in the diagnosis of syncope in children and adolescents. *Pediatrics* 1998; 101(2): e6.

36. Asensio E, Oseguera J, Loría A et al. Clinical findings as predictors of positivity of head-up tilt table test in neurocardiogenic syncope. *Arch Med Res* 2003; 34(4): 287–291.

37. Kim BG, Cho SW, Lee HY et al. Reduced systemic vascular resistance is the underlying hemodynamic mechanism in nitrate-stimulated vasovagal syncope during head-up tilt-table test. *J Arrhythm* 2015; 31: 196–200.

38. Forleo C, Guida P, Iacoviello M et al. Head-up tilt testing for diagnosing vasovagal syncope: A meta-analysis. *Int J Cardiol* 2013; 168(1): 27–35.

39. Sheldon RS, Grubb BP 2nd, Olshansky B et al. 2015 Heart rhythm society expert consensus statement on the diagnosis and treatment of postural tachycardia syndrome, inappropriate sinus tachycardia, and vasovagal syncope. *Heart Rhythm* 2015; 12(6): e41–e63.

40. Brignole M, Menozzi C, Del Rosso A et al. New classification of haemodynamics of vasovagal syncope: Beyond the VASIS classification. Analysis of the pre-syncopal phase of the tilt test without and with nitroglycerin challenge. Vasovagal Syncope International Study. *Europace* 2000; 2(1): 66–76.

CATHETER ABLATION TECHNIQUES

ABLATION OF SVT (AVNRT AND AVRT)

Kushwin Rajamani and Patrick Tchou

CONTENTS

CATHETER ABLATION OF AVNRT

In the common form of typical AtrioVentricular Nodal Reentrant Tachycardia (AVNRT), anterograde conduction occurs through the slow AV nodal pathway, typically localized along the tricuspid annulus just anterior to the coronary sinus (CS) os, while retrograde conduction occurs through the fast pathway localized more superiorly along the mid to anterior part of the septum. Earlier attempts at ablation targeted the fast AV nodal pathway,[1,2] proved to be effective in 80%–90% of patients. However, the risk of complete AV block ranged up to 22% due to its close proximity to the compact AV node. Therefore fast pathway ablation is rarely performed now, especially in the context of the safer approach of slow pathway ablation. There are rare and unusual circumstances when fast pathway ablation may be necessary. Those would be described later in the chapter.

SLOW PATHWAY ABLATION
There are two approaches to slow AV nodal pathway ablation. One is called an anatomic approach while the other uses electrogram characteristics to guide ablation. In reality, both approaches use electrogram guidance as well as anatomic landmarks.

ANATOMIC APPROACH
This was first proposed by Jazayery et al.[3] and ablation is performed using only anatomic landmarks (Figure 20.1). Ablation has been primarily performed using 4-mm non-irrigated catheters. Contact force ablation catheter with slow flow irrigation is an appealing alternative, which provides good feedback on adequate tissue. The triangle of Koch from the CS os to the His bundle is divided into three regions called the posterior, mid, and anterior regions. Since the tricuspid valve, one of the borders of the triangle, is almost vertically oriented, these three zones can also be anatomically considered inferior, mid, and superior segments along the septal portion of the tricuspid valve. The ablation catheter is placed along the septal edge of the tricuspid annulus just anterior to the CS os (posterior zone) to obtain an AV ratio of 0.1–0.5. The need for fluoroscopy is significantly reduced with the advent of electro-anatomic mapping systems. Furthermore, the inferior boundary of the His could be tagged (His cloud) which serves as a visual marker if encroached during ablation. If AVNRT is still inducible, further RF ablation is applied adjacent to the previous site with a higher AV ratio. This slightly higher ratio moves the catheter slightly away from the tricuspid annulus so as to transect the tail of the AVN—the slow pathway. If unsuccessful, the catheter is moved toward the mid and superior positions again targeting a small AV ratio. initially, this approach achieves a success rate of

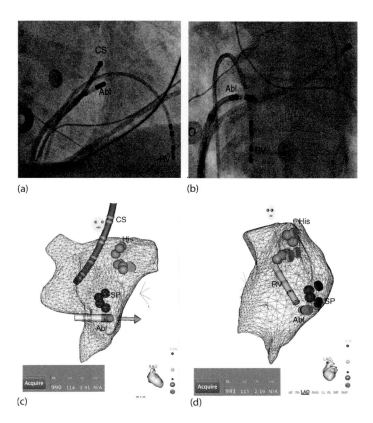

Figure 20.1 Fluroscopic images in RAO (a) confirming ablation catheter is anterior the coronary sinus catheter while slow pathway mapping. Confirmation of catheter is septally and inferiorly oriented in the LAO (b) view. Electro-anatomic images (c, d) in RAO and LAO views with the ablation catheter at the site of the slow pathway. CS, coronary sinus; Abl, ablation catheter; SP, slow pathway; RV, right ventricular catheter.

95%–99% with an extremely low risk of AV block of 0.6%–0.9%. In rare cases, the slow pathway has left-sided extensions and interrogation of either the proximal coronary sinus or the septal mitral annulus via a transeptal access may be required.

ELECTRO-ANATOMIC APPROACH

This electro-anatomic approach utilizes both endocardial potentials and anatomic markers to guide RF ablation (Figure 20.1). Sun[4] described sharp atrial electrograms following a low amplitude atrial electrogram during sinus rhythm. This is recorded around the CS os, usually just anterior to it. Jais[5] described the potential recorded at the mid or posterior septum, anterior to the CS. The potential is variable, from sharp to slow with a common AV ratio of 0.5–0.7. Both of these potentials can be recorded simultaneously in the same patient: the sharp potential more inferiorly and the slow potential more superiorly (Figure 20.2). Occasionally, an overlapping zone near the CS os where both potentials can be recorded is present.

In unusual cases, the slow pathway may be located along the mitral annulus or the AV node may have slow pathway extensions along both the tricuspid and mitral annuli. The mitral annular extensions can sometimes be targeted via the anterior wall of the proximal coronary sinus. When ablation along the tricuspid annulus and the proximal coronary sinus fails, the slow pathway may be located along the mitral annulus. Ablating this pathway may require access to the left atrium via a transeptal approach. Locating the site of ablation is

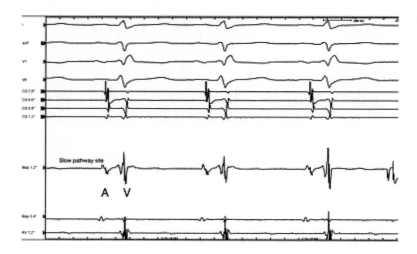

Figure 20.2 Mapping of putative slow pathway site with a fractionated atrial potential (A) and a ventricular potential (V) seen on mapping catheter, with an A–V ratio of 0.5–0.7.

similar to the right side approach. The annulus is mapped anatomically. The sites of ablation typically have a smaller A than V electrogram. The compact node near the His bundle should be avoided. The inferior end of the septal mitral annulus should be targeted first with gradual migration of the ablation site superiorly as needed to achieve slow pathway ablation. Junctional rhythm should be monitored during RF application to assure persistence of retrograde conduction, just as during ablation on the right side.

FAST PATHWAY ABLATION

When the slow pathway ablation is not properly targeted, one may generate a situation where typical AVNRT is so readily initiated that it becomes incessant. This scenario occurs when the antegrade fast pathway becomes injured and blocks readily with any premature beat or even during sinus rhythm in a Wenkebach pattern. Alternatively, the antegrade fast pathway may be non-conducting at all. In such circumstances, the retrograde conduction via the fast pathway may still be robust enough to maintain AVNRT. When this occurs, exclusive conduction via the slow pathway can readily initiate AVNRT. The PR Interval in sinus rhythm may well be prolonged already, consistent with slow pathway conduction. Under these circumstances, ablation of the AVNRT would necessitate targeting the fast pathway as eliminating slow pathway conduction would very likely result in high degree AV block if not complete AV block. Mapping of the earliest atrial activation during tachycardia would identify the retrograde fast pathway connection to the atrium. Ablation would typically start at this site using low power at first and applying incremental power. The ablation can be performed either during tachycardia or in sinus rhythm. But, the proceduralist should be aware that retrograde conduction via the fast pathway during accelerated junctional rhythm may not occur as the target of the ablation is the retrograde fast pathway. If retrograde fast pathway conduction is not eliminated with the first targeted site, the catheter tip is moved just slightly towards the tricuspid annuls and His bundle and the ablation power again applied. This approach has a higher risk of generating complete heart block and should be performed at a center with significant experience in ablation of AVNRT, preferably by an operator with prior experience in pursuit of fast pathway ablation.

CATHETER PLACEMENT AND ELECTROPHYSIOLOGIC STUDY

Generally, a catheter with four or more poles is positioned in the His bundle region, a second multi-polar catheter is placed in the CS, and a 4 pole catheter is placed at the right ventricular apex. The presence of a separate lateral right atrial catheter is desirable, but not necessary. The His bundle catheter or the RV catheter can be moved to the RA to define atrial activation sequences if needed (Figure 20.3).

The electrophysiology study is performed to document the fast pathway refractory period when possible, 1:1 AV conduction cycle lengths through the slow pathway, maximum AH intervals during 1:1 AV conduction, and inducibility of AVNRT. Isoproterenol, or atropine infusion, or both may be required if basal conditions are not yielding. The ablation catheter is withdrawn inferiorly from the His bundle region along the atrial edge of the tricuspid annulus. The use of a long sheath may be considered to improve catheter stability, for example if a funnel-shaped CS is suspected. Positioning of the catheter at the slow pathway region can be performed in either the right atrial oblique (RAO) or left atrial oblique (LAO) view. In the LAO view, the septal position of the catheter can be readily appreciated. Deviations of the catheter to the right or into the CS os can be easily detected. However, the annular location of the catheter has to be assessed using the AV electrogram ratios. In the RAO view, the location of the catheter along the tricuspid annulus can be readily appreciated. However, the septal position of the catheter has to be guided by rotating the catheter until it touches the septum. An LAO view is used with the catheters placed in the His bundle region and curled down along the septal annulus towards the CS os. The most common area where a slow potential can be recorded occurs in the inferior third of the axis from the His bundle to the CS os. The sharp potential described by Jackman[4] is usually recorded by moving the catheter slightly anteriorly from the CS os towards the tricuspid annulus. Frequently an overlapping zone with both sharp and slow potential exists anterior to the CS os. With the use of electro-anatomic mapping systems, the need to use fluoroscopy can be minimized and a simultaneous LAO and RAO view of the map can be readily displayed. A short period of time needed to generate the anatomic map with such a system may well be worthwhile in providing a clear view of catheter position during application of ablation energy without the need to constantly be looking at fluoroscopic images.

To minimize the risk of AV block, it is best to start the RF application at a low power output such as 20–30 W and a temperature setting of 50°C. The power and the temperature can be gradually increased during the RF application toward 50 W and 60°C, while the occurrence of fast junctional rhythm is closely monitored. It is infrequent that temperatures above 60°C are needed. A slow junctional acceleration is usually seen when the slow pathway is heated. The cycle length of this junctional rhythm can be just above sinus rate to around 600 ms. Cycle lengths shorter than 500 ms should be a warning sign that the more distal portion of the AVN is being heated. Retrograde atrial conduction via the fast pathway should be closely monitored during this acceleration. Any evidence of retrograde block should prompt immediate termination of the RF application as this is another sign that the distal AV node may be affected by the RF. Absence of any junctional acceleration usually indicates that the ablation lesion was ineffective in eliminating the slow pathway. Electrical endpoints, including non-inducibility of AVNRT, increase in the AV nodal refractory period consistent with elimination of the slow pathway, an increase in the 1:1 AV nodal conduction cycle length, as well as a decrease in the maximum AH interval achieved during 1:1 AV conduction, are all signs of successful slow pathway ablation. Use of isoproterenol and/or atropine infusion may be necessary if those drugs were needed to induce tachycardia prior to ablation. At times, following ablation, a single AV nodal echo beat can still be induced with premature atrial stimulation. This may be an acceptable outcome (perhaps even an optimal outcome) if no AVNRT could be induced following isoproterenol challenge. Usually, when such an echo beat is still present in the absence of inducible AVNRT, the antegrade AV nodal slow pathway refractory period is longer and/or the longest achievable AH interval during premature atrial stimulation is shorter than before ablation. This indicates that modification of the slow pathway had occurred during ablation such that the longest conducting slow pathway fibers, those likely involved in the AVNRT, had been eliminated. Shorter conducting slow pathway fibers may still be present, but those are unable to sustain the AVNRT.

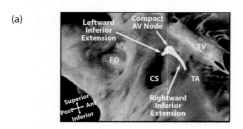

(a)

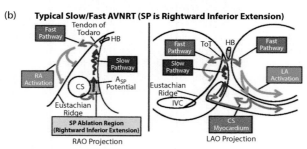

(b) **Typical Slow/Fast AVNRT (SP is Rightward Inferior Extension)**

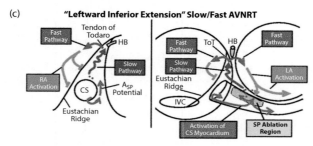

(c) **"Leftward Inferior Extension" Slow/Fast AVNRT**

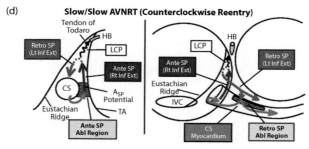

(d) **Slow/Slow AVNRT (Counterclockwise Reentry)**

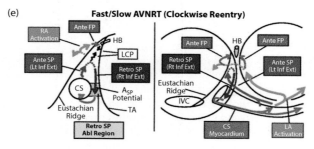

(e) **Fast/Slow AVNRT (Clockwise Reentry)**

Figure 20.3 (A) Anatomic location of the compact AV node and the rightward and leftward inferior extensions of the AV node. (B–E) Schematic representations of AVNRT reentrant circuits. (From Nakagawa, H. and Jackman, WM., *Circulation*, 116, 2465-2478, 2007.)

COMPLICATIONS

The dreaded complication in AV nodal pathway ablation is atrioventricular block, a complication seen at a much higher incidence in fast AV nodal pathway ablation. If present, atrioventricular block usually occurs immediately at the time of RF application. However, it may occur later, usually within the first 24–48 h, although even late occurrences have been reported.[6]

Damage to the compact AV node or His bundle can occur if RF energy was delivered in anatomic sites near them. In such cases, positioning of the catheter at the slow pathway region is usually not very stable. Changes of position can occur readily with heart beat movement or with breathing. Thus, close monitoring of the catheter position during RF application is important in minimizing this complication. The presence of a faster accelerated junctional tachycardia, PR prolongation, and/or retrograde block of junctional ectopy during RF application are markers predictive of complete permanent AV block.[7] Abrupt PR or AH interval lengthening during RF ablation should be a warning that the RF lesions are being applied closer to the fast pathway than the slow pathway. RF application should be stopped immediately. Transient AV block that occurs during RF ablation usually indicates that the targeted site may be dangerously close to the compact AV node, especially if the block persists for a short period of time after termination of RF application. Prolongation of the PR Interval may persist for a variable amount of time. However, even if antegrade conduction reverts to baseline after an observation period, the patient should be observed post procedure for 24–48 h to assure that later development of AV block does not occur, possibly related to edema from the heated tissues. In these circumstances, a short course of corticosteroids may be helpful in minimizing inflammation and edema at the ablated tissue.

CRYOABLATION

Although the risk of AV block is very low when the electro-anatomic approach is adopted, it is nonetheless a severe and at times a permanent complication. The use of cryoablation may mitigate this risk. While cooling of the tissue would quickly result in cessation of function, the creation of permanent tissue ablation with cryoablation usually takes much longer application. Thus, it is recommended that these lesions be applied for up to 4 min. Close monitoring of the development of functional AV block during cooling usually provides adequate warning that an ablation site could result in permanent AV block. If ablation is stopped immediately upon detection of rapid AV prolongation or even AV block, the block is totally reversible. Another advantage is the possibility of applying reversible cooling at 0°C, thereby allowing assessment of the functional effect of any prospective lesion before permanent damage is inflicted. However, close monitoring of AV block should still be performed during application of maximal cooling for the ablation. During cryoablation, no junctional rhythm is observed, unlike that of RF ablation. Below 0°C, the catheter is stuck to the atrial endocardium facilitating stability. This allows stimulation of the atrium to test the modification or disappearance of dual AV node physiology, non-inducibility of AVNRT, or interruption of the AVNRT due to slowing down followed by block of conduction over the slow pathway; or modification of the fast pathway ERP. If one or more of these criteria are met without changes in the basal AV conduction during ice mapping, then the temperature is maximally lowered for 4 min, creating a permanent lesion.

While elimination of slow pathway conduction during cooling indicates that the catheter tip is near the slow pathway, it does not guarantee that the ablation will be successful. This is due to the large tissue temperature difference needed to interrupt function with cooling versus that needed to permanently kill the tissue. Another advantage of using cryoablation is the adhesion of the catheter tip to the atrial endocardium. This prevents any inadvertent catheter dislodgement during application. The disadvantage of this approach is that it frequently takes more time as the lesions have to be applied for up to 4 min at each location. Applying a second lesion at the successful site may add assurance that the tissue is permanently ablated. The lesion may also have to be applied at a location that appears closer to the compact AV node than during RF application. In most cases, these lesions have to be applied close enough to the compact node to note mild PR prolongation during the application which reverses after completion of the lesion application. The occurrence of marked PR prolongation or AV block should prompt immediate termination of the cryothermal application. While AV block and PR prolongation may persist for several seconds, and sometimes up to 30 seconds, it typically reverses if the application is terminated promptly at the development of the block.

CONCLUSION

AVNRT can be cured with the ablation of either the fast or slow AV nodal pathway. The approach of choice would be to target the slow AV nodal pathway ablation. The techniques described for slow pathway ablation have a reasonably high percentage of success. The development of electro-anatomic mapping systems and contact force ablation catheters has improved procedural safety and effectiveness. There should be no immediate or late AV block if there is no impairment of either anterograde or retrograde conduction via the fast pathway during lesion application. However, a small percentage of late AV block has been seen with RF ablation. The use of cryoablation may further reduce the risk of this complication.

CATHETER ABLATION OF AVRT

CATHETER PLACEMENT AND ELECTROPHYSIOLOGIC STUDY

Catheters are placed in the high right atrium, His bundle region, right ventricle, and coronary sinus. ECG localization of manifest accessory pathways will provide an important clue to where mapping needs to be performed and also help in preparation for the additional catheters and sheaths that may be required. Knowledge of the anatomic locations of the various accessory pathways is important (Figure 20.4). Programmed electrical stimulation is then performed to initiate SVT. The following electrophysiologic features are used to identify the anatomic site of an AP:

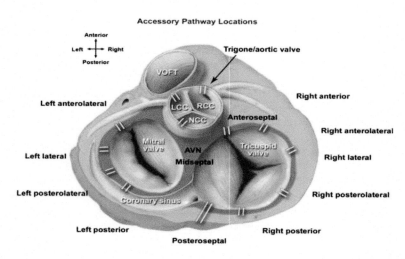

Figure 20.4 Trial ventricular accessory pathways may occur anywhere along the atrial ventricular annulus. Note the posteroseptal region is not part of the true septum. Also note the position of the aortic annulus interspersed between the right and left anteroseptal regions. Midseptal pathways are among the most difficult to ablate because of the proximity of the AV mode. VOFT = ventricular outflow tract; LCC = left coronary cusp; RCC = right coronary cusp; NCC = noncoronary cusp; AVN = AV node.

1   *Earliest ventricular and atrial potentials:* In manifest AP, the earliest local ventricular potential of pre-excited beats is mapped. Atrial pacing can be performed to enhance pre-excitation and the site of earliest ventricular excitation identifies the ventricular insertion site. In both concealed and manifest AP capable of retrograde conduction, the earliest local atrial potential during orthodromic AVRT or ventricular stimulation identifies the atrial insertion site. Some cautions: the sites of shortest VA or AV intervals should not be confused with the site of earliest A or V activation. While the sites of accessory pathway insertion usually have short activation intervals, they may not be the shortest. The VA or AV interval is an activation interval and does not necessarily indicate conduction time. This is due to the oblique course of most accessory pathways (Figure 20.5). Caution should be utilized when mapping the earliest atrial activation during ventricular pacing. One must be aware that retrograde conduction can occur via both the accessory pathway and the AV node. For pathways near the septal regions, both of these two potential pathways could activate the atrium during ventricular pacing and therefore may be difficult to distinguish. Thus, mapping atrial activation during orthodromic tachycardia is the best way to confirm that the site of earliest atrial activation is the accessory pathway insertion site. If a septal pathway needs to be mapped during ventricular pacing, efforts should be made to pace near the AV annulus on the ventricular side so as to minimize VA conduction time via the accessory pathway and maximize the VA conduction time via the AV node.

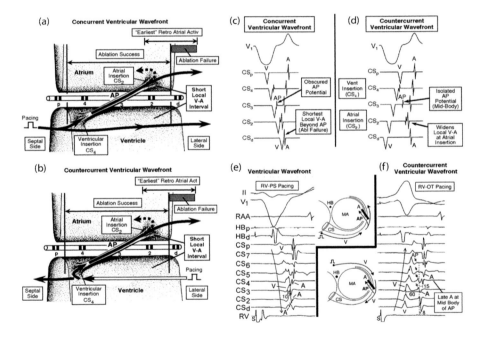

Figure 20.5 Effects of the oblique course in a left free-wall accessory pathway on the timing of ventricular (V), atrial (a), and AP potentials by reversing the direction of the ventricular wave front. (a–d) Schematic representations. (e and f) Recordings from a patient with a left lateral accessory pathway. Reversing the ventricular wave front from the concurrent direction (e: posteroseptal basal RV pacing [RV-PS]) to the countercurrent direction (f: distal RV outflow tract pacing [RV-OT]) increased the local VA interval at the site in the coronary sinus of earliest atrial activation (electrogram CS_3) from 10 to 60 ms and exposed the AP potential. The ventricular insertion (left) was located 15 mm septal to the atrial insertion (right), RAA indicates right atrial appendage. ([c–f] From Otomo, K. et al., *Circulation*, 104, 550–556, 2001.)

2 *Atrioventricular and ventriculoatrial interval:* Local atrioventricular and ventriculoatrial intervals are close to each other at sites of earliest activation. These potentials are seen in bipolar recordings. The gain of the recordings should be adjusted such that the entire electrogram can be seen. The onset of the rapid deflection of the electrogram should be marked as the beginning of local activation at the catheter tip. At high gains, low amplitude low frequency signals can frequently be seen preceding the rapid component. These represent the far field approach of the wave front and should not be used to mark the local activation time. In unipolar recordings at sites of earliest ventricular activation, a QS morphology identifies the endocardial breakout of the pre-excited V electrogram.

3 *Atrioventricular pathway potential:* An AP potential can be recorded at times during anterograde and retrograde conduction (Figure 20.6). However, the AP potential is less frequently identified during retrograde conduction as this often super-imposes onto the ventricular potential. Varying the site of ventricular pacing may facilitate observation of the AP potential. Similarly, varying the atrial pacing site might offer the same facilitation. The use of ventricular extrastimuli can be used to confirm the origin of an antegrade AP potential: a late extrastimulus advances the local ventricular potential without advancing the AP potential and an early extrastimulus advances the AP potential without advancing the local atrial potential.

ABLATION OF LEFT-SIDED FREE WALL PATHWAYS

Either a retrograde aortic or a trans-septal approach can be adopted. In the retrograde aortic approach, the mapping catheter is advanced across the aortic valve by accessing the femoral artery. It can be placed just underneath the mitral valve on its ventricular aspect to map the ventricular insertion of the AP. At this position, the movement of the catheter tip is in concert with the ventricular motion. The atrial to ventricular (A/V) potential amplitude is less than 1. Alternatively, it can be further advanced across the mitral annulus to map the atrial insertion of the AP. At this position, the wagging motion of the catheter tip is dissociated from the ventricular motion. The A/V potential ratio is 1 or greater and increases as the catheter tip is advanced away from the annulus. In either approach, atrial potential amplitude beat-to-beat variation of less than 20% reflects catheter stability. However, mapping of the atrial insertion site is probably best achieved using a trans-septal approach. In the transseptal antegrade approach, the atrial septum is crossed to map and ablate the atrial insertion

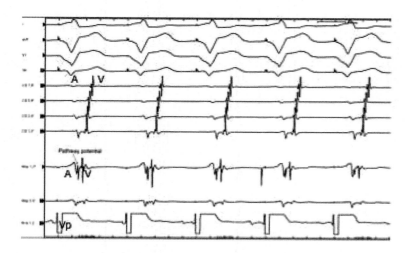

Figure 20.6 Mapping catheter near left lateral accessory pathway with sharp pathway potential seen at earliest atrial potential (A) during right ventricular pacing (Vp).

of the AP. Long directional sheaths can be used to offer greater catheter stability. Deflectable long sheaths are now available which allow for greater reach and stability.

Left-sided APs can be ablated with a success rate of 95% and a low recurrence rate of 5%. Recurrence usually occurs early, within 1–2 weeks, but may occur as late as 6 months following ablation. In cases of early recurrence, a repeat ablation is not advisable until 6–8 weeks after the initial ablation as some pathways that were damaged by the initial ablation may eventually lose conduction. Risk of myocardial perforation of friable tissue created by the initial ablation is higher should repeat ablation be attempted soon. Additionally, the presence of edema, a reaction of the ablated tissue, may distort the local electrograms and impede energy delivery for efficient ablation.

ABLATION OF RIGHT-SIDED FREE WALL ACCESSORY PATHWAYS

The initial success of right-sided AP ablation is lower than that of left-sided AP. However, the complication risk is lower and myocardial perforation with cardiac tamponade is less common than left-sided ablation. Rare cases of paradoxical emboli through a patent foramen ovale and right coronary artery occlusion have been reported.[8]

The lower success rate can be attributed to the challenges associated with mapping right-sided accessory pathways:

1   *Difference in mitral and tricuspid annuli:* The tricuspid annulus is larger in size, averaging 11 cm in circumference.[9] The tricuspid valve is less of a complete fibrous ring and may have gaps where atrial or ventricular muscles are in continuity. Furthermore, right-sided APs often penetrate the annulus and may consist of a broad band of tissues. Though the prevalence of APs is lower in this region, multiple pathways are slightly more prevalent. Unlike the mitral annulus, which can be marked by placing a catheter in the CS, there is no analogous venous structure to mark the tricuspid annulus. If needed, a thin angioplasty wire or six French multi-electrode catheter can be placed in the right coronary artery to delineate portions of the tricuspid annulus.

2   *Catheter stability:* It can be difficult to maintain catheter stability during ablation of right-sided APs. The lateral aspect of the tricuspid annulus has a large spatial excursion during ventricular systole. In addition, the approach to the tricuspid annulus from the inferior vena cava results in a more acute turn than the trans-septal approach to the mitral annulus. This more acute angle and the large movement of the lateral tricuspid annulus towards the RV apex during systole render catheter tip stability on the annulus more precarious. Long vascular sheaths with preformed curves that aim the catheter in the appropriate directions within the right atrium can improve the stability and facilitate appropriate delivery of RF energy on the atrial side of the annulus. An approach from the superior vena cava can be adopted for APs localized on the anterolateral aspect of the tricuspid annulus to provide better stability. Alternatively, a ventricular approach can offer much better stability during systole. However, a curved sheath and a smaller catheter curve may be needed to achieve a retroflexed contact at the ventricular end of the tricuspid annulus.

ABLATION OF SEPTAL ACCESSORY PATHWAYS

APs in this area are commonly classified as anteroseptal, midseptal, and posteroseptal, as described in the early part of this chapter. Precise mapping and localization of all APs is mandatory to avoid impairment of AV nodal conduction during RF ablation. Understanding the anatomy of the conduction system in relationship to structures at the AV groove is critical for achieving successful ablation with minimal complication rates. As mentioned above, the AV node runs along the atrial edge of the tricuspid annulus in a cranial direction with a slight anterior tilt. At the central fibrous body, the compact node transition to the His bundle and crosses the tricuspid annulus. Just anterior and superior to the compact node is the membranous septum. The His bundle runs along the inferior border of the membranous septum along a ridge of ventricular myocardium. Thus, in anteroseptal accessory pathways there is always a small distance, no more than 5 mm, that separates the His bundle from the nearest myocardial connections to the tricuspid annulus. On the other hand, true septal pathways may have virtually no separation from the AV node. Cryoablation is a good alternative to RF ablation if there is concern for potential damage to the normal conduction system, as permanent injury is rarely seen with this method. Furthermore, the catheter adheres to the tissue once a certain threshold temperature is reached allowing for better catheter stability.

ANTEROSEPTAL APs

These are classically defined as para-Hisian or anteroseptal if the earliest AP activation site also shows a His potential. It is safest to ablate these pathways from the atrial side of the annulus as this position optimizes the distance from the His bundle and the AV node. Use of a sheath may help stabilize the catheter contact with the annular tissue. Optimally, RF energy should only be applied during narrow QRS rhythm in order to minimize the potential of ablating the normal conduction pathway. In cases where sinus rhythm is associated with marked pre-excitation, initial RF lesions may need to be applied to during orthodromic tachycardia. Application of RF energy should be in a graded manner, paying close attention to onset of rapid junctional tachycardia, indicating heating of the compact AV node, or the development of right bundle branch block, indicating heating of the right-sided surface of the His bundle. When applying energy during orthodromic tachycardia, block in the AP is associated with sudden slowing of the rhythm to sinus rhythm. This may cause the catheter to dislodge. The map location of the catheter tip may also change significantly due to changes in cycle lengths. Thus, atrial pacing at a rate similar to the tachycardia may need to be instituted immediately to maintain contact and to assess stability of catheter tip location. A slow accelerated junctional rhythm can be seen at times due to the proximity of RF application to the compact AV node. This indicates that there is mild heating of the AV node tissue. However, more rapid junctional acceleration should prompt immediate cessation of RF application, similar to the approach during slow pathway ablation. Cryoablation can also be utilized in this region. Its advantages and disadvantages are similar to those in ablation of AVNRT. During orthodromic tachycardia the rapid movement of the heart may make catheter stability in the anteroseptal region difficult to achieve. At times, stable catheter position may only be achievable during sinus rhythm. After carefully mapping the earliest site of ventricular activation, one can start ablation slightly lateral to the earliest activation site and gradually encroach upon this site using low energies and gradually incrementing this energy. Careful attention should be given to the disappearance of ventricular pre-excitation to distinguish sinus rhythm with absence of accessory pathway from the onset of accelerated junctional rhythm which would also generate a QRS complex without pre-excitation. The latter would reflect heating of the AV node rather than cessation of accessory pathway conduction and could herald the onset of AV node block. An atrial approach should be used when ablating during sinus rhythm to minimize the possibility of damage to the His or right bundle as such damage may not be accompanied by accelerated junctional rhythms.

MIDSEPTAL APs

The AP potential can be recorded in an area along the tricuspid annulus defined by the His bundle anteriorly and coronary sinus ostium posteriorly, either on the right or left side of the atrial septum. Care should be taken in mapping either side as the AV node is in close proximity to the atrial insertion site, especially in the midseptal location. Application of RF energy is best directed on the ventricular side of the annulus, aiming to ablate the ventricular insertion, as the AV node is on the atrial side. This would minimize the chance of causing damage to the AV node. In left-sided midseptal APs, catheters are positioned at the His bundle and coronary sinus to mark the area. The ablation catheter is then moved along the mitral or tricuspid annulus bounded by these two catheters. Electro-anatomic mapping systems should be used whenever available to facilitate accurate location of these pathways.

POSTEROSEPTAL APs

Posteroseptal APs traverse the pyramidal space posterior to the septum. This region of the cardiac anatomy is complex and understanding the relationships of the mitral and tricuspid annular regions to the CS and the basal LV septum is crucial to locating the accessory pathway properly. The septal and inferior portions of the tricuspid annulus, the triangle of Koch, the anterior superior regions of the proximal CS abutting the mitral annulus, and the proximal CS venous branches should all be carefully mapped to reveal the atrial and ventricular connections of the AP. Left-sided mapping of the atrial septum and ventricular side along the mitral annulus should be considered. The right posteroseptal AP inserts along the tricuspid annulus in the vicinity of the CS ostium. The left posteroseptal AP may be located at a subepicardial site around the proximal CS or the middle cardiac vein. In such instances, the ablation catheter may be advanced into the CS to search for early activation sites or an AP potential to target RF application. At other times, the left posteroseptal AP may be located at a subendocardial site along the posteromedial aspect of the mitral annulus. The ventricular end of this location can also be approached from the retrograde direction. The septal portion of the mitral annulus is directly inferior to the aortic outflow and can best be reached by clocking the catheter tip from a mid-ventricular septal position while holding a gentle curve. Again, application of RF lesions in these areas, especially in the midseptal region, should be done during narrow QRS antegrade conduction whenever possible to minimize inadvertent ablation of the normal conduction pathway. Cryoablation, of course, can also be used if available. The use of cryoablation may be particularly desirable in the smaller venous branches originating from the proximal CS as it has greater safety in minimizing potential damage to the nearby arteries.

ABLATION OF EPICARDIAL ATRIOVENTRICULAR PATHWAYS

The incidence of epicardial AP is approximately 0.5% of patients referred for RF ablation of AP. In right-sided epicardial AP, small or no AP potentials can be recorded. A thin multipolar catheter can be placed in the right coronary artery for epicardial mapping. Endocardial ablation can be guided by both location and recordings from the epicardial electrode. Because the right atrium and the right ventricle are relatively thin, transmural ablation is usually feasible from an endocardial approach. However, there are rare instances where the pathway connects from the right atrial appendage to the epicardial ventricular surface somewhat removed from the annulus. If this site has heavy endocardial trabeculations, transmural ablation may not be achieved. A transcutaneous epicardial approach for ablation has been described[10] and can be used in these rare instances. Ablation of accessory pathways along the annulus from an epicardial approach may be difficult as it could be hindered by the close proximity of the right coronary artery. The presence of epicardial fatty tissue around the AV groove also limits RF ablation efficacy.

A left-sided epicardial AP is characterized by a large AP potential along the CS or its tributaries. These pathways typically connect to the epicardial ventricular surface. Ablation can be successfully and safely achieved by delivering RF applications within the CS or its tributaries with a lower power between 10 and 15 W.[11] Cryoablation via a CS approach may also be used in these circumstances. It has a lesser propensity to cause venous stenosis and has a lower risk of damaging the nearby arteries that frequently travel close to the veins. In rare circumstances, there may be AP connections from the left atrial appendage to the LV epicardial surface. These may need an epicardial approach to achieve successful ablation.

ABLATION OF ATRIOVENTRICULAR PATHWAYS WITH SLOW DECREMENTAL CONDUCTION

These AP variants were originally described as nodoventricular or Mahaim pathways. Clinically, these arrhythmias exhibit a wide QRS tachycardia, usually with a left bundle branch block pattern. While nodal connections of these pathways have been postulated, the vast majority of these pathways are atrio-fascicular or atrioventricular in nature, with slow decremental conduction characteristics suggestive of a node-like properties.[12] The ventricular insertion sites of atrioventricular and atrio-fascicular fibers can be localized by mapping the local AP potential. Early ventricular activation may not reveal the true site of accessory pathway in the atrio-fascicular variety. A His-like potential can frequently be identified in these cases just under the anterolateral portion of the tricuspid annulus. Distal connection to the myocardium may occur via the Purkinje fibers or possibly even directly into the right bundle, yielding rapid retrograde conduction into the conduction system. Mechanical block of the AP by catheter manipulation can occur during manipulation of the catheter tip on either side of the tricuspid annulus. These pathways typically conduct only in the antegrade direction. Thus activation mapping of the atrial insertion site cannot be accomplished. Pace mapping on the atrial side of the tricuspid annulus can facilitate localization of the atrial end of the pathway. The shortest stimulus to QRS or RV interval of maximally pre-excited beats during atrial pacing should identify the atrial end of the pathway. Once a site has been identified, RF ablation can be delivered during pre-excited SVT or during atrial pacing with maximal pre-excitation. If successful, the SVT will terminate. In many cases, pre-excited accelerated rhythms occur during RF ablation due to heating of excitable node-like tissue. Left-sided decremental accessory pathways can also occur, but are much less frequently seen than the right-sided variety. Ablation can be approached in the same manner, but using left-sided approaches on the ventricular side of the mitral annulus or even along the aortic root.[13]

True nodal ventricular conduction is indeed rare and their existence controversial. These pathways have been suggested in reports where ablation of the slow AV nodal pathway had eliminated a pre-excited decremental AV conduction.[14] In some instances, the earliest ventricular activation of pre-excited beats was recorded at the ventricular aspect of the annulus, suggesting a ventricular insertion rather than a fascicular insertion site. Given these observations, it is not clear if these fibers originate from the AV node or course the annulus in close proximity to the AV node. When these occur, distinguishing these pathways from septal accessory pathways with decremental conduction can be difficult. However pathways conducting from the ventricle to the AV node or proximal His bundle have been reported. Tachycardia involving these pathways have a narrow QRS and can mimic typical forms of AVNRT. Instances of "AVNRT" with intermittent or persistent VA dissociation may well involve this type of pathways.[15]

ABLATION OF PERMANENT JUNCTIONAL RECIPROCATING TACHYCARDIA (PJRT)

PJRT is characterized by sustained tachycardia (12 h/day) with a narrow QRS complex. This tachycardia commonly appears in infants and children and may persist into adulthood. It is usually refractory to drug therapy and is frequently not associated with clinical symptoms. It may go undetected in young people due to its relatively slow rate in the range of 100–150. The rates can vary depending on sympathetic or even vagal tone as antegrade conduction of this reentrant rhythm is typically via the fast AV nodal pathway. However, it can cause tachycardia-mediated cardiomyopathy. Studies indicate that a concealed AP with slow and decremental retrograde conduction properties is involved in the initiation and maintenance of this type of orthodromic AVRT.[16] Due to the atrial insertions of these pathways and their slow conducting properties, they can mimic atypical AVNRT (antegrade fast and retrograde slow pathway). Standard EP testing maneuvers should distinguish PJRT from atypical AVNRT. The AP is usually localized to the septal tricuspid annulus close to or just inside the CS os in 80% of cases, and along the posterior right or left free wall in the remaining cases.

CONCLUSION

Catheter ablation of AP has been a preferred therapy given its low procedural risk and its excellent success rate. However, a clear understanding of the anatomy at the various sites of ablation is important in generating successful outcomes and minimizing risks. Careful mapping of APs with modern mapping equipment can be very useful, especially in complex anatomic areas of the heart. Use of alternative energy sources to RF may enhance the safety of these procedures in special circumstances. In addition, percutaneous epicardial access may allow ablation of pathways that are inaccessible from the endocardial side. Although the need for such an approach is rare, this approach may spare surgical ablation in such an unusual circumstance.

REFERENCES

1. Haissaguerre M, Warin JF, Lemetayer P et al. Closed chest ablation of retrograde conduction in patients with atrioventricular nodal reentrant tachycardia. *N Engl J Med* 1989; 320: 426–433.

2. Epstein LM, Scheinman MM, Langberg JJ et al. Percutaneous catheter modification of the atrioventricular node: A potential cure for atrioventricular nodal reentrant tachycardia. *Circulation* 1989; 80: 757–768.

3. Jazayeri MH, Hempe SL, Sra JS et al. Selective transcatheter ablation of fast and slow pathways using radiofrequency energy in patients with atrioventricular nodal reentrant tachycardia. *Circulation* 1992; 85: 1318–1328.

4. Sun Y, Arruda M, Otomo K et al. Coronary sinus-ventricular accessory connections producing posteroseptal and left posterior accessory pathways: incidence and electrophysiological identification. *Circulation* 2002; 106(11): 1362–1367.

5. Jais P, Haissaguerre M, Shah DC et al. Successful radiofrequency ablation of a slow atrioventricular nodal pathway on the left posterior atrial septum. *Pacing Clin Electrophysiol* 1999; 22(3): 525–527.

6. Elhag O, Miller HC. Atrioventricular block occurring several months after radiofrequency ablation for the treatment of atrioventricular nodal reentrant tachycardia: A report of two cases. *Heart* 1998; 79(6): 616–618.

7. Thakur RK, Klein GJ, Yee R. Junctional tachycardia: A useful marker during radiofrequency ablation for atrioventricular node reentrant tachycardia. *J Am Coll Cardiol* 1993; 22(6): 1706–1710.

8. Khanal S, Ribeiro PA, Platt M et al. Right coronary artery occlusion as a complication of accessory pathway ablation in a 12 year old treated with stenting. *Cathet Cardiovasc Interv* 1999; 46: 59–61.

9. Davies MJ. *Pathology of Cardiac Valves.* Butterworths, London, UK, 1980: 71.

10. Yamane T, Jais P, Shah DC et al. Efficacy and safety of an irrigated tip catheter for the ablation of accessory pathways resistant to conventional radiofrequency catheter ablation. *Circulation* 2000; 102: 2565–2568.

11. Giorgberidze I, Saksena S, Krol RB, Matthew P. Efficacy and safety of radiofrequency catheter ablation of left sided accessory pathways through the coronary sinus. *Am J Cardiol* 1995; 76: 359–365.

12. Tchou P, Lehmann MH, Jazayeri M, Akhtar M. Atriofascicular connection or a nodoventricular Mahaim fiber? Electrophysiologic elucidation of the pathway and associated reentrant circuit. *Circulation* 1988; 77(4): 837–848.

13. Wilsmore BR, Tchou PJ, Kanj M et al. Catheter ablation of an unusual decremental accessory pathway in the left coronary cusp of the aortic valve mimicking outflow tract ventricular tachycardia. *Circ Arrhythm Electrophysiol* 2012; 5(6): e104–e108.

14. Grogin HR, Randall JL, Kwasman M et al. Radiofrequency catheter ablation of atriofascicular and nodofascicular Mahaim tracts. *Circulation* 1994; 90: 272–281.

15. Bassiouny M, Kanj M, Tchou PJ. *Ablation of Atriofascicular Accessory Pathways and Variants in Catheter Ablation of Cardiac Arrhythmias*, 3rd ed. Huang SKS and Miller JM (eds.). Elsevier Saunders, Philadelphia, PA, 2015.

16. Gaita F, Haissaguerre M, Giustetto C et al. Catheter ablation of permanent reciprocating tachycardia with radiofrequency current. *J Am Coll Cardiol* 1995; 25: 655–664.

MANAGEMENT AND ABLATION OF ATRIAL FLUTTER

Carola Gianni, Amin Al-Ahmad, and Andrea Natale

CONTENTS

INTRODUCTION

Atrial flutter (AFL) is a macro-reentrant atrial tachycardia (AT) that propagates around an obstacle (anatomical, functional, or both), regardless of the atrial cycle length (CL). AFLs are characterized by a regular atrial rate and a constant P-wave morphology and, according to their mechanism, are usually classified as[1]:

- Cavotricuspid isthmus (CTI)-dependent flutters:
    - Typical flutter (counterclockwise rotation around the tricuspid valve—TV—annulus)
    - Reverse-typical flutter (clockwise rotation around the TV annulus)
    - Lower loop re-entry
    - Partial isthmus re-entry
- Non CTI-dependent flutters (or atypical)
    - Right atrial (RA) flutters:
        - Upper loop re-entry
        - Dual loop re-entry
        - Right atrial free-wall re-entry (including scar-related)
        - Scar-related (e.g., atriotomy, atrial septal patch, RF ablation)
    - Left atrial (LA) flutters:
        - Peri-mitral re-entry (around the mitral valve—MV–annulus)
        - Roof-dependent re-entry (peri-pulmonary vein—PV—ostia)
        - Peri-septal re-entry
        - Scar-related (e.g., RF ablation, Maze, atriotomy)

In this chapter, we will discuss the acute and chronic management of AFLs, particularly focusing on catheter ablation.

Acute treatment of AFL depends on the hemodynamic status of the patient (presence of ischemic chest pain, dyspnea at rest, altered mental status, or systolic blood pressure <90 mmHg) (Figure 21.1).[2]

- *Hemodynamically unstable* patients require immediate cardioversion:
  - Usually by means of direct current (DC) synchronized shock (50–200 J biphasic).
  - Pharmacological cardioversion with antiarrhythmic drugs (AADs) can be attempted (less effective, risk of proarrhythmia → usually reserved for stable patients—see below).
  - While waiting for electrical cardioversion, in patients with a permanent pacemaker or implantable cardioverter-defibrillator (ICD) or with temporary epicardial atrial pacing after cardiac surgery, rapid atrial overdrive pacing can be performed:
    - Use a CL 5%–10% faster than the AFL CL for at least 15 s.
    - Can be repeated at incrementally faster CLs until sinus rhythm or atrial fibrillation (AF–easier to rate control).
- *Hemodynamically stable* patients can be managed either with rhythm or rate control (Table 21.1):
  - *Rhythm control* can be achieved with:
    - Synchronized DC cardioversion (50–200 J biphasic shock).
    - Overdrive pacing (see above).
    - Pharmacologic cardioversion:
      - Class III AADs are the drugs of choice, prolonging the refractory period without slowing conduction velocity.
        - o Intravenous (IV) ibutilide is the most effective (success rate ~ 60%)[3]; it prolongs the QT, causing torsades de pointes (TdP) in 2%–5% (more frequently in low LVEF, low serum Mg/K, or concomitant QT prolonging drugs) → continuous ECG monitoring for at least 4–6 h after administration, or until the QT returns to baseline.
        - o Oral dofetilide is an alternative, with the same precautions.
  - *Rate control*, more difficult to achieve than in AF, can be attempted with:
    - IV AV-nodal blocking agents, such as beta-blockers, diltiazem, or verapamil; they are negative inotropic drugs and their main side effect is hypotension → contraindicated in patients with low blood pressure or systolic heart failure.
    - IV amiodarone can be used as an alternative, as it acutely slows AV-nodal conduction and prolongs AV-nodal refractoriness. Although unlikely, amiodarone may convert AFL to sinus → caution in inadequately anticoagulated patients with AFL lasing ≥48 h.
    - In case of pre-excitation, given the risk of precipitation to ventricular fibrillation (VF) with rate control, electrical cardioversion is the strategy of choice.

Of note, regardless of the treatment strategy, antithrombotic therapy is recommended, as AFL increases the risk of thromboembolism,[4] and should be instituted following the same risk-based recommendations for AF.[5]

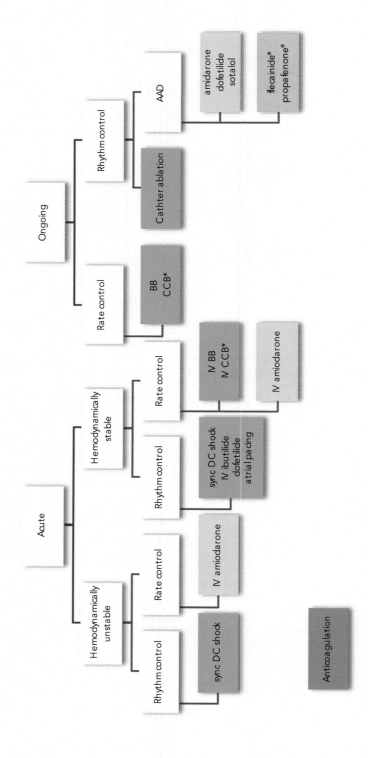

Figure 21.1 Management of atrial flutter. *diltiazem or verapamil; °patients without structural heart disease. Based on reference[2]: green, class I recommendation; yellow, class IIa recommendation; orange, class IIb recommendation. AAD, antiarrhythmic drugs; BB, beta-blockers; CCB, calcium channel-blockers; DC, direct current; IV, intravenous.

Table 21.1 Drug therapy for atrial flutter (acute setting)

Drug	Loading dose	Maintenance dose	Major adverse effects
Rate control			
Esmolol IV	500 µg/kg over 1 min	25–300 µg/kg/min infusion, titrating by 25–50 µg/kg/min q5–10 min	↓ BP ↓ HR Bronchospasm HF
Atenolol IV	5 mg over 5 min	Repeat q10–15 min once	Same as above
Metoprolol IV	2.5–5 mg over 2 min	Repeat q5 min up to a total dose of 15 mg	Same as above
Diltiazem IV	0.25 mg/kg over 2 min	Repeat 0.35 mg/kg q15 min once, followed by 5–15 mg/h infusion for up to 24 h	↓ BP ↓ HR HF Hepatic toxicity
Verapamil IV	2.5–5 mg over 2 min	Repeat q15–30 min up to a total dose of 20 mg	↓ BP ↓ HR HF
Rhythm control			
Ibutilide IV	≥60 kg: 1 mg over 10 min <60 kg: 0.01 mg/kg over 10 min	Repeat q10 min once	QT prolongation, TdP
Dofetilide OS	CrCl > 60 mL/min: 500 µg CrCl 40–60 mL/min: 250 µg CrCl 20–40 mL/min: 125 µg CrCl < 20 mL/min: contraindicated	NA	Same as above
Amiodarone[a] IV	5 mg/kg over 30–60 min, diluted in at least 250 mL dextrose 5% in water	1 mg/min infusion over 6 h, followed by 0.5 mg/min over 18 h	↓ BP ↓ HR Phlebitis QT prolongation
Anticoagulation			

Abbreviations: BP, blood pressure; CrCl, creatinine clearance; GI, gastrointestinal; HF, heart failure; HR, heart rate; IV, intravenous; NA, not available; OS, oral; min, minutes; TdP, torsades de pointes.
[a] Used for rate control in the acute setting, but cardioversion possible.

ONGOING MANAGEMENT

For chronic management, beside antithrombotic prophylaxis per CHA_2DS_2-VASc/HAS-BLED score, the choice is that of rhythm control vs rate control (Figure 21.1) (Table 21.2).[2]

- *Rhythm control*:
  - Best accomplished with catheter ablation.
  - Alternatively, in case of contraindications (i.e., comorbidities) or patient preference, AADs and electrical cardioversion can be used to manage and prevent AFL recurrences.
    - AADs act by suppressing ectopic beats that trigger AFL or by preventing AFL maintenance.[6]
    - AAD choice usually depends on underlying heart disease and comorbidities.
    - Class Ic drugs (namely flecainide or propafenone) may lengthen the AFL CL resulting in 1:1 AV nodal conduction (in some patients the associated marked QRS widening secondary to Na-blocking in the ventricular myocardium can make this look like ventricular tachycardia) → to reduce the

Table 21.2   Drug therapy for atrial flutter (ongoing management)

Drug	Initial dose	Maximal dose	Common major adverse effects
Rate control			
Atenolol OS	25 mg OD	100 mg OD	↓ BP ↓ HR Bronchospasm HF
Metoprolol OS	25 mg BID 50 mg OD (ER)	100 mg BID 400 mg OD (ER)	Same as above
Bisoprolol OS	2.5 mg OD	10 mg OD	Same as above
Carvedilol OS	3.125 mg BID	25 mg BID	Same as above
Diltiazem OS	120 mg OD (ER)	300 mg OD (ER)	↓ BP ↓ HR HF Hepatic toxicity
Verapamil OS	180 mg OD (ER)	480 mg OD (ER)	↓ BP ↓ HR HF
Rhythm control			
Flecainide OS	50 mg BD	200 mg BD	1:1 AFL ↓ HR PR, QRS prolongation
Propafenone OS	150 mg TID 225 mg BD	200 mg TID 425 mg BD	1:1 AFL ↓ HR PR, QRS prolongation Bronchospasm
Amiodarone OS	400–600 mg OD for 2–4 weeks (loading), followed by 100 mg OD (maintenance)	200 mg OD (maintenance)	↓ HR QT prolongation Photosensitivity Lung, liver, thyroid toxicity Eye complications
Dofetilide OS	CrCl > 60 mL/min: 500 µg BID CrCl 40–60 mL/min: 250 µg BID CrCl 20–40 mL/min: 125 µg BID CrCl < 20 mL/min: contraindicated	NA	QT prolongation, TdP
Sotalol OS	80 mg BID	160 mg BID	QT prolongation, TdP ↓ HR HF Bronchospasm
Anticoagulation			

Abbreviations: AFL, atrial flutter; CrCl, creatinine clearance; ER, extended release; HF, heart failure; HR, heart rate; IV, intravenous; OS, oral; TdP, torsades de pointes.

risk of 1:1 AFL (usually poorly tolerated due to the fast ventricular rate), an AV nodal blocking agent can be added.

- *Rate control* with oral beta-blockers, diltiazem, or verapamil
  - Reasonable strategy in some circumstances of persistent refractory AFL or in those with infrequent well-tolerated episodes.
  - It is often more difficult to achieve compared to AF, because of the paradoxical effect of a slower atrial rate: concealed AV nodal conduction is less and this results in faster AV conduction with higher ventricular rates.

CATHETER ABLATION

Catheter ablation is the strategy of choice to manage recurrent AFLs.[2] The ability to identify the macro-reentrant circuit by activation mapping with consequent reliable elimination of its critical isthmus makes radiofrequency (RF) ablation of AFL a safe and curative with >90% long-term success rate.

In general, ablation of AFLs can be performed with the patient on therapeutic oral anticoagulation. Of note, despite successful AFL ablation, oral anticoagulation should be continued long-term (per CHA_2DS_2-VASc/HAS-BLED score) unless high-intensity rhythm monitoring (implantable loop recorder or 7-day ECG Holter every 3 months) confirms sinus rhythm, given the high incidence of AF in this population (~60% over 5 years).[7]

CAVOTRICUSPID ISTHMUS-DEPENDENT ATRIAL FLUTTER

CTI-dependent flutters (typical counterclockwise, reverse typical clockwise, and lower loop and partial isthmus) are flutters in which the CTI is the predominant area of slow conduction. They can be reliably and successfully treated with CTI ablation.

ANATOMY

The CTI extends between the TV annulus and the inferior vena cava (IVC)/eustachian ridge (ER); the base of the triangle of Koch lies medially (septal), and the lower end of the crista terminalis (CT) laterally (Figure 21.2).[8] The CTI is usually subdivided in three portions: septal (between 4 and 5 o'clock in the left anterior oblique–LAO—projection), central (6 o'clock), and lateral (starting at 7 o'clock). The anatomy of the CTI is highly variable. Its length from few millimeters to more than 3 cm, with the septal portion being relatively narrow compared to the lateral end. The central isthmus is the thinnest portion, ranging from an average of 3.5 mm anteriorly (near the TV) in the muscular portion to 0.8 mm centrally in the fibro-fatty portion.[9] CTIs can be flat, uneven (with prominent ERs and pectinate muscles), concave, and commonly have one or more distinct pouches (usually sparing the lateral third).

During typical AFL, the activation wavefront exits the medial CT, ascends the atrial septum (bounded posteriorly by the fossa ovalis) and then descent laterally between the CT and the TV, entering the lateral CTI (Figure 21.3).[10] Reverse typical AFL runs in the same circuit, just in an opposite direction. The circuit of lower-loop re-entry is around the ostium of the IVC, while in partial isthmus flutter, the circuit runs posteriorly in the CTI, through the ER and posterior to the CS os, by-passing the medial CTI (Figure 21.4).[11]

DIAGNOSIS

The surface 12-lead ECG is diagnostic for typical AFL, in which an inverted sawtooth F wave is observed in the inferior leads II, III, aVF, and an upright F wave in V_1 (Figure 21.5). By contrast, in reverse typical, lower loop re-entry, and partial isthmus, the ECG is less specific (as in typical flutter after extensive ablation in the left atrium, the so-called pseudo-atypical flutter),[12] and a formal electrophysiologic study (EPS) demonstrating macro-reentrant RA activation with the entire CL covered in the RA and concealed entrainment from the CTI is needed for definite diagnosis.

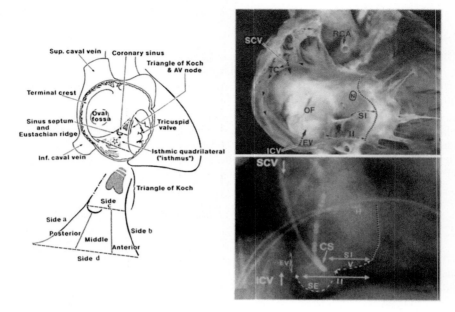

Figure 21.2 Anatomy of the CTI. EV, eustachian valve; H, His bundle catheter; I, inferior or lateral isthmus; ICV, inferior vena cava; N, atrioventricular node; OF, fossa ovalis; RCA, right coronary artery; SCV, superior vena cava; SE, subeustachian sinus or pouch; SI, septal isthmus; TC, crista terminalis; V, vestibular or anterior isthmus. (From Cabrera, J.A. et al.: The architecture of the atrial musculature between the orifice of the inferior caval vein and the tricuspid valve: The anatomy of the isthmus. *Journal of Cardiovascular Electrophysiology.* 1998. 9. 1186–1195. Copyright Wiley-VCH Verlag GmbH & Co. KGaA. Reproduced with permission.)

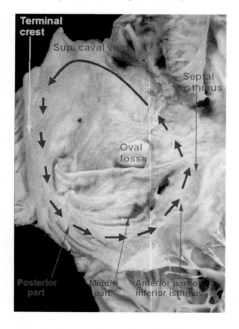

Figure 21.3 Wavefront of typical counterclockwise atrial flutter. (Courtesy of Medtronic, Inc., Minneapolis, MN.)

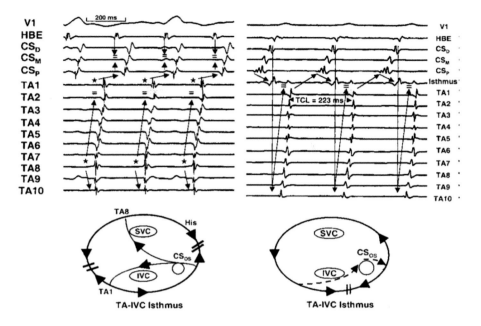

Figure 21.4 Intracardiac electrograms and schematics of lower loop (left) and partial isthmus (right) re-entry. (Adapted from Yang, Y. et al., *Circulation*, 103, 3092–3098, 2001. With permission of Wolters Kluwer Health.)

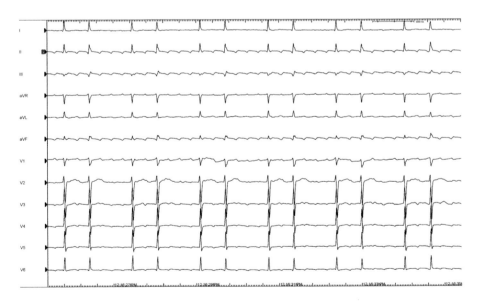

Figure 21.5 12 lead ECG of typical counterclockwise atrial flutter.

ELECTROPHYSIOLOGIC STUDY AND ABLATION

Before ablation:

- Activation mapping, performed with:
  - Multielectrode catheters:
    - One positioned in the lateral RA (CT) and one in the CS
      - Commonly, a 20-electrode Halo mapping catheter is positioned around the TV annulus (spanning the septum, roof, and lateral wall) along with a separate CS catheter (Figure 21.6).
      - The 20-electrode catheter can be positioned to cross the CTI, with the distal part advanced into the CS, obviating the need for a separate CS catheter.
      - Alternatively, a 10-electrode mapping catheter positioned in the lateral wall along with a separate CS catheter.
    - Additionally, a His bundle catheter may be used to mark the AV node location, for safety purposes.
  - Alternatively, tridimensional (3D) electro-anatomical mapping systems (Figure 21.7):
    - Establish the circuit.
    - Delineate the anatomic landmarks (e.g., the His cloud).
    - Guide the lesion set.
    - Reduce radiation exposure.[13]

Ablation:

- For RF ablation, large-curve catheters with an irrigated or large (8–10 mm) tip are preferred to standard 4-mm tip catheters: procedure and ablation times are shorter and acute and long-term success rates are higher.[14,15]
  - Large-tip catheters are most useful for flat CTIs.
    - Power is usually set at 70 up to 100 W, with a target temperature of 50°C–70°C (note: two grounding pads are needed to avoid skin burns).
  - Irrigated-tip can be helpful in the presence of pouches.
    - Power is usually set at 35–50 W power.
  - Occasionally, a long sheath with a fixed distal curve can be used to improve reach (e.g., RAMP) and stability (e.g., SR0) across the entire CTI.

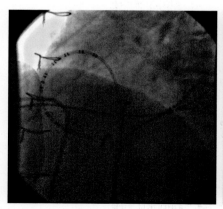 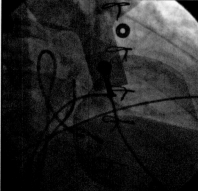

Figure 21.6 Fluoroscopy—LAO (left) and RAO (right) projections—showing a Halo mapping catheter, along with CS and His catheters; the ablation catheter is positioned at 6 o'clock along the CTI.

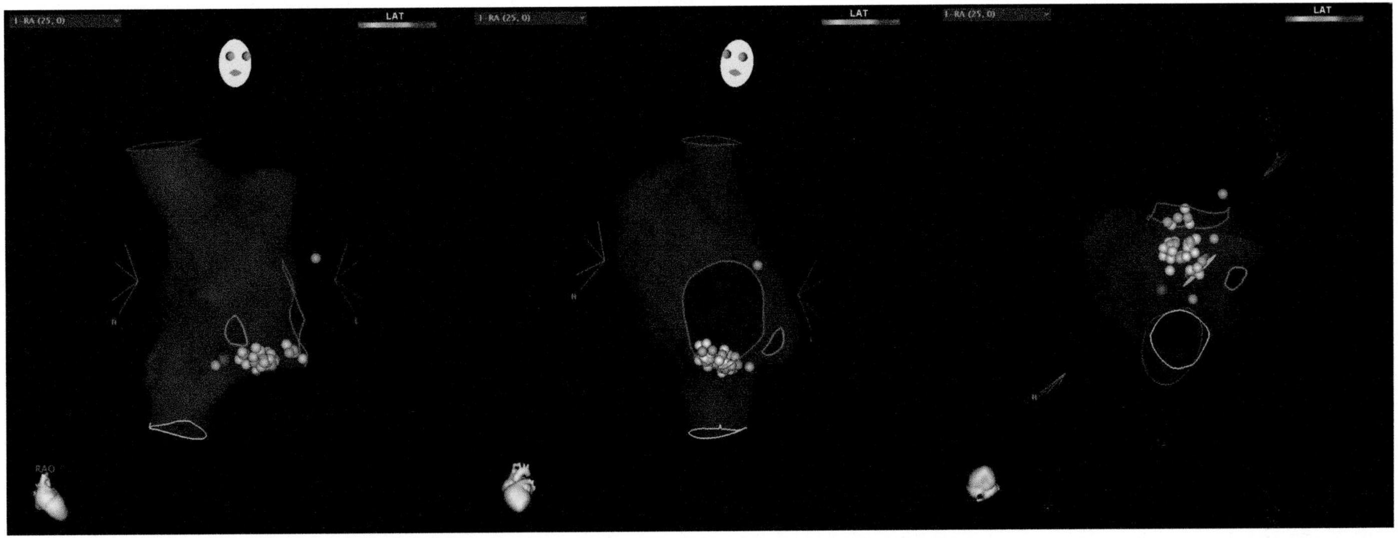

Figure 21.7 3D electro-anatomical map—LAO (left) and RAO (right) projections—of the right atrium showing the His bundle region (yellow dot) and the ablation line (red dots) along the CTI.

- Target is the central CTI, located at 6 o'clock in the LAO projection (Figure 21.6):
  - Start at the level of TV annulus (anterior in the right anterior oblique—RAO–view), with an A:V ratio of 1:2 to 1:4 on the distal ablation electrode; a linear set of lesions spanning across the CTI are then created either with a succession of point-by-point applications or by continuous application while withdrawing the ablation catheter towards the IVC.
  - With every successful lesion, the local distal electrogram (EGM) decreases in voltage with fragmentation and the ablation catheter is withdrawn until a sharp atrial EGM is seen.
  - As the catheter approaches the IVC (no atrial EGMs in the proximal electrodes of the ablation catheter), the curve should be slightly released so that the tip rests on the isthmus without abruptly slipping off into the IVC.
  - If a mapping catheter traverse the isthmus, the ablation catheter should go underneath it to ensure adequate tissue contact and effective ablation.
  - To avoid pouches or thick pectinate muscles, a more lateral or medial ablation line (respectively) might be necessary.
- Can be performed either in AFL or in SR (usually with proximal CS pacing at a CL ~600 ms)
  - AFL termination during RF ablation is only a proof of its isthmus dependency: in more than half of the patients, isthmus conduction persists after the termination and further ablation in necessary.
  - During pacing on either side of the isthmus, conduction gaps can be mapped, looking for single or fractionated potentials bounded by split EGMs across the line.[16]

ABLATION ENDPOINT

Bidirectional CTI conduction block is the endpoint of CTI ablation. There are several methods to confirm CTI block:

- Atrial activation sequence:
  - *Medial-to-lateral CTI block*: With pacing from the medial aspect of the CTI (e.g., proximal CS) (Figure 21.8):
    - Before ablation there is collision of the cranial and caudal RA wavefronts in the mid-lateral RA.
    - With block the lateral RA is activated in a strictly cranio-caudal pattern.
  - *Lateral-to-medial CTI block*, With pacing from the lateral aspect of the CTI (e.g., distal Halo):
    - Before ablation there is collision of the cranial and caudal RA wavefronts in the mid-superior septum.
    - With block the septum is activated in a strictly cranio-caudal pattern.
- Transisthmus conduction time:[17]
  - With pacing from the medial or lateral aspect of the CTI and measuring the conduction time on the opposite side, ≥50% increase in conduction time from baseline (Figure 21.9).
  - There is no definite number that confirms conduction block, however, bidirectional conduction times of >130 ms are typically considered to be indicative of block.
- Split potentials:[16]
  - Double EGMs separated by an isoelectric line with an interval of ≥90 ms across the whole ablation line (Figure 21.10).
- Differential pacing:[18]
  - With pacing from the medial or lateral aspect of the CTI and measuring the conduction time on the opposite side, when the pacing site is moved away from the ablation line conduction time shortens with block, the opposite occurring if there is still conduction through the CTI.

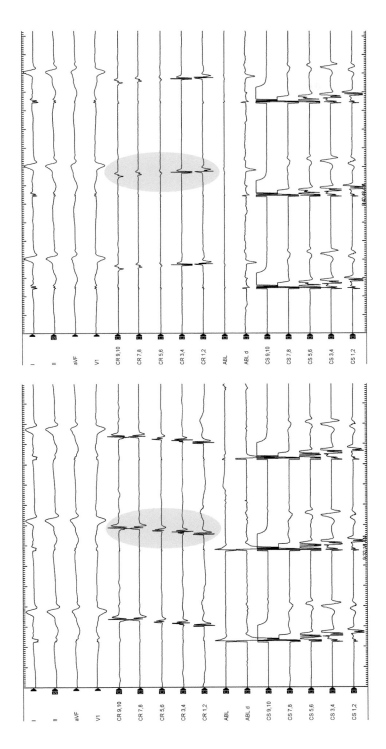

Figure 21.8 Change in crista terminalis activation sequence with medial-to-lateral CTI block.

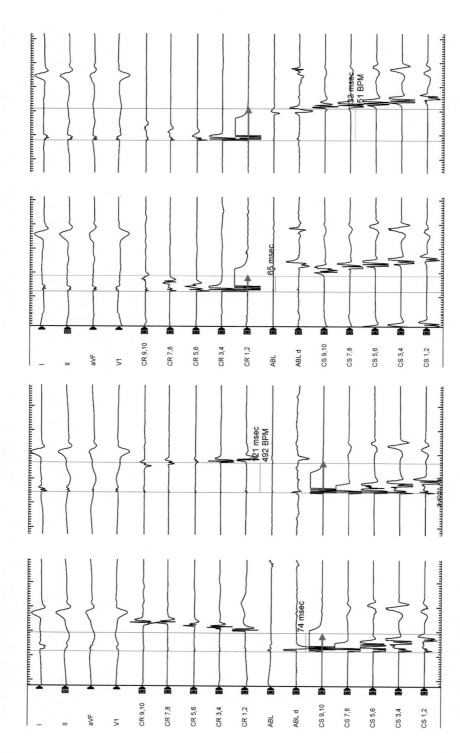

Figure 21.9 CTI block as shown by increase in transisthmus conduction time with pacing from the medial (CS os) and lateral (low HRA) aspect of the CTI.

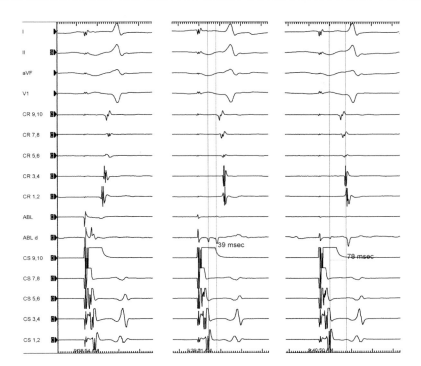

Figure 21.10 Split potentials with incomplete and complete block.

- EGM polarity:[19,20]
  - *Unipolar EGM*: With pacing from the medial or lateral aspect of the CTI and recording the unipolar EGM on the opposite side, change from biphasic to positive monophasic with block.
  - *Bipolar EGM*: With pacing from the medial or lateral aspect of the CTI and recording the unipolar EGM on the opposite side, change of polarity with block.
- Inferior leads P-wave morphology:[21]
  - With pacing from the lateral aspect of the CTI, P-wave morphology in the inferior leads (mainly determined by the direction of septal activation) change from negative to positive with clockwise block (Figure 21.11).

SUCCESS RATES AND COMPLICATIONS

With large- or irrigated-tip ablation catheters, acute success is high (>95%) with a low rate of recurrences (~10%).[2] Despite this, incidence of atrial fibrillation (AF) or atypical AFL is high in this population (up to 60% over 5 years).[7] Indeed, evidence suggests that these arrhythmias share the same electrophysiological triggers and anatomic substrate.[22] This has implications for long-term anticoagulation (as discussed above) and rhythm control strategies. In this regard, recent studies have shown that AF ablation at the time of AFL ablation should be considered.[23–25]

RF ablation of CTI is safe, with complication rates ~3%, the most common being peripheral vascular injury,[7] which can be greatly reduced with ultrasound-guided venous access. Serious complications are rare (~0.5%),[2] and include AV block (the most common – best avoided with careful His mapping and targeting a non-septal line), tamponade, myocardial infarction (due to right coronary artery injury and consequent acute thrombosis) and thromboembolic events (pulmonary embolism and stroke).

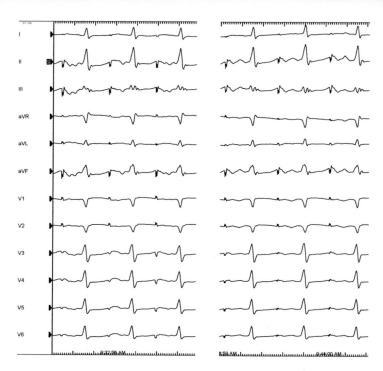

Figure 21.11 Inferior leads P-wave morphology before and after CTI block.

ATYPICAL ATRIAL FLUTTER

Atypical AFLs are an heterogeneous group of AFLs, more often associated with structural heart diseases (including congenital heart disease) or previous surgical and/or ablation procedures.

Generally, a routine anatomic ablation is not feasible because of the multiple possible circuits that can sustain these atypical AFLs and careful mapping (ideally 3D electro-anatomical mapping using multipoles catheters to acquire simultaneous multiple points) is required to determine the precise flutter circuit and define its critical isthmus that is amenable for ablation.

ANATOMY

Anatomical structures (TV annulus, CT, SVC, IVC, ER, fossa ovalis, MV annulus, PV ostia), scars from previous surgeries/ablation, and natural scars all offer a substrate for a flutter to circulate around.

RA atypical flutters are usually associated with prior atrial surgery (atriotomy scar, suture line, septal patch) (Figure 21.12) or after RF ablation, but scar (areas of low or no voltage) can be found also in patients without prior cardiac interventions, usually with a posterolateral or lateral distribution.[26] An exception is upper loop re-entry, in which the circuit is around the SVC with CT serving as the area of slow conduction. Dual-loop re-entry in the RA encompasses every combination of two RA flutters, either two atypical AFLs or one atypical AFL in conjunction with typical AFL or lower loop re-entry.

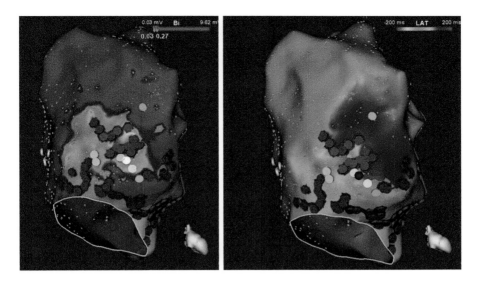

Figure 21.12 3D electro-anatomic map showing voltage (left) and activation (right) in a patient who had previous cardiac surgery for congenital heart disease.

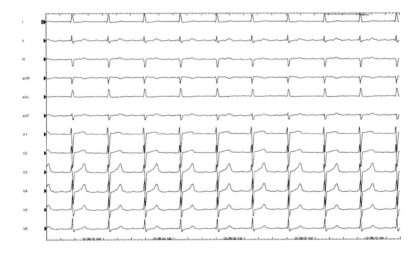

Figure 21.13 12 lead ECG of atypical atrial flutter.

LA atypical flutters are frequently related to AF. They might follow surgical or catheter ablation of AF, but can also be found in patients without prior ablation, in which areas of patchy scar (usually found in the posterior wall, roof, or antero-septum) reflects the underlying atrial myopathy. In these patients, the circuit usually revolves around either the MV annulus (peri-mitral) or homolateral PV ostia (roof-dependent) (Figures 21.13 and 21.14). Given the complex substrate, dual-loop and multiple-loop and multiple circuits are common. A rare form of LA flutter is the peri-septal AFL, in which the circuit is around the fossa ovalis: it usually occurs in patients without prior interventions, with atrial dilation and AADs facilitating re-entry by means of intra-atrial conduction prolungation.[27]

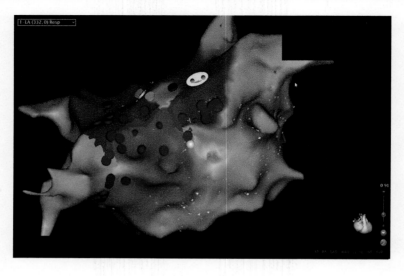

Figure 21.14 3D electro-anatomic map showing activation of an atypical roof-dependent atrial flutter in a patient who had a previous RF ablation for atrial fibrillation (same patient as Figure 21.12).

DIAGNOSIS

Atypical flutters can be either RA or LA. A combination of patient history, ECG, and activation/entrainment mapping are helpful to localize the chamber in which the re-entry takes place.

- *Patient history*:
  - Associated structural heart diseases.
  - Detailed description of previous surgical/ablative procedures.
    - RA: prior atriotomy, congenital heart disease (with or without surgical correction), prior cardiac surgery (e.g., TV surgery, atrial septal).
    - LA: structural left heart disease (e.g., hypertrophy, dilated cardiomyopathy, MV disease), prior AF ablation or Maze surgery, prior cardiac surgery (e.g., left atriotomy).
- *ECG*:
  - P-wave morphology is usually of limited value in itself, especially because the associated electro-anatomical anomalies modify the atrial wavefront propagation in an unpredictable manner.
  - In the absence of prior interventions, V_1 can be helpful:
    - RA: negative/negative-positive P-wave.
    - LA: positive/positive-negative P-wave.
- *CL variation*:
  - Large CL variations in the RA with a relative fixed CL in the LA (through the CS catheter) can be seen with flutters of LA origin as a result of LA/RA dissociation.
- *Activation mapping*:
  - Quick activation mapping in the RA can point to a diagnosis of LA AFL (→ need of trans-septal catheterization).
    - CS activation proximal-to-distal is indicative of a RA AFL, with two major exceptions:
      - A superior RA AFLs, in which LA can be passively activated through the Bachmann's bundle.
      - Counterclockwise peri-mitral AFL, in which CS typically activates in a proximal-to-distal direction).

- Timing span from the earliest to the latest of at least 10 evenly distributed sites in the RA < 50% of the tachycardia CL (TCL) is indicative of a LA AFL; exceptions would be a small re-entry circuit in the RA or extensive RA scarring.
- *Entrainment mapping*:
  - Begin by excluding CTI-dependent flutters with atypical ECGs (pseudo-atypical flutter) by means of entrainment mapping at the CTI.
  - Post-pacing interval (PPI)—TCL >30 ms at multiple sites in the RA (usually high RA, mid-lateral RA, and CTI, excluding the septum and CS as the LA would be captured) rules out RA AFL.

ELECTROPHYSIOLOGIC STUDY AND ABLATION

Before ablation:

- 3D electro-anatomical mapping is performed with the goal is to identify the three key components of re-entry (Figures 21.12 and 21.14).
  - Barriers:
    - Substrate mapping:
      - Anatomical barriers: RA → IVC, SVC, CS os, TV annulus; LA → MV annulus, PVs.
      - Acquired barriers: Dense scar → bipolar voltage <0.2 mV and no capture with pacing at 20 mA; lines of block → split EGMs.
  - Circuit (i.e., the shortest distance of continuous activation encompassing the whole TCL)
    - Activation mapping:
      - ≥100 points homogenously distributed accounting for ≥90% of the TCL
      - Continuous activation with an early-meets-late area.
    - Entrainment mapping:
      - Manifest fusion of the atrial activation sequence.
      - PPI—TCL < 30 ms.
  - Critical Isthmus (i.e., conductive myocardium within the circuit, usually located between two barriers, essential for AFL propagation):
    - Activation mapping:
      - Mid-diastolic EGMs (Figure 21.15).
      - With 3D electro-anatomic mapping, if the onset of the window of interest is set between two P waves, the isthmus is located in the early-meets-late area.
    - Entrainment mapping (Figure 21.16)
      - Concealed fusion of the atrial activation sequence.
      - PPI—TCL < 30 ms.
- Identify and tag anatomical landmarks to avoid during ablation, such as the SA node, AV node/His bundle, and phrenic nerve.
- In case of short-lived or non-reproducibly induced AFLs:
  - Voltage mapping can be performed in sinus rhythm to identify barriers.
  - Noncontact mapping may be used for fast identification of the circuit/critical isthmus.
- For atypical RA flutters, conventional mapping with multi-electrode catheters might be useful: Despite incomplete mapping, an empiric ablation line connecting two barriers encompassing the putative critical isthmus can be attempted.

Ablation

- RF ablation is usually performed with irrigated tip ablation catheter:
  - Power is usually set up to 40–45 W.
  - Parallel tip-tissue orientation.
  - The specific curve catheter and/or need of long preformed sheaths depend on the specific site of ablation.

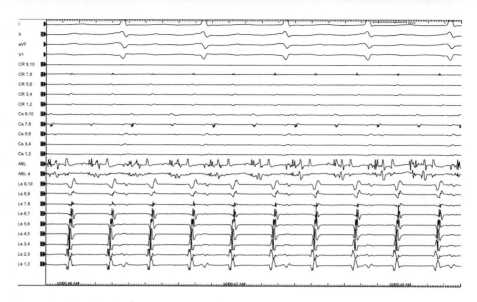

Figure 21.15 Mid-diastolic atrial activity at the site of the critical isthmus.

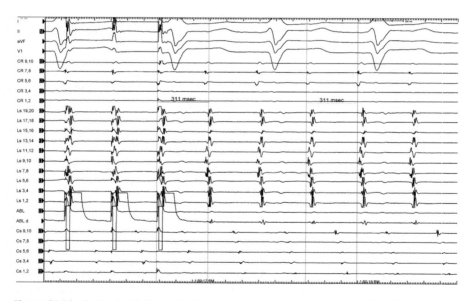

Figure 21.16 Pacing inside the critical isthmus shows concealed fusion and PPI−TCL = 0.

- RF lesions should target the critical isthmus, while forming a line between two barriers:
  - *Scar-related flutters*: From the patient-specific barrier (e.g., atriotomy, atrial septal patch, RF ablation area, etc.) to the closest anatomic barrier.
  - *RA flutters*:
    - Upper loop re-entry: SVC to TV annulus.
    - Right atrial free-wall re-entry: Patient-specific barrier (e.g., scar, atriotomy, suture line) to either IVC, TV annulus, or SVC.

- *LA flutters*:
  - *Peri-mitral re-entry*: MV annulus to either left inferior PV (lateral mitral isthmus line), roof line/a superior PV (anterior line), or a right PV (septal line).
    - *Note*: A mitral isthmus line often requires epicardial ablation within the distal CS, usually starting with power settings of 20 W and an irrigation flow rate ≥17 mL/min, discontinuing RF in case of a rapid change in impedance or rise in temperature.
  - *Roof-dependent re-entry*: Between the two superior PVs (roof line).
  - *Peri-septal re-entry*: Fossa ovalis to either MV annulus or a right PV.
- The line should be continuous, and can be formed either with sequential point-by-points RF applications or while withdrawing the catheter during a single continuous RF application.
- For each ablation site, RF energy should be maintained until the local atrial EGM splits into a double potential, indicating an effective lesion leading to local conduction block.
- During RF energy delivery, the AFL can terminate, ideally after some CL lengthening (Figure 21.17), but—again—this is not a reliable ablation end-point.
- In atypical AFLs following AF ablation, it is also important to confirm the persistence of PV antral isolation as well as address other non-PV triggers (i.e., LA posterior wall, SVC, CS, CT, interatrial septum, LAA, etc.) depending on the underlying substrate (see relative chapter).

ABLATION ENDPOINT

Non-inducibility can be used only if the AFL was easily and reliably induced before ablation. Gold standard remains documentation of bidirectional block across the ablation line, although this might be challenging. Usually, this is done with a combination of looking for continuous split potentials all along the line and evaluating differences of transisthmus conduction time, with or without differential pacing (Figure 21.18).

As an example, validation of lateral mitral isthmus block can be done with the CS catheter in combination with one catheter positioned in the superior-lateral LA (usually left atrial

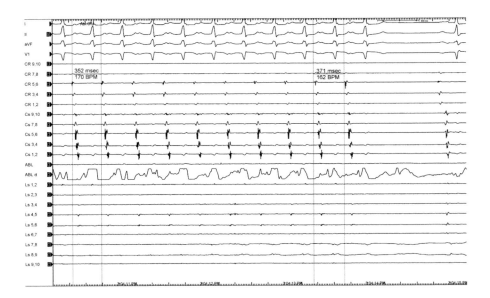

Figure 21.17   AFL termination with slowing during RF ablation.

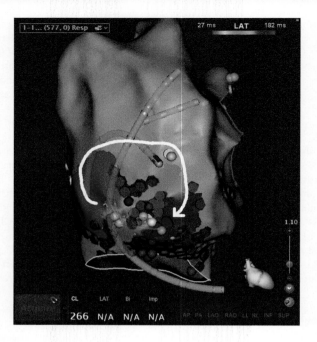

Figure 21.18 While pacing on one side of the ablation line, the electrical activation is very late just across the line suggesting electrical conduction block across the line (same patient as Figure 21.10).

appendage—LAA), allow pacing and recording on either side of the ablation line. Specific criteria are the following:

- Atrial activation sequence:
  - *Medial-to-lateral block*, With pacing from the septal aspect of the MI (e.g., distal CS):
    - Before ablation there is early activation in the LAA.
    - With block the LAA is activated late (following proximal CS)
  - *Lateral-to-medial block*, With pacing from the lateral aspect of the MI (e.g., LAA):
    - Before ablation CS activates from distal-to-proximal.
    - While with block the CS is activated in a strictly proximal-to-distal pattern.
- Split potentials:
  - Double EGMs separated by an isoelectric line with an interval of ≥150 ms across the whole ablation line.
- Differential pacing:
  - With pacing from the medial or lateral aspect of the MI and measuring the conduction time on the opposite side:
    - With block, when the pacing site is moved away from the ablation line conduction time shortens.
    - If there is still conduction through the MI, when the pacing site is moved away from the ablation line conduction time lengthens.

SUCCESS RATES AND COMPLICATIONS

Acute success rates are high (~73%–100%), with a moderate rate of recurrences (~7%–53%).[2] This variability mostly depends on the site of the circuit, underlying substrate, and experience of the operator. Repeat procedures are often needed and is not uncommon that recurrences actually represent different arrhythmias (either other atypical AFLs or AF).

For RA atypical flutters, complications are rare (see CTI). Specifically, right phrenic nerve injury can occur when ablating in the anterior aspect of the SVC and lateral LA. This is best avoided with pacing at high output (≥ 10 mA) from the distal ablation catheter before delivering RF energy to demonstrate lack of capture of the phrenic nerve; alternatively, a dedicated catheter can be positioned in the SVC to capture the phrenic nerve during RF ablation, stopping its delivery in case of reduced/absent diaphragmatic motion.

For LA atypical flutters, the risks are similar to those of AF ablation (reported rates up to 7%).[2] Most importantly, to reduce thromboembolic events, the procedure should be performed after adequate and with uninterrupted anticoagulation to prevent the formation of LAA clots; moreover, during the procedure IV heparin should be administered ideally before or immediately after transseptal access (goal ACT $\geq$ 300 s) and LA sheaths continuously flushed with a flow of 2–4 mL/min with pressurized heparinized-saline bags.

REFERENCES

1. Saoudi N, Cosío F, Waldo A et al. A classification of atrial flutter and regular atrial tachycardia according to electrophysiological mechanisms and anatomical bases. *Eur Heart J.* 2001;22(14):1162–1182. doi:10.1053/euhj.2001.2658.

2. Page RL, Joglar JAA, Caldwell MA et al. 2015 ACC/AHA/HRS guideline for the management of adult patients with supraventricular tachycardia. *J Am Coll Cardiol.* 2015. doi:10.1016/j.jacc.2015.08.856.

3. Stambler BS, Wood MA, Ellenbogen KA et al. Efficacy and safety of repeated intravenous doses of ibutilide for rapid conversion of atrial flutter or fibrillation. Ibutilide Repeat Dose Study Investigators. *Circulation.* 1996;94(7):1613–1621. doi:10.1161/01.CIR.94.7.1613.

4. Ghali WA, Wasil BI, Brant R et al. Atrial flutter and the risk of thromboembolism: A systematic review and meta-analysis. *Am J Med.* 2005;118(2):101–107. doi:10.1016/j.amjmed.2004.06.048.

5. January CT, Wann LS, Alpert JS et al. AHA/ACC/HRS guideline for the management of patients with atrial fibrillation: A report of the American college of cardiology/American heart association task force on practice guidelines and the heart rhythm society. *Circulation.* 2014;130(23):e199–e267. doi:10.1161/CIR.0000000000000041.

6. Wellens HJJ. Contemporary management of atrial flutter. *Circulation.* 2002; 106(6):649–652. doi:10.1161/01.CIR.0000027683.00417.9A.

7. Pérez FJ, Schubert CM, Parvez B et al. Long-term outcomes after catheter ablation of cavo-tricuspid isthmus dependent atrial flutter: A meta-analysis. *Circ Arrhythmia Electrophysiol.* 2009;2(4):393–401. doi:10.1161/CIRCEP.109.871665.

8. Cabrera JA, Damian S-Q, Ho SY et al. The architecture of the atrial musculature between the orifice of the inferior caval vein and the tricuspid valve: The anatomy of the isthmus. *J Cardiovasc Electrophysiol.* 1998;9(11):1186–1195.

9. Cabrera JA, Sánchez-Quintana D, Farré J et al. The inferior right atrial isthmus: Further architectural insights for current and coming ablation technologies. *J Cardiovasc Electrophysiol.* 2005;16(4):402–408. doi:10.1046/j.1540-8167.2005.40709.x.

10. Tai C-TT, Huang J-LL, Lee P-CC et al. High-resolution mapping around the crista terminalis during typical atrial flutter: New insights into mechanisms. *J Cardiovasc Electrophysiol.* 2004;15(4):406–414. doi:10.1046/j.1540-8167.2004.03535.x.

11. Yang Y, Cheng J, Bochoeyer A et al. Atypical right atrial flutter patterns. *Circulation.* 2001;103(25):3092–3098.

12. Chugh A, Latchamsetty R, Oral H et al. Characteristics of cavotricuspid isthmus-dependent atrial flutter after left atrial ablation of atrial fibrillation. *Circulation.* 2006;113(5):609–615. doi:10.1161/CIRCULATIONAHA.105.580936.

13. Hindricks G, Willems S, Kautzner J et al. Effect of electroanatomically guided versus conventional catheter ablation of typical atrial flutter on the fluoroscopy time and resource use: A prospective randomized multicenter study. *J Cardiovasc Electrophysiol.* 2009;20(7):734–740. doi:10.1111/j.1540-8167.2009.01439.x.

14. Atiga WL, Worley SJ, Hummel J et al. Prospective randomized comparison of cooled radiofrequency versus standard radiofrequency energy for ablation of typical atrial flutter. *Pacing Clin Electrophysiol {PACE}.* 2002;25(8):1172–1178. doi:10.1046/j.1460-9592.2002.01172.x.

15. Scavée C, Jaïs P, Hsu L-FF et al. Prospective randomised comparison of irrigated-tip and large-tip catheter ablation of cavotricuspid isthmus-dependent atrial flutter. *Eur Heart J.* 2004;25(11):963–969. doi:10.1016/j.ehj.2004.03.017.

16. Tada H, Oral H, Sticherling C et al. Double potentials along the ablation line as a guide to radiofrequency ablation of typical atrial flutter. *J Am Coll Cardiol.* 2001;38(3):750–755.

17. Oral H, Sticherling C, Tada H et al. Role of transisthmus conduction intervals in predicting bidirectional block after ablation of typical atrial flutter. *J Cardiovasc Electrophysiol.* 2001;12(2):169–174.

18. Shah D, Haïssaguerre M, Takahashi A et al. Differential pacing for distinguishing block from persistent conduction through an ablation line. *Circulation.* 2000;102(13):1517–1522.

19. Villacastin J, Almendral J, Arenal A et al. Usefulness of unipolar electrograms to detect isthmus block after radiofrequency ablation of typical atrial flutter. *Circulation.* 2000;102(25):3080–3085.

20. Tada H, Oral H, Sticherling C et al. Electrogram polarity and cavotricuspid isthmus block during ablation of typical atrial flutter. *J Cardiovasc Electrophysiol.* 2001;12(4):393–399.

21. Hamdan MH, Kalman JM, Barron HV, Lesh MD. P-wave morphology during right atrial pacing before and after atrial flutter ablation: A new marker for success. *Am J Cardiol.* 1997;79(10):1417–1420. doi:10.1016/S0002-9149(97)00156-2.

22. Waldo AL, Feld GK. Inter-relationships of atrial fibrillation and atrial flutter mechanisms and clinical implications. *J Am Coll Cardiol.* 2008;51(8):779–786. doi:10.1016/j.jacc.2007.08.066.

23. Navarrete A, Conte F, Moran M et al. Ablation of atrial fibrillation at the time of cavotricuspid isthmus ablation in patients with atrial flutter without documented atrial fibrillation derives a better long-term benefit. *J Cardiovasc Electrophysiol.* 2011;22(1):34–38. doi:10.1111/j.1540-8167.2010.01845.x.

24. Steinberg JS, Romanov A, Musat D et al. Prophylactic pulmonary vein isolation during isthmus ablation for atrial flutter: The PReVENT AF Study I. *Heart Rhythm.* 2014;11(9):1567–1572. doi:10.1016/j.hrthm.2014.05.011.

25. Mohanty S, Natale A, Mohanty P et al. Pulmonary vein isolation to reduce future risk of atrial fibrillation in patients undergoing typical flutter ablation: Results from a randomized pilot study (REDUCE AF). *J Cardiovasc Electrophysiol.* 2015;26(8):819–825. doi:10.1111/jce.12688.

26. Fiala M, Chovančík J, Neuwirth R et al. Atrial macroreentry tachycardia in patients without obvious structural heart disease or previous cardiac surgical or catheter intervention: Characterization of arrhythmogenic substrates, reentry circuits, and results of catheter ablation. *J Cardiovasc Electrophysiol.* 2007;18(8):824–832. doi:10.1111/j.1540-8167.2007.00859.x.

27. Marrouche NF, Natale A, Wazni OM et al. Left septal atrial flutter: Electrophysiology, anatomy, and results of ablation. *Circulation.* 2004;109(20):2440–2447. doi:10.1161/01.CIR.0000129439.03836.96.

RADIOFREQUENCY ABLATION OF ATRIAL FIBRILLATION

Jorge Romero, Carola Gianni, Sanghamitra Mohanty,
Chintan Trivedi, Domenico G. Della Rocca,
Andrea Natale, and Luigi Di Biase

CONTENTS

INTRODUCTION

- AF ablation aims to eliminate triggers or alter the substrate:
  - AF triggers frequently originate from the thoracic veins (pulmonary veins—PVs, superior vena cava—SVC, coronary sinus—CS). AF ablation aims to electrically "disconnect" these veins from the rest of the left and right atria. Other common AF triggers include the left atrial (LA) posterior wall, crista terminalis (CR), left atrial appendage (LAA), interatrial septum (IAS), ligament of Marshall (LoM), and mitral or tricuspid valve annuls.
  - Substrate-based AF ablation aims to alter the arrhythmic substrate. This is obtained by compartmentalizing the left atrium with linear lesions, targeting areas of complex electrograms (such as the CFAE), autonomic ganglionated plexi (GP), or AF drivers (such as rotors or focal impulses), and scar homogenization.
- In our center, AF ablation is trigger-based and includes the following:
  - Empirical electrical isolation of the entire PV antra, including the LA PW (Figure 22.1).[1] This is guided by a circular mapping catheter (CMC) and intracardiac echocardiography (ICE) to confirm isolation and avoid PV stenosis.
  - SVC isolation is usually performed empirically in both paroxysmal and non-paroxysmal AF.[2]
  - Additional trigger ablation is guided by their induction with high-dose isoproterenol.
  - More extensive ablation is necessary for persistent or long-standing persistent AF, extending PW isolation down to the mitral valve annulus ("floor" of the LA), anterior wall, and mid-IAS (anterior to the antra of the right PVs); it might also include empirical isolation of the CS and LAA.[3,4]

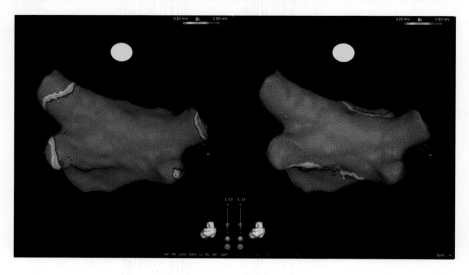

Figure 22.1   Posterior view of the LA showing voltage maps before and after PVAI.

- AF catheter ablation is useful for symptomatic AF patients refractory or intolerant to class I or III antiarrhythmic drugs (AAD).
- A baseline standard 2D transthoracic echocardiogram is useful to assess LA dimensions, interatrial septum morphology, left ventricular ejection fraction, and other gross abnormalities.
- Computerized tomography (CT) or magnetic resonance imaging (MRI) can also be performed for a better definition of LA anatomy, which can be integrated with the mapping system at the time of the ablation procedure (Figure 22.2); however, CT/MRI are not required to perform the procedure, mostly due to the utility of ICE.

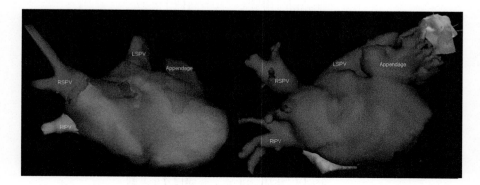

Figure 22.2   Volume map of the LA and corresponding CT scan.

- To minimize embolic risk:
  - All patients are required to undergo at least 4 weeks of therapeutic oral anticoagulation prior to the procedure.
  - If INR is subtherapeutic or non-adherence to novel oral anticoagulants (NOACs) is suspected, a trans-esophageal echocardiography (TEE) is performed to rule out LAA thrombosis.
  - The ablation procedure should be performed on uninterrupted therapeutic warfarin or factor Xa inhibitors.[5]

PROCEDURE

Catheter Selection
- A circular mapping catheter CMC is used as a roving catheter for mapping and directing the ablation catheter throughout the procedure.
  - It should be small enough to move within the chamber easily but of a large enough diameter that it does not readily fall deep inside the PVs: in most adults, a 20-mm 10-pole CMC is used.
  - CMC-guided ablation allows for efficient targeting of electrical potentials and it is the most effective way to confirm complete PVI.
- RF energy delivery with open irrigated catheters is the standard of care in performing PVAI.
  - Our catheter of choice is a unidirectional open-irrigated 3.5-mm tip catheter with an F or J curve (according to the LA size).
- Additionally, to map non-PV triggers, a 20-pole catheter is placed in the CS.
  - The distal 10 poles record CS electrograms while the proximal 10 poles record RA electrograms.

Before Transseptal Access
- All patients undergo ablation under general anesthesia to control respiration and patient movements, thus improving catheter stability; of note, paralytic agents should not be used or discontinued before ablation in proximity of the phrenic nerve(s).[6]
- An esophageal temperature probe is inserted orally in all patients to monitor esophageal location and luminal temperatures during ablation in the posterior aspect of the LA.
- Central venous access is obtained with real-time ultrasound to avoid vascular complications.[7] Access is as follows:
  - Two 8-French sheaths in the right femoral vein
    - These are later replaced with the transseptal sheaths.
  - One 11-French sheath in the left femoral vein for placement of the ICE catheter
    - The ICE catheter is placed in the RA/right ventricle to assess for baseline effusion, assist with performing transseptal punctures, guiding catheter location and manipulation within the LA, as well as monitoring for complications.
  - One 7-French sheath is also placed in the right jugular vein and used to pass a 20-pole deflectable catheter.
  - In most cases, an arterial line is not necessary and leads to hematomas in anticoagulated patients; non-invasive intermittent blood pressure monitoring (every 2–5 min) is usually sufficient.
- A heparin bolus is given before the transseptal puncture (usually 100 U/kg up to 10.000 U with warfarin, or 12.000–15.000 U with factor Xa inhibitors) to achieve an ACT of 350–500 s.
  - ACT is checked every 15 min during the procedure, and repeat small boluses might be necessary to keep the ACT at goal.

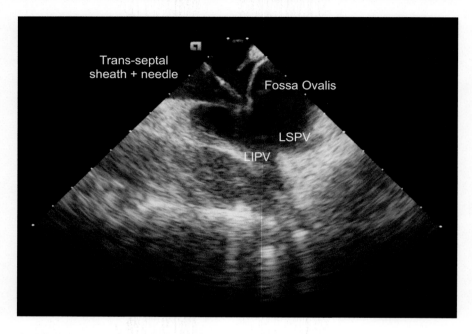

Figure 22.3 ICE view during transseptal access.

Transseptal Access

- Left atrial catheterization is then performed under ICE guidance through two transseptal punctures at the mid to posterior IAS (e.g., the left-sided PVs should be visible on ICE; Figure 22.3).
  - To advance the transseptal needle, manual pressure can be used; to facilitate access, radiofrequency (RF) is frequently used (either using an electrocautery pen set to cut at 20–40 W and applied externally near the metal hub or using a dedicated RF-powered transseptal needle).
  - A successful transseptal puncture is confirmed with visualization of contrast or bubbles in the LA on fluoroscopy or ICE, respectively.
  - Although a second transseptal sheath can be introduced via wire exchange, a separate transseptal puncture minimizes sheath-to-sheath interaction.
  - LA access can be obtained using a variety of transseptal sheaths; sheaths with a moderate primary curve and no secondary curve (such as the SLO 50° for the ablation catheter and a LAMP 90° for the circular mapping catheter—CMC) allow easier catheter maneuverability in the posterior aspect of the LA.

Mapping and Ablation

- Before ablation, it is useful to create an accurate volume map of the LA using the CMC and ablation catheter and the electro-anatomical mapping (EAM) system of choice (Carto, NavX EnSite, Rhythmia; Figure 22.2).
  - The use of ICE during mapping facilitates locating the four PVs and LAA, making sure that the CMC is not advanced far into the PV (Figure 22.4).
    - The left-sided PVs can be seen with clockwise rotation of the ICE catheter a few degrees past the LAA and the mitral valve annulus.
    - The right PVs, the ICE catheter is advanced slightly and further rotated clockwise.
  - While maneuvering the CMC, care should be taken not to displace it anteriorly, as this can result in its entrapment in the mitral valve apparatus.

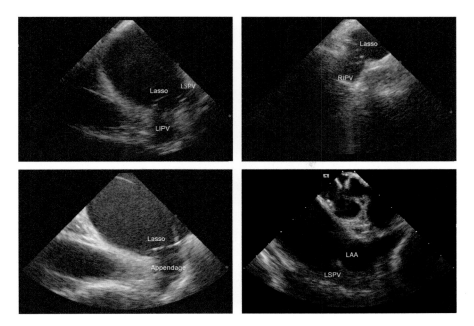

Figure 22.4 ICE views of the PVs and LAA obtained from the RA and RVOT.

- When using fluoroscopy, the AP view is commonly used for all purposes; an orthogonal view is often helpful when CMC-ablation catheter contact is not clear: RAO for the left-sided PVs, LAO for the right-sided PVs.
- Using the open-irrigated tip ablation catheter, a power of 40 W is typically used (the temperature cut-off varies according to the type of ablation catheter) with the goal of local potential abatement.
  - Occasionally, on the anterior aspect of the PVs (e.g., a thick ridge), a higher power is needed (generally, not exceeding 45 W).
  - With these power settings, when using contact-force sensing ablation catheters, the contact force goal is 7–15 g.
  - As for duration, when using 40 W applied with 7–15 g, RF energy is delivered for approximately 10–20 s per lesion site, until the electrical signals have diminished.
  - Of note, in areas near the esophagus, energy delivery should be limited to up to 10 s per lesion site, and the ablation catheter should move frequently to different/distant areas during ablation to prevent esophageal heating.
    - It is very important to monitor the esophageal temperature, readjusting the position esophageal probe so that it is close to the ablation area.
    - As a general rule, esophageal temperatures greater than 38°C–39°C should be avoided to minimize the risk of deep tissue injury.
    - The esophagus is wider than the temperature probe, therefore sometimes no or minimal temperature change is recorded, despite ablating over the esophagus, as assessed by ICE or fluoroscopy with esophageal contrast (Figure 22.5).
    - If real-time imaging of the esophagus is not available, it is important to move quickly whenever ablating in the posterior aspect of the left atrium regardless of the location of the esophageal probe.

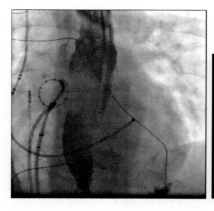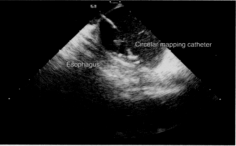

Figure 22.5 Fluoroscopy with contrast injection or ICE to delineate the course of the esophagus.

- The endpoint of PVAI is to achieve PVI and eliminate electrical signals in the antra of the PVs.
  - Under CMC-guidance, lesions are delivered throughout the antral surface, including the areas between and around the PVs and the roof of the LA.
  - Electrical potentials are identified with the roving CMC, and the ablation catheter is maneuvered to these targets (Figure 22.6).
  - We usually begin with ablation of the electrical potentials surrounding each PV.
    - Complete PV electrical isolation is confirmed by entrance and exit block.
    - Entrance block is confirmed by the absence of electrical signals where these signals had been previously observed (Figure 22.7).
    - Occasionally, dissociated PV potentials can be recorded to confirm exit block (Figure 22.7); in addition, pacing from within the PV can be performed, although this is not necessary.
  - Once PVI is achieved, we focus on the remaining antral areas, including the LA posterior wall/roof and interatrial septum anterior to the right PVs.
    - The CMC is useful for identifying additional electrical potentials along the PW and roof of the LAA.
    - The ablation catheter is maneuvered to the CMC poles, where the potentials are observed, and RF energy is delivered.
- PVAI can be performed either in AF or sinus rhythm; when patients remain in AF at the end of the ablation, cardioversion is performed.
- With patients in sinus rhythm, 20–30 mcg/kg/min of isoproterenol are infused to assess for PV reconnection and elicit non-PV triggers.
  - The 10-pole CMC is positioned in the left superior PV recording the far-field LAA activity (thus avoiding mechanical induction of LAA arrhythmias); the ablation catheter in the right superior PV that records the far-field IAS; the 20-pole catheter records activity from the SVC to the CS (Figure 22.8).
  - If non-PV triggers are consistent (repetitive PACs, PACs triggering atrial flutter/AF, focal atrial tachycardia), their sites of origin are further targeted with ablation.
    - When triggers from either the SVC, CS, or LAA are observed, isolation of these structures is the best endpoint.
    - SVC isolation is performed at the end of the procedure (see below).

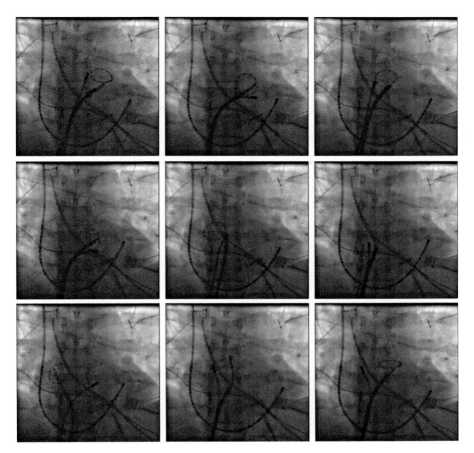

Figure 22.6   CMC position to perform PVAI.

- CS isolation is achieved by ablating the structure endocardially in the LA (at the level of the mitral valve annulus) and epicardially inside the CS.
- LAA isolation is isolated similarly to PVI, by targeting the breakthrough recorded on the CMC during sinus rhythm; the myocardium surrounding the LAA is thicker, therefore longer RF application times and/or higher power are usually necessary.

- Once ablation in the LA is completed, catheters and sheaths are pulled back in the RA and protamine (40 mg are usually sufficient) can be given to reverse heparin-induced anticoagulation.
- SVC isolation (empirical or isoproterenol-driven) is performed at the end of the procedure.
  - It is achieved similarly to PVI, by positioning the CMC at the level of the RA-SVC junction and targeting early potentials.
  - Phrenic nerve mapping (see complications) should be performed when ablating non-septal segments and ablation avoided if capture is present.
  - Sinus node injury can occur when ablating the anterior segments: If sinus rhythm accelerates, RF should be promptly interrupted.

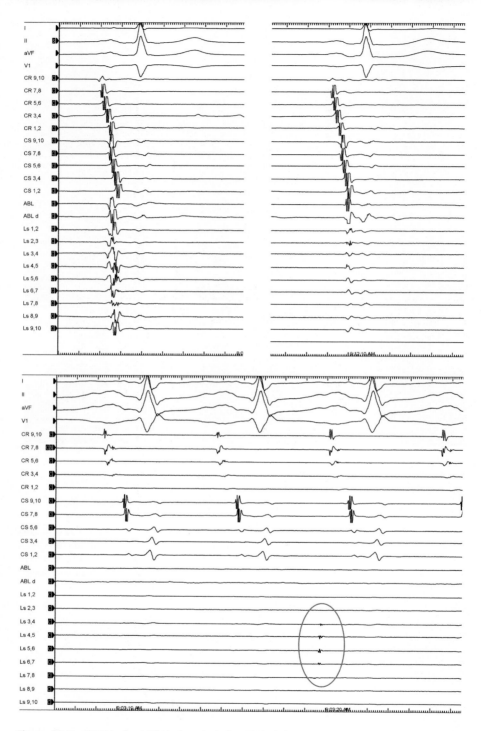

Figure 22.7 CMC in the LSPV before and after PV isolation; CMC in the LSPV showing dissociated firing during high-dose isoproterenol.

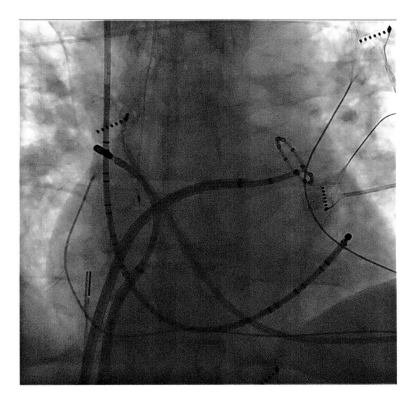

Figure 22.8 Catheter position during isoproterenol infusion.

POST-PROCEDURE CARE AND FOLLOW-UP

- Access sheaths can be pulled once the ACT is <180 s; alternative, vascular access closure devices can be used.
- Many patients will have a large net positive fluid balance when non-low flow irrigated-tip catheters are used, and diuretics should be administered accordingly.
- Patients will typically lie flat for 4–6 h after sheaths are pulled and are usually discharged the following day, after being monitored overnight for peri-procedural complications.
- All patients receive oral anticoagulation for at least 3 months, irrespective of their baseline thromboembolic risk; the decision to discontinue oral anticoagulation thereafter is taken on an individual basis, and it depends on the patient's thromboembolic and bleeding risk as well as the success of the procedure (assessed with intense ECG monitoring).[8]
  - If LAA isolation is performed, it is mandatory to assess its mechanical function during sinus rhythm with TEE (usually 6 months post ablation): if poor LAA contractility/low LAA systolic flow velocities (<0.4 m/s), either oral anticoagulation should be continued indefinitely or LAA occlusion taken into consideration.
- Patients typically follow the pre-ablation antiarrhythmic regimen during the first 2–3 months, with the decision to discontinue, continue, or change AADs depending on the arrhythmia burden thereafter.

COMPLICATIONS

- Vascular complications (hematomas, pseudoaneurysm, and arteriovenous fistulas) these can be easily prevented using real-time ultrasound when obtaining central venous access.
- To reduce periprocedural thromboembolic events, the procedure should be performed under uninterrupted oral anticoagulation and heparin administered transseptal access with goal ACT ≥ 350 s.
- To prevent air embolism, transseptal sheaths should be continuously flushed with 2–4 mL/min of heparinized-saline using pressure bags set at 300–400 mmHg.
- A drop in blood pressure, both sudden and gradual, should be evaluated carefully.
    - A vagal response to ablation near the ganglionic plexi may result in transient sudden hypotension, usually associated with bradycardia (sinus arrest or atrioventricular block); if there is no immediate recovery, cardiac tamponade should be assumed until proven otherwise.
    - Cardiac tamponade should be suspected after a difficult transseptal puncture (especially without ICE guidance), a steam pop, or inadvertent application of excess pressure in the LAA or the roof of the LA.
        - Early diagnosis of cardiac tamponade is important not to delay pericardiocentesis: a quick assessment can be performed with ICE; if this is not available, fluoroscopy usually demonstrates a reduction in the excursion of the cardiac silhouette in the LAO view.
- Atrio-esophageal fistulas can present in the weeks following ablation; though exceedingly rare, they are frequently fatal therefore prevention and early diagnosis/treatment (surgical repair) are important to reduce mortality.
    - During ablation, temperature monitoring as well as limitation of the duration of energy delivery when ablating in the posterior aspect of the LA (down to the CS) is vital to avoid excessive heating of the esophagus.
    - A short course of prophylactic proton pump inhibitors and sucralfate can be prescribed.
    - During follow-up, patient and physician awareness is key: patients should be instructed to immediately contact the electrophysiology service if fever, chest pain, neurological symptoms, dysphagia, hematemesis, or melena occur.
- Phrenic nerve injury can be right sided, when ablating in the right superior PV or performing isolation of the SVC, or left sided, when ablating inside the LAA.
    - To prevent phrenic nerve injury, it is important to avoid ablation inside the PVs or LAA, and to perform phrenic nerve mapping when isolating the SVC.
    - Patients with phrenic nerve paralysis are usually asymptomatic, but they can present with dyspnea on exertion; there is no treatment, but the condition is usually transient, so observation is all that is needed.
- PV stenosis is a rare occurrence after true PVAI, since RF energy is not delivered ostial or inside the PVs.
    - Positioning the CMC at the level of the PV antrum (as assessed by ICE) and targeting potentials proximal to it helps to avoid RF delivery inside the PV ostia.
    - Patients are usually asymptomatic, but severe stenosis can lead to dyspnea, with or without cough or hemoptysis.
    - Severe or symptomatic PV stenosis might require intervention (venoplasty and stenting).

REFERENCES

1. He X, Zhou Y, Chen Y et al. Left atrial posterior wall isolation reduces the recurrence of atrial fibrillation: A meta-analysis. *J Interv Card Electrophysiol.* 2016;46(3):267–274. doi:10.1007/s10840-016-0124-7.

2. Corrado A, Bonso A, Madalosso M et al. Impact of systematic isolation of superior vena cava in addition to pulmonary vein antrum isolation on the outcome of paroxysmal, persistent, and permanent atrial fibrillation ablation: Results from a randomized study. *J Cardiovasc Electrophysiol.* 2010;21(1):1–5. doi:10.1111/j.1540-8167.2009.01577.x.

3. Chang H, Lo L, Lin Y et al. Long-term outcome of catheter ablation in patients with atrial fibrillation originating from the superior vena cava. *J Cardiovasc Electrophysiol.* 2010;68(9):955–961. doi:10.1111/j.1540-8167.2012.02337.x.

4. Di Biase L, Burkhardt JD, Mohanty P et al. Left atrial appendage isolation in patients with longstanding persistent AF undergoing catheter ablation: BELIEF trial. *J Am Coll Cardiol.* 2016;68(18):1929–1940. doi:10.1016/j.jacc.2016.07.770.

5. Zhao Y, Yang Y, Tang X et al. New oral anticoagulants compared to warfarin for perioperative anticoagulation in patients undergoing atrial fibrillation catheter ablation: A meta-analysis of continuous or interrupted new oral anticoagulants during ablation compared to interrupted or co. *J Interv Card Electrophysiol.* 2017;48(3):267–282. doi:10.1007/s10840-016-0221-7.

6. Di Biase L, Conti S, Mohanty P et al. General anesthesia reduces the prevalence of pulmonary vein reconnection during repeat ablation when compared with conscious sedation: Results from a randomized study. *Hear Rhythm.* 2011;8(3):368–372. doi:10.1016/j.hrthm.2010.10.043.

7. Wu S, Ling Q, Cao L et al. Real-time two-dimensional ultrasound guidance for central venous cannulation: A meta-analysis. *Anesthesiology.* 2013;118(2):361–375. doi:10.1097/ALN.0b013e31827bd172.

8. Themistoclakis S, Corrado A, Marchlinski FE et al. The risk of thromboembolism and need for oral anticoagulation after successful atrial fibrillation ablation. *J Am Coll Cardiol.* 2010;55(8):735–743. doi:10.1016/j.jacc.2009.11.039.

VENTRICULAR ARRHYTHMIAS IN THE STRUCTURALLY NORMAL HEART

Andres Enriquez and Fermin Garcia

CONTENTS

INTRODUCTION

Ventricular tachycardia (VT) most often occurs in the context of structural heart disease, such as coronary artery disease (CAD), severe valvular heart disease, or idiopathic dilated cardiomyopathy. However, ventricular arrhythmias (VAs) may also occur in individuals with no apparent structural heart disease. These arrhythmias are termed idiopathic VTs and account for 10% of all VT diagnoses.[1] Although the prognosis is typically favorable, they may be associated with invalidating symptoms, and patient with a high burden of VAs may develop a reversible form of cardiomyopathy.[2] In rare cases, they can trigger ventricular fibrillation (VF) and be a cause of sudden cardiac death in a normal structural heart.[3,4]

Various classifications have been proposed, based on different criteria such as clinical presentation, underlying mechanism, site of origin, and response to pharmacological interventions. From a mechanistic point of view, idiopathic VTs can be divided into two groups: focal VTs, which are predominantly triggered or automatic arrhythmias, and fascicular VTs (verapamil-dependent VT or Belhassen VT), which are predominantly re-entrant arrhythmias that involve the Purkinje system.[5] Outflow tract (OT) VT is the most common form of focal VT and originates in 70%–80% of cases from the right ventricular OT (RVOT),[6,7] explaining its typical electrocardiographic (ECG) appearance characterized by left bundle branch block (LBBB) pattern and inferior axis.

OT VTs are a subgroup of focal VTs that are predominantly localized in and around the right and left ventricular (LV) outflow tracts (Figure 23.1) and are easily recognized by a positive QRS in inferior leads. In a large series including 265 patients with idiopathic OT VTs referred for catheter ablation, the successful ablation site was the RVOT in 75%, the aortic root in 17%, the basal LV endocardium in 4%, the LV epicardium in 1%, and the pulmonary artery (PA) in 1%.[7] VTs originating in the RVOT show a predilection for females, whereas VTs originating in the aortic cusps are more common in men.[8,9]

Clinical presentations include repetitive monomorphic ectopy (the most common), nonsustained monomorphic VT, and exercise-induced sustained VT.[10] Patients are typically aged 30–50 years and the most common symptom is palpitations, however it may also present with fatigue, chest pain, dyspnea, and occasionally presyncope or heart failure.[11] Some patients, on the other side, may be completely asymptomatic.

As demonstrated by Lerman et al., the mechanism of OT VT is triggered activity due to delayed after-depolarizations that are determined by intracellular calcium overload.[12,13] Catecholamine stimulation of the β-adrenergic receptor results in a rise in intracellular cyclic AMP, producing an increase in the levels of intracellular calcium and release of calcium from the sarcoplasmic reticulum. This process then gives rise to delayed after-depolarizations and VT. Focal VTs can be induced with catecholamines and rapid pacing, but not usually with programmed ventricular stimulation. Adenosine exerts an inhibitory effect on AC and cAMP, reversing intracellular calcium overload; thus, termination by adenosine is a signature of idiopathic OT VTs.[14]

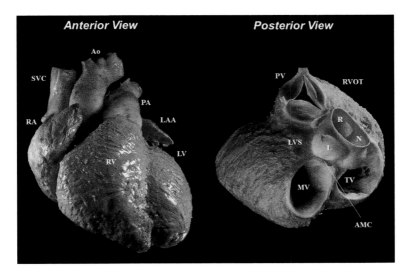

Figure 23.1 Anatomy of the outflow tract region. The anterior view is mostly dominated by the RVOT wrapping around the aorta. In the posterior view the complex relationship of all the structures of the RVOT and LVOT becomes evident. AMC = aortomitral continuity; Ao = aorta; L = left coronary cusp; LAA = left atrial appendage; LV = left ventricle; LVS = left ventricular summit; MV = mitral valve; N = noncoronary cusp; PA = pulmonary artery; PV = pulmonic valve; R = right coronary cusp; RA = right atrium; RV = right ventricle; SVC = superior vena cava; TV = tricuspid valve. (Courtesy of Dr. K. Shivkumar, UCLA Cardiac Arrhythmia Center, Wallace A. McAlpine Collection.)

The prognosis is usually benign and patients with no or minimal symptoms may only need reassurance without specific therapy. In case of significant symptoms or PVC-mediated cardiomyopathy, treatment options include pharmacological therapy and catheter ablation. First-line antiarrhythmic therapy is usually a beta-blocker, which is effective in less than 50% of patients.[11] Other options include class I antiarrhythmic agents, such as flecainide or propafenone, or class III antiarrhythmic agents, such as sotalol and amiodarone.[11,15,16] Catheter ablation is a safe and effective alternative to antiarrhythmic medication and is considered a first line therapy for symptomatic patients with RVOT VT/PVCs.[17] In these patients success rates exceed 90%–95%.[18] Ablation at other sites can be more challenging and is associated with lower success rates.

GENERAL APPROACH FOR ECG LOCALIZATION

A systematic approach to ECG analysis is helpful for predicting the likely site of arrhythmia origin, which is important for preprocedural planning and patient counseling regarding risks and success rates. All OT VAs share an inferiorly directed QRS axis, with positive forces in leads II, III, and aVF. Additional elements allow a more precise localization, including the bundle branch pattern, precordial transition, and frontal plane axis.[19]

A first initial step is to discriminate between origin from the RVOT or LVOT regions. Typically, RVOT VAs exhibit a LBBB configuration with precordial R/S transition at or after lead V3. By contrast, LVOT VT usually manifests either a right bundle branch block (RBBB) or a LBBB with precordial R/S transition at or before lead V3. This can be better understood if we imagine that the RVOT is anterior in the chest and the precordial leads register anterior to posterior (front to back) (Figure 23.2). Thus, as we move progressively more posterior from the RVOT free wall to the lateral mitral annulus, the precordial transition becomes progressively earlier

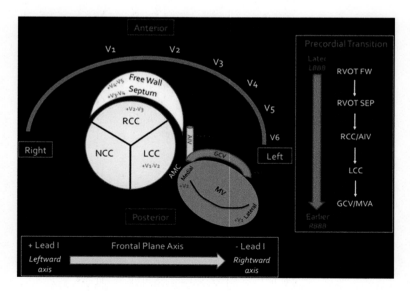

Figure 23.2 Attitudinally-based schema to understand the ECG patterns of outflow tract ventricular arrhythmias. (From Hutchinson, M. and Garcia, F., *J. Cardiovasc Electrophysiol.* 24, 1189–1197, 2013.)

(V4–V5 for RVOT free wall, V3–V4 for RVOT septum, V2–V3 for right coronary cusp [RCC]), and finally transforms from an LBBB to a RBBB configuration at the top of the mitral valve (MV) or left coronary cusp (LCC). Differentiation between RVOT/LVOT may be challenging when the R/S transition is in V3, as this pattern can be seen both in VAs from the posteroseptal RVOT or the LVOT (especially RCC), and some ECG criteria have been proposed to predict the site of origin in these cases. One algorithm compares the precordial transition during VT/premature ventricular complexes (PVCs) and sinus rhythm.[20] When VT/PVC transition occurs later than the sinus rhythm transition, the PVC origin is the RVOT (100% specificity). If the VT/PVC transition occurs at or earlier than the sinus rhythm transition, then the so-called V2 transition ratio is measured. This is calculated as the percentage R-wave during VT/PVC divided by the percentage R-wave during sinus rhythm. A ratio ≥0.6 predicts an LVOT origin with a sensitivity of 95% and a specificity of 100%. Another ECG criteria are the indexes of R wave duration (QRS duration divided by the longer R wave duration in V1 or V2) and R/S wave amplitude (greater R/S wave amplitude ratio) in leads V1 and V2.[21] A longer R wave duration index (>0.5) and higher R/S wave amplitude index (>0.3) suggests an LVOT origin.

Another important element to consider is the frontal plane QRS axis, reflected by the bipolar limb lead I and by the relative S wave amplitude in aVL compared to aVR (Figure 23.3). A positive QRS complex in lead I and a more negative aVR compared to aVL suggests an origin on the right side of midline. Such structures include the posterior RVOT, RCC, tricuspid valve (TV), the parahisian region, and the posterior LV. In contrast, a negative QRS complex in lead I and a more negative aVL than aVR suggest an origin on the left side of midline, including: anterior RVOT, LCC, MV, and LV summit (LVS). The right-left cusp junction can have characteristics of either the right or left side of the midline and its behavior in the frontal plane is less predictable, however a notch in the downstroke of V1 is suggestive of origin from this structure.[22]

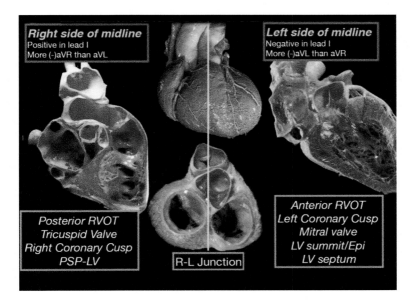

Figure 23.3 Determination of frontal plane axis to rapidly localize the site of origin of outflow tract ventricular arrhythmias. Ventricular arrhythmias are divides in those that are positive in lead I versus the ones that are negative in lead I. The R–L junction could be in either group, however the signature "W" pattern in V1 helps guide mapping. (Courtesy of Dr. K. Shivkumar, UCLA Cardiac Arrhythmia Center, Wallace A. McAlpine Collection.)

MAPPING

The procedure should be performed under conscious sedation to avoid suppression of the clinical VT/PVCs. A quadripolar catheter is positioned at the RV apex for pacing and a phased-array intra-cardiac echocardiography (ICE) catheter is advanced into the right atrium (RA). When an LVOT or LVS origin is suspected based on ECG features, an additional quadripolar or decapolar catheter (4 or 6 French) should be placed within the coronary sinus (CS) and advanced as distally as possible to compare activation time of the great cardiac vein (GCV)/anterior interventricular vein (AIV) region with other sites within the LVOT. CS cannulation with a long sheath may facilitate catheter advancement and manipulation. For mapping the RVOT, the use of deflectable sheaths (Agilis, St. Jude Medical, St. Paul, MN) allows to improve catheter maneuverability and contact. For aortic root and basal LV arrhythmias, a long sheath (SL1 or SR0) is also helpful for enhanced catheter stability. For LV mapping and ablation, heparin is administered to maintain an ACT > 250 s.

Given the focal mechanism of these VAs, activation mapping is the preferred technique in patients with spontaneous or inducible VT/PVCs. At the site of successful ablation, the local bipolar electrogram recorded from the distal electrode usually precedes the QRS onset by about 20–40 ms and the unipolar electrogram records a QS signal. In the absence of spontaneous arrhythmia, induction of VT or PVCs is attempted with isoproterenol or dobutamine infusion and ventricular or atrial burst pacing.

Electro-anatomic mapping is very helpful and further enhances precise localization by permitting three-dimensional (3D) reconstruction of intracardiac anatomy. We use the CARTO 3D mapping system (Biosense Webster, Inc., Diamond Bar, CA) complemented with phased-array ICE (AcuNav, Siemens Medical Solutions, Mountain View, CA). We usually start by creating a detailed anatomic reconstruction of both ventricles and the aortic cusp region. The CARTOSOUND module (Biosense Webster, Diamond Bar, CA) permits the rapid construction of a 3D shell by integration of real-time two-dimensional (2D) contours. Important anatomic landmarks, such as the His, the tricuspid annulus, pulmonic annulus, and the ostia of the coronary arteries, are identified and tagged in the 3D map. Other integration techniques with 3D mapping systems are also available using pre adquired, offline cardiac MRI, or CT scan reconstruction.

Pace mapping may be used as an adjunct to activation mapping or as the primary mapping strategy if PVCs/VTs are infrequent. Pacing is performed at the diastolic threshold to avoid farfield capture and at a rate similar to the tachycardia cycle length. The goal is to achieve an identical match (12 of 12 leads) between the clinical arrhythmia and the paced beat. Pace mapping is particularly valuable for RVOT arrhythmias, but is less useful for VAs from the LVOT and aortic cusps because of the close proximity of the different structures, preferential conduction across the ventricular septum or the inability to obtain myocardial capture despite high pacing current.[23] Automated algorithms have been incorporated within recording and mapping systems to increase the accuracy of pace mapping. These algorithms quantify the similarity between the paced beat and a stored template of the clinical VT/PVC and the matching score is expressed as a percentage.[24-26]

In case of nonsustained arrhythmias or infrequent PVCs despite provocation techniques, there is a role for non-contact mapping system and multielectrode catheters. Non-contact mapping (EnSite Array, St. Jude Medical, St. Paul, MN) can create a full activation map from a single tachycardia beat. Use of commercially available multi-electrode catheters enables rapid high-density activation mapping through simultaneous multiple-point acquisition.

In the majority of cases, we use a 3.5-mm open-irrigated tip ablation catheter. In the RVOT, a maximum power setting of 30–35 W is used. For the LVOT and aortic cusp region, the typical maximal power setting is 30 W; however, in select cases with late termination of PVCs or suppression and recurrence of ectopy, powers of up to 50 W are used. When ablating in the aortic cusps, we start with low power (20 W) and gradually increase to no more than 30–35 W.

As mentioned, targets for radiofrequency (RF) delivery include earliest local bipolar activation preceding the QRS and the presence of a QS pattern in the unipolar electrogram of the ablation catheter, usually associated with good pace mapping. The bipolar electrogram usually has a sharp rapid initial deflection, and may demonstrate reversal of a late component present during sinus rhythm.

Ablation at the successful site usually results in early termination of the VT ($\leq$15 s), in some cases preceded by increase in arrhythmia frequency likely due to stimulatory effect of RF energy in proximity to the arrhythmia focus. If VT/PVC suppression or acceleration occurs in the first 10 s, RF delivery is continued for a total of 60 s. An impedance drop of approximately 10 Ω is desired. If no effect is observed after 15–20 s, RF delivery is terminated and the catheter repositioned.

Acute ablation success is defined as the absence of the clinical VT/PVC at 30 min after the last RF delivery, both with and without isoproterenol, and confirmed by continuous cardiac telemetry in the subsequent 24 h of inpatient care.

RVOT TACHYCARDIAS

The RV is the most anterior cardiac chamber, lying immediately behind the sternum, and wraps around the aorta, so its anterior aspect becomes the most leftward and highest OT structure. Beginning at the level of the TV, the RV is divided into 2 parts: an inflow tract or "sinus", highly trabeculated, particularly at the apex, and an outflow tract or "infundibulum (conus)", relatively glabrous. Both portions are separated by the crista supraventricularis, a prominent muscular ridge that extends from the interventricular septum to the RV free wall, becoming the moderator band (MB).[27] The RVOT region is defined superiorly by the pulmonic valve and inferiorly by the level of the superior aspect of the TV. Although the RV inflow and the TV lie to the right and anterior to the LV inflow and MV, the RVOT crosses the LVOT anteriorly and therefore the upper portion and the pulmonic valve lies to the left of the aortic valve.[28] The pulmonary trunk continues leftward and divides in a right and left PA, the right of which will course below the aortic arch. The posterior wall of the infundibulum is in continuity with the LVOT and adjacent anterior interventricular septum, while its more distal portion is immediately adjacent to the left aortic cusps. The anatomical relationship between the RVOT and LVOT can be better understood if one imagines that the RVOT wraps around the LVOT, so that the posteroseptal aspect starting in the septal leaflet of the TV continues wrapping around the RCC and finishes in the septal pulmonic valve (Figure 23.3). The anteroseptal aspect of the RVOT is adjacent to the LCC, in close proximity to the left anterior descending (LAD) and AIV.

For the purpose of mapping, the RVOT can be divided in 3 zones, named 1 to 3 from posterior to anterior, each of which is subdivided into a septal and free wall site (Figure 23.4).[6] Most RVOT VAs originate from the anterosuperior aspect of the septum below the pulmonic valve (septal sites 2 and 3). VAs originated from the RVOT typically have a LBBB configuration with an inferior axis. Free wall RVOT sites can be differentiated from septal sites by a smaller voltage in lead II and III, later precordial transition (V4–V5 versus V3–V4), a wider QRS duration (>140 ms), and the presence of characteristic "notching" in the inferior leads. In addition, the QRS morphology in lead I helps to distinguish posterior from anterior

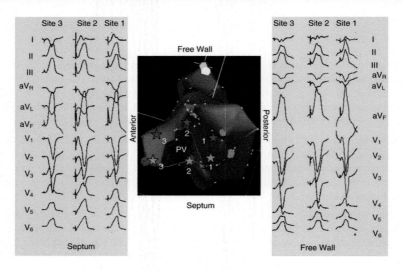

Figure 23.4 Twelve-lead ECG pacemaps from sites 1, 2, and 3 along the septum and free wall of the RVOT showing characteristic features. PV = pulmonic valve. (From Dixit, S. et al., *Heart Rhythm.*, 2, 485–491, 2005.)

sites along the septum and free wall, with posterior locations (site 1) demonstrating a positive polarity in lead I (R wave) and more negative aVR than aVL, while anterior locations (site 3) exhibit a negative polarity in lead I (QS pattern) and more negative aVL than aVR.[6] Intermediate sites (site 2) demonstrate either a biphasic or multiphasic QRS pattern (rs, qrs) or an isoelectric segment preceding a small q or r wave.

Mapping the RVOT is facilitated by the use of a deflectable sheath (Agilis, St. Jude Medical, St. Paul, MN). The catheter is advanced through the sheath into the PA and then slowly withdrawn into the RV. The point where the ventricular electrogram appears as the catheter is withdrawn is marked as valve point. Within the RVOT, counterclockwise torque moves the catheter tip towards the septal aspect, while clockwise torque moves the catheter tip towards the free wall. Catheter deflection brings the catheter tip posteriorly and release of deflection moves it anteriorly.

In approximately 4%–6% of patients with RVOT tachycardia, the site of origin may be above the plane of the pulmonic valve, likely from strands of myocardial tissue extending into the PA.[29,30] ECG characteristics of these arrhythmias include a strong right inferior axis with tall R waves in II, III, and aVF; negative QRS in lead I, and deeper S waves in aVL than aVR. These findings are explained by the fact that the site of origin within the PA is higher, more anterior, and more leftward compared to most RVOT VAs. It is important to acknowledge that the LAD runs at the same level of the pulmonic valve in the interventricular sulcus and ablation above the pulmonic valve could injure the proximal LAD with catastrophic consequences. Therefore, any attempt of ablation above the level of the valve should be preceded by careful definition of the coronary circulation.

LVOT TACHYCARDIAS

LVOT tachycardias represent approximately 20% of OT idiopathic VTs.[7] These arrhythmias include those originating from the left parahisian region, the aortomitral continuity (AMC), and the MV. Aortic cusp and epicardial OT VTs will be discussed separately.

Anatomically, the LVOT corresponds to the opening of the LV, also termed the LV ostium by McAlpine.[31] This has an elliptical shape and is covered by the aorto-ventricular membrane, a fibrous structure that is perforated by the aorta anteriorly, and the mitral valve posteriorly and laterally (Figure 23.4). In contrast to the RV infundibulum, which is comprised entirely of muscle, the ventriculo-aortic junction is composed of a fibrous portion and a muscular portion.[32,33] The muscular portion, more extensive, corresponds to the interventricular muscular septum and is under the right coronary sinus and the anterior half of the left coronary sinus. The fibrous portion corresponds to the AMC, a curtain of fibrous tissue that extends between the anterior leaflet of the MV and the noncoronary and left coronary leaflets of the aortic valve.

VAs from the left parahisian region are characterized by a LBBB morphology with a QS or Qr pattern in V1, early precordial transition (≤V3), higher amplitude in lead II than lead III, and predominantly positive forces (R or Rs morphology) in lead I. VAs ablated from the AMC shows a RBBB pattern in the majority of cases, with a positive vector in V1. Using pace mapping, Dixit et al. demonstrated that a qR pattern in lead V1 is relatively specific for pacing at the AMC,[6] but the sensitivity of this finding is <50%.[34,35] VAs ablated from the MV annulus represent a 5% of all idiopathic VTs/PVCs.[36–38] Most common location is anterolateral, followed by the posteroseptal and posterior regions. The ECG typically shows a RBBB pattern and an S wave in lead V6. Precordial R wave transition usually occurs by V1 (positive concordance in precordial leads), but in some VTs mapped to the posteroseptal region transition may occur between leads V1 and V2.[36–38] Compared to septal sites, anterolateral and lateral sites exhibit a longer QRS duration along with predominantly negative forces in lead I. For mapping and ablation, access to the MV can be retrograde, via transeptal puncture or epicardial via the CS.

For mapping LVOT sites we use a retrograde aortic approach. First, planes of mitral and aortic valves are defined.[39] For outlining the MV, the mapping catheter is positioned in the basal LV such that the distal electrode pair records a large ventricular electrogram preceded by a smaller or equal size atrial electrogram. In this orientation, three different points (medial, lateral, and superior or inferior) are acquired to create the valve plane. Next, the catheter is retracted into the aorta and then advanced down to the aortic valve, where the individual cusps (left, right, and noncoronary), as determined by distinct catheter locations on orthogonal fluoroscopy, are tagged. Then, the catheter is readvanced with a curve into the LV and, without releasing the curve, the catheter is pulled against the different structures of the LVOT to take activation points and perform pace mapping. ICE is very helpful to confirm accurate anatomical location of the catheter in this region. Clockwise rotation will move the tip towards the septum, whereas counterclockwise rotation allows to map more lateral structures. Figure 23.5 shows a short axis view of the LV ostium, demonstrating the different structures to be mapped as we rotate the catheter in a clockwise fashion. Starting top and laterally, the first structure encountered is the MV annulus (lateral and anterior aspects). VAs from this region can be mapped from below the valve or epicardially from the GCV. If we continue in a clockwise direction, the following structures are, in order, the left fibrous trigone and AMC, the LCC, the right-left cusp junction, and the RCC. The epicardial region opposite to the LCC corresponds to the LVS, and arrhythmias from this region can be mapped from the LCC, from below the valve in the LV or epicardially from the AIV (see below). VAs from the more medial ventricular muscle can be mapped from the right-left cusp junction or from below the valve, and VAs from the anterior and septal portion of the LV ostium (parahisian region) can be mapped from the RCC. Further clockwise rotation will take us to the membranous interventricular septum. This portion is devoid of muscle and therefore cannot be a source of VAs. Even further clockwise rotation leads us to the posterior-superior process of the LV. This is the most inferior and posterior aspect of the LV and is adjacent of the inferior and medial aspect of the right atrium.[40] VAs from the posterior-superior process of the LV can be mapped from the LV endocardium below the NCC or from the adjacent

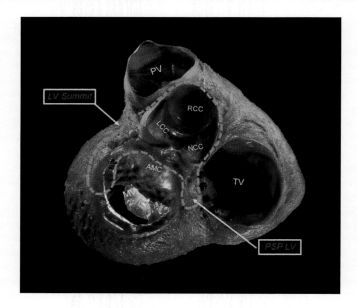

Figure 23.5 Short-axis view of the LVOT, showing the different structures. See text for details. (Courtesy of Dr. K. Shivkumar, UCLA Cardiac Arrhythmia Center, Wallace A. McAlpine Collection.)

RA. Particular care should be taken when mapping the area below the junction of the RCC and NCC. This corresponds to the central fibrous body, where the penetrating His bundle crosses the interventricular septum and ablation here carries an imminent risk of atrio-ventricular block.[41]

AORTIC CUSPS VENTRICULAR ARRHYTHMIAS

According to a series, PVC/VTs ablated from the aortic root represent a 71% of LVOT VAs and 17% of all idiopathic Vas.[7] The aortic valve occupies a central position within the heart and is composed of 3 cusps, each of one with relevant anatomical relationships. From an attitudinal perspective, the RCC is the most anterior and inferior cusp relative to the sternum, the NCC is posterior and rightward, and the LCC is posterior and leftward.[28] The RCC is in close proximity to the posteroseptal aspect of the RVOT, while the LCC is adjacent to the anterior aspect of the LV ostium, in close proximity to the LAD and AIV/GCV junction from the epicardial surface. On the other side, the NCC is in relationship to both the left and right atria separated by the interatrial septum. Below the commissure between the RCC and NCC lies the membranous ventricular septum, where the penetrating bundle of His is located.

The base of the RCC and LCC lies in direct contact to the myocardium of the LV ostium, and sleeves of myocardial tissue may extend into the aortic root, serving as a source of these VAs. In our experience, most VAs ablated from the aortic root are targeted at the junction between the RCC and LCC.[22] VAs from the RCC have a LBBB configuration with a QS pattern in V1 and precordial transition at V2 or V3, while those arising from the LCC have a predominant R wave in V1, often with a multiphasic pattern (M or W).[42] VAs successfully ablated from the right-left cusp junction typically demonstrate a QS complex with notching of the downstroke in lead V1,

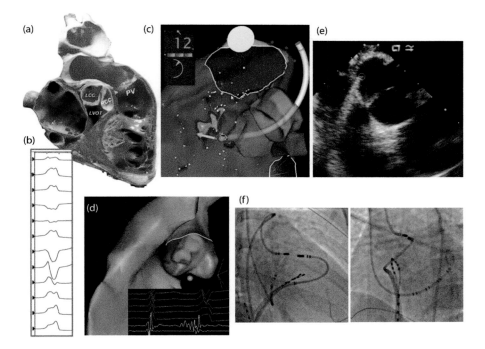

Figure 23.6 Ablation of PVC from the RCC. (a). Anatomical altitudinal section showing the relationships of the posterior RVOT. (b). PVC morphology of a posterior outflow tract PVC with transition in V3. Initially mapped early and ablated in the RVOT, but with early recurrence. As such, attention was turned to the neighboring RCC, where the PVC was eliminated by RF. (c). Tip of the ablation catheter in the RCC with good contact force and vector orientation towards the septum. (d). PVC activation map on the ICE-guided reconstruction of the aortic root. (e). ICE section of the coronary cusps and ablation catheter positioned to the RCC (green circle denotes the ICE plane cutting the tip of the catheter in the mapping system ICE software integration). (f). Two ablation catheters placed at the posterior RVOT and RCC simultaneously (RAO and LAO projections).

and precordial transition by lead V3.[22] VAs originating from the NCC are extremely rare due to the absence of muscular fibers in this region.[43]

For mapping the aortic cusps, a retrograde approach through the femoral artery is used (Figures 23.6 and 23.7). The catheter location at each valve cusp is confirmed by a combination of fluoroscopy, intracardiac electrograms, and ICE. The LCC is located at the most leftward aspect of the aortic root in the LAO view and mid position in RAO, while the RCC is anterior in the RAO view and rightward in the LAO view. The NCC is located at the most inferior and posterior aspect of the aortic root in the RAO view, in close proximity to the interatrial septum and His bundle recording, and is mid position in LAO. At the NCC, an A/V relationship >1 is typically recorded due to close proximity to the interatrial septum; on the contrary, at the RCC and LCC, a large ventricular electrogram and a small far-field atrial electrogram are recorded. When ICE is used, the best view for mapping this region is the short axis image of the aortic cusp region with its characteristic trileaflet appearance ("Mercedes-Benz sign"). This is obtained by advancing the ICE catheter into the RVOT base, followed by clockwise rotation.

Before RF delivery, coronary angiography must be performed to ensure that the tip of the ablation catheter is >5 mm from a coronary vessel. However, a coronary angiogram is

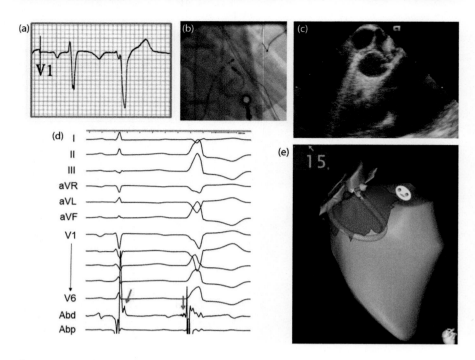

Figure 23.7 Ablation of PVC mapped to the right-left cusp junction. (a). Classic pattern in lead V1. (b). RAO fluoroscopy image with the typical curve used for placing the catheter in the right-left cusp junction. (c). ICE-guided positioning of the ablation catheter. (d). At the site of successful ablation, an electrogram is recorded in the final portion of the QRS in sinus rhythm and becomes early during the PVC. (e). The mapping system shows the catheter in contact with vector orientation and contact force at the successful site.

not always necessary if ICE clearly shows a safe distance of the ablation catheter tip to the coronary ostia.[44] The catheter tip should be deflected towards the myocardium rather than the valve leaflet to ensure good contact and avoid valve damage. As mentioned, RF is delivered with a maximum temperature of 50°C and stepwise incremental of energy application, starting at 20 W and titrating up to a maximum power of 30–35 W, with a goal of 8–10 Ω impedance drop.

LEFT VENTRICULAR SUMMIT ARRHYTHMIAS

The term LVS describes the highest portion of the LV epicardium, above the upper end of the anterior interventricular sulcus[31] (Figure 23.6). It is a triangular region bounded by the bifurcation between the LAD and the left circumflex (LCx) coronary arteries.[45] It is bisected laterally by the GCV in 2 regions: a medial and more superior region, close to the apex of the triangle, that is inaccessible to catheter ablation due to close proximity to the major coronary vessels (the inaccessible area), and a more lateral and inferior region, toward the base of the triangle, that may be suitable for catheter ablation (the accessible area).

LVS arrhythmias usually have a RBBB pattern with inferior axis and larger R waves in lead III than lead II, but VAs from the inaccessible area may also exhibit a LBBB with inferior axis and early transition (V2 or V3). An epicardial origin is suspected by prominent pseudo-delta waves.[45–47]

Despite their epicardial origin, LVS arrhythmias rarely can be ablated from the pericardial space due to close proximity to the major coronary vessels and the presence of a thick layer of epicardial fat.[48] Instead, they are more often targeted from the coronary venous system (GCV-AIV), and because the origin could be intramural below the epicardial LVS, they can also be ablated from adjacent structures such as the LCC, LVOT endocardium, or anteroseptal RVOT (Figure 23.8).[47] To decide the optimal site of ablation, we also map the intramural component of the LVS by advancing a guidewire into the septal perforator branches of the AIV. If the arrhythmia focus is epicardial (earliest activation in the GCV/AIV), we attempt ablation from the coronary venous system; on the other side, if the focus is intramural (earliest activation in the wire) we favor ablation from the LV endocardium. Also, if earliest activation is epicardial, but ablation within the coronary venous system is limited by proximity to coronary vessels, impedance rise, or inability to advance the catheter, endocardial ablation still can be successful in a significant proportion of patients. The use of irrigated catheters is mandatory to deliver adequate power in the low-flow venous system and stepwise incremental of RF energy if possible (to a target 20–40 W) is recommended. The upper impedance limit is sometimes turned off to allow adequate RF delivery.

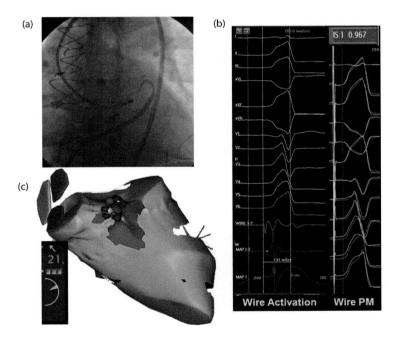

Figure 23.8 Ablation of PVC mapped to the LV summit. (a). After suspecting an LV summit origin, the coronary sinus was cannulated using a deflectable sheath and a mapping unipolar wire was placed inside a septal perforator vein. (b). Earliest activation was documented at the mapping wire, suggesting origin from an intramural site. Pace mapping from the same wire showed an excellent match (96.7%). (c). Because of the inability to ablate from inside of the septum, the ablation catheter was placed in the basal LVOT, opposite to the wire guided by fluoroscopy and ICE, where RF application resulted in permanent PVC elimination. This is a 3D reconstruction of the LV, showing the location of the ablation catheter at the site of successful ablation.

Ventricular Arrhythmias in the Structurally Normal Heart 283

PAPILLARY MUSCLE VENTRICULAR ARRHYTHMIAS

The LV papillary muscles (PMs) have been reported to be a source of idiopathic VAs in patients without structural heart disease.[49-51] In addition, PVCs arising from the PMs may play a role as triggers of VF.[4,52] PM VT is usually exercise induced and is catecholamine sensitive, requiring isoproterenol or epinephrine for induction. The mechanism is typically focal in nature and not re-entrant.[49] This VT cannot be entrained and has a lack of late potentials at the site of ablation.

The PM VAs have distinct electrocardiographic characteristics.[49-53] VT/PVCs arising from the posteromedial PM (most common) show a RBBB morphology, left superior axis (positive in I and aVL, negative in aVR, negative in II and III), and transition at V3–V5. VT/PVCs from the anterolateral PM typically demonstrate a RBBB morphology, right axis (negative in I and aVL, positive in aVR), transition at V3–V5, and frequently inferior lead discordance (negative II and positive III). Differences with fascicular VT include a wider QRS duration, a qR or R morphology in V1 (compared with rsR' for fascicular VT), and absence of Q waves in leads I and aVL.[54,55]

Ablation is challenging due to the PM complex anatomy and high motion during the cardiac cycle. A retro-aortic or trans-septal access to the LV may be used. In our experience, the posteromedial PM and the medial aspect of the anterolateral PM are best approached with a retro-aortic access, while the lateral aspect of the anterolateral PM is best approached in a trans-septal fashion.[53] ICE is essential to ensure adequate catheter-tissue contact and correct orientation of the catheter tip during mapping and ablation. Changes in the QRS morphology can occur during RF delivery, suggesting a change in the exit site, and several RF lesions on different parts of the PM are often required to completely eliminate the VT/PVC. When catheter stability is an issue, cryoablation is an alternative, as the cryocatheter adherence to the tissue limits mobility and improves contact.[56,57]

OTHER RIGHT VENTRICULAR ARRHYTHMIAS

Approximately 10% of RV arrhythmias may arise from other sites than the RVOT, according to a large series of patients ($n = 278$) from our center.[58] In this series, 14 (48%) were from the TV annulus, 8 (28%) from the basal RV, and 7 (24%) from the apical RV segments. An important consideration in patients with non-OT RV arrhythmias and in those with multiple PVC/VT foci is to rule out arrhythmogenic RV cardiomyopathy and cardiac sarcoidosis prior to ablation. Cardiac magnetic resonance imaging (MRI) and cardiac positron emission tomography (PET) may be helpful in this regard.

VT/PVCs from the TV annulus always have a LBBB morphology, with a late transition and variable axis depending on location. Septal sites are more common than free wall sites in a series reported by Tada et al. (74% and 26%, respectively).[59] A free wall origin was suggested by a longer QRS duration, later precordial transition, more frequent QRS notching, and an rS pattern in lead V1 (as opposed to a QS pattern in VT/PVCs arising from the septal portion of the annulus). Those VT/PVCs from the anteroseptal and midseptal regions ascribe to the group of parahisian VAs. When mapping TV arrhythmias, stability is particularly challenging on the superior and lateral region.[41]

A relatively under-recognized source of VA is the MB. This is a prominent muscular trabeculation that crosses from the septum to the free wall of the RV and provides support to the anterior PM of the TV. The spectrum of MB arrhythmias includes PVC/nonsustained VT, sustained monomorphic VT, and PVC-triggered VF.[60] VT/PVCs from the MB typically demonstrate a LBBB morphology, left superior axis, and late transition (≥V4). Catheter ablation is facilitated by ICE guidance and the use of deflectable sheaths enhances catheter stability. In a series of 10 patients reported by Sadek et al., ablation was acutely successful in all patients, but 6 patients required a second procedure for arrhythmia recurrence.[60]

CRUX VENTRICULAR ARRHYTHMIAS

The crux of the heart is an epicardial location near the junction of the middle cardiac vein (MCV) and the CS. Crux VAs typically demonstrate a LBBB pattern, early precordial transition, and superior axis with a QS pattern in the inferior leads.[61] Due to their epicardial origin, the QRS is relatively wide, with a pseudo-delta wave and delayed intrinsicoid deflection.[62] Typically, an early ventricular activation is recorded within the MCV or proximal CS. Ablation can be attempted within the coronary venous system using an irrigated catheter. If unsuccessful, epicardial mapping via a subxiphoid pericardial approach should be performed. Coronary angiography is recommended prior to RF delivery to ensure a safe distance (>5 mm) between the ablation catheter and the posterior descending artery.

REFERENCES

1. Brooks R, Burgess JH. Idiopathic ventricular tachycardia: A review. *Medicine* (Baltimore) 1988;67:271–94.

2. Lee GK, Klarich KW, Grogan M, Cha YM. Premature ventricular contraction-induced cardiomyopathy: A treatable condition. *Circ Arrhythm Electrophysiol*. 2012;5(1):229–36.

3. Haïssaguerre M, Shoda M, Jaïs P, et al. Mapping and ablation of idiopathic ventricular fibrillation. *Circulation*. 2002;106(8):962–7.

4. Van Herendael H, Zado ES, Haqqani H, et al. Catheter ablation of ventricular fibrillation: Importance of left ventricular outflow tract and papillary muscle triggers. *Heart Rhythm*. 2014;11(4):566–73.

5. Roberts-Thomson KC, Lau DH, Sanders P. The diagnosis and management of ventricular arrhythmias. *Nat Rev Cardiol*. 2011;8(6):311–21.

6. Dixit S, Gerstenfeld EP, Lin D, et al. Identification of distinct electrocardiographic patterns from the basal left ventricle: Distinguishing medial and lateral sites of origin in patients with idiopathic ventricular tachycardia. *Heart Rhythm*. 2005;2(5):485–91.

7. Yamada T, McElderry HT, Doppalapudi H, et al. Idiopathic ventricular arrhythmias originating from the aortic root prevalence, electrocardiographic and electrophysiologic characteristics, and results of radiofrequency catheter ablation. *J Am Coll Cardiol*. 2008;52(2):139–47.

8. Callans DJ, Menz V, Schwartzman D, et al. Repetitive monomorphic tachycardia from the left ventricular outflow tract: Electrocardiographic patterns consistent with a left ventricular site of origin. *J Am Coll Cardiol*. 1997;29(5):1023–7.

9. Nakagawa M, Takahashi N, Nobe S, et al. Gender differences in various types of idiopathic ventricular tachycardia. *J Cardiovasc Electrophysiol*. 2002;13(7):633–8.

10. Kim RJ, Iwai S, Markowitz SM, et al. Clinical and electrophysiological spectrum of idiopathic ventricular outflow tract arrhythmias. *J Am Coll Cardiol*. 2007;49(20):2035–43.

11. Buxton AE, Waxman HL, Marchlinski FE, et al. Right ventricular tachycardia: Clinical and electrophysiologic characteristics. *Circulation*. 1983;68(5):917–27.

12. Lerman BB, Belardinelli L, West GA, et al. Adenosine sensitive ventricular tachycardia: Evidence suggesting cyclic AMP-mediated triggered activity. *Circulation*. 1986;74(2):270–80.

13. Lerman BB, Stein K, Engelstein ED, et al. Mechanism of repetitive monomorphic ventricular tachycardia. *Circulation*. 1995;92(3):421–9.

14. Lerman BB, Ip JE, Shah BK, et al. Mechanism-specific effects of adenosine on ventricular tachycardia. *J Cardiovasc Electrophysiol*. 2014;25(12):1350–8.

15. Gill JS, Mehta D, Ward DE, Camm AJ. Efficacy of flecainide, sotalol, and verapamil in the treatment of right ventricular tachycardia in patients without overt cardiac abnormality. *Br Heart J*. 1992;68(4):392–7.

16. Goy JJ, Tauxe F, Fromer M, et al. Ten-years follow-up of 20 patients with idiopathic ventricular tachycardia. *Pacing Clin Electrophysiol*. 1990;13(9):1142–7.

17. Al-Khatib SM, Stevenson WG, Ackerman MJ, et al. 2017 AHA/ACC/HRS Guideline for management of patients with ventricular arrhythmias and the prevention of sudden cardiac death: Executive summary: A report of the American College of Cardiology/American Heart Association Task Force on Clinical Practice Guidelines and the Heart Rhythm Society. *Circulation*. 2018;138(13):e210–e271.

18. Scheinman MM, Huang S. The 1998 NASPE prospective catheter ablation registry. *Pacing Clin Electrophysiol*. 2000;23(6):1020–8.

19. Hutchinson MD, Garcia FC. An organized approach to the localization, mapping, and ablation of outflow tract ventricular arrhythmias. *J Cardiovasc Electrophysiol*. 2013;24(10):1189–97.

20. Betensky BP, Park RE, Marchlinski FE, et al. The V(2) transition ratio: A new electrocardiographic criterion for distinguishing left from right ventricular outflow tract tachycardia origin. *J Am Coll Cardiol*. 2011;57(22):2255–62.

21. Ouyang F, Fotuhi P, Ho SY, et al. Repetitive monomorphic ventricular tachycardia originating from the aortic sinus cusp: Electrocardiographic characterization for guiding catheter ablation. *J Am Coll Cardiol*. 2002;39(3):500–8.

22. Bala R, Garcia FC, Hutchinson MD, et al. Electrocardiographic and electrophysiologic features of ventricular arrhythmias originating from the right/left coronary cusp commissure. *Heart Rhythm*. 2010;7(3):312–22.

23. Yamada T, Murakami Y, Yoshida N, et al. Preferential conduction across the ventricular outflow septum in ventricular arrhythmias originating from the aortic sinus cusp. *J Am Coll Cardiol*. 2007;50(9):884–91.

24. Moak JP, Sumihara K, Swink J, et al. Ablation of the vanishing PVC, facilitated by quantitative morphology-matching software. *Pacing Clin Electrophysiol*. 2017;40(11):1227–33.

25. Kuteszko R, Pytkowski M, Farkowski MM, et al. Utility of automated template matching for the interpretation of pace mapping in patients ablated due to outflow tract ventricular arrhythmias. *Europace*. 2015;17(9):1428–34.

26. Kosiuk J, Portugal G, Hilbert S, et al. In vivo validation of a novel algorithm for automatic premature ventricular contractions recognition. *J Cardiovasc Electrophysiol*. 2017;28(7):828–33.

27. James TN. Anatomy of the crista supraventricularis: Its importance for understanding right ventricular function, right ventricular infarction and related conditions. *J Am Coll Cardiol*. 1985;6(5):1083–95.

28. Asirvatham SJ. Correlative anatomy for the invasive electrophysiologist: Outflow tract and supravalvar arrhythmia. *J Cardiovasc Electrophysiol*. 2009;20(8):955–68.

29. Tada H, Tadokoro K, Miyaji K, et al. Idiopathic ventricular arrhythmias arising from the pulmonary artery: Prevalence, characteristics, and topography of the arrhythmia origin. *Heart Rhythm*. 2008;5(3):419–26.

30. Sekiguchi Y, Aonuma K, Takahashi A, et al. Electrocardiographic and electrophysiologic characteristics of ventricular tachycardia originating within the pulmonary artery. *J Am Coll Cardiol*. 2005;45(6):887–95.

31. McAlpine WA. *Heart and Coronary Arteries*. New York: Springer-Verlag;1975.

32. Piazza N, de Jaegere P, Schultz C, et al. Anatomy of the aortic valvar complex and its implications for transcatheter implantation of the aortic valve. *Circ Cardiovasc Interv*. 2008;1(1):74–81.

33. de Kerchove L, El Khoury G. Anatomy and pathophysiology of the ventriculo-aortic junction: Implication in aortic valve repair surgery. *Ann Cardiothorac Surg*. 2013;2(1):57–64.

34. Steven D, Roberts-Thomson KC, Seiler J, et al. Ventricular tachycardia arising from the aortomitral continuity in structural heart disease: Characteristics and therapeutic considerations for an anatomically challenging area of origin. *Circ Arrhythm Electrophysiol*. 2009;2(6):660–6.

35. Kumagai K, Fukuda K, Wakayama Y, et al. Electrocardiographic characteristics of the variants of idiopathic left ventricular outflow tract ventricular tachyarrhythmias. *J Cardiovasc Electrophysiol*. 2008;19(5):495–501.

36. Tada H, Ito S, Naito S, et al. Idiopathic ventricular arrhythmia arising from the mitral annulus: A distinct subgroup of idiopathic ventricular arrhythmias. *J Am Coll Cardiol*. 2005;45(6):877–86.

37. Wasmer K, Köbe J, Dechering DG, et al. Ventricular arrhythmias from the mitral annulus: Patient characteristics, electrophysiological findings, ablation, and prognosis. *Heart Rhythm*. 2013;10(6):783–8.

38. Kumagai K, Yamauchi Y, Takahashi A, et al. Idiopathic left ventricular tachycardia originating from the mitral annulus. *J Cardiovasc Electrophysiol*. 2005;16(10):1029–36.

39. Huang S, Miller J. *Catheter Ablation of Cardiac Arrhythmias* (3rd ed.) Philadelphia, PA: Elsevier Saunders; 2015.

40. Santangeli P, Hutchinson MD, Supple GE, et al. Right atrial approach for ablation of ventricular arrhythmias arising from the left posterior-superior process of the left ventricle. *Circ Arrhythm Electrophysiol*. 2016;9(7). https://doi.org/10.1161/CIRCEP.116.004048

41. Enriquez A, Tapias C, Rodriguez D, et al. How to map and ablate parahisian ventricular arrhythmias. *Heart Rhythm*. 2018;15(8):1268–1274.

42. Lin D, Ilkhanoff L, Gerstenfeld E, et al. Twelve-lead electrocardiographic characteristics of the aortic cusp region guided by intracardiac echocardiography and electroanatomic mapping. *Heart Rhythm*. 2008;5(5):663–9.

43. Yamada T, Lau YR, Litovsky SH, et al. Prevalence and clinical, electrocardiographic, and electrophysiologic characteristics of ventricular arrhythmias originating from the noncoronary sinus of Valsalva. *Heart Rhythm*. 2013;10(11):1605–12.

44. Enriquez A, Saenz L, Rosso R, et al. Use of Intracardiac Echocardiography in Interventional Cardiology: Working with the anatomy rather than fighting it. *Circulation*. 2018;137(21):2278–94.

45. Yamada T, McElderry HT, Doppalapudi H, et al. Idiopathic ventricular arrhythmias originating from the left ventricular summit: Anatomic concepts relevant to ablation. *Circ Arrhythm Electrophysiol*. 2010;3(6):616–23.

46. Jauregui Abularach ME, Campos B, Park KM, et al. Ablation of ventricular arrhythmias arising near the anterior epicardial veins from the left sinus of Valsalva region: ECG features, anatomic distance, and outcome. *Heart Rhythm*. 2012;9(6):865–73.

47. Enriquez A, Malavassi F, Saenz LC, et al. How to map and ablate left ventricular summit arrhythmias. *Heart Rhythm*. 2016 Sep 21. pii: S1547–5271(16)30801–3.

48. Santangeli P, Marchlinski FE, Zado ES, et al. Percutaneous epicardial ablation of ventricular arrhythmias arising from the left ventricular summit: Outcomes and electrocardiogram correlates of success. *Circ Arrhythm Electrophysiol*. 2015;8(2):337–43.

49. Doppalapudi H, Yamada T, McElderry HT, et al. Ventricular tachycardia originating from the posterior papillary muscle in the left ventricle: A distinct clinical syndrome. *Circ Arrhythm Electrophysiol* 2008;1:23–9.

50. Yamada T, McElderry HT, Okada T, et al. Idiopathic focal ventricular arrhythmias originating from the anterior papillary muscle in the left ventricle. *J Cardiovasc Electrophysiol*. 2009;20(8):866–72.

51. Yamada T, Doppalapudi H, McElderry HT, et al. Idiopathic ventricular arrhythmias originating from the papillary muscles in the left ventricle: Prevalence, electrocardiographic and electrophysiological characteristics, and results of the radiofrequency catheter ablation. *J Cardiovasc Electrophysiol*. 2010;21(1):62–9.

52. Santoro F, Di Biase L, Hranitzky P, et al. Ventricular fibrillation triggered by PVCs from papillary muscles: Clinical features and ablation. *J Cardiovasc Electrophysiol* 2014;25:1158–64.

53. Enriquez A, Supple GE, Marchlinski FE, Garcia FC. How to map and ablate papillary muscle ventricular arrhythmias. *Heart Rhythm*. 2017;14(11):1721–28.

54. Good E, Desjardins B, Jongnarangsin K, et al. Ventricular arrhythmias originating from a papillary muscle in patients without prior infarction: A comparison with fascicular arrhythmias. *Heart Rhythm* 2008;5:1530–7.

55. Deyell MW, Man JP, Supple GE, et al. ECG differentiation of ventricular arrhythmias arising from the left posterior fascicle and postero-medial papillary muscle. *Heart Rhythm* 2012;9(5S):S474.

56. Rivera S, Ricapito Mde L, Tomas L, et al. Results of cryoenergy and radiofrequency-based catheter ablation for treating ventricular arrhythmias arising from the papillary muscles of the left ventricle, guided by intracardiac echocardiography and image integration. *Circ Arrhythm Electrophysiol* 2016;9:e003874.

57. Gordon J, Zado E, Hutchinson M, et al. Effectiveness of cryoablation on papillary muscle PVCs and VT after radiofrequency has failed. *Heart Rhythm* 2016;13:PO06–150.

58. Van Herendael H, Garcia F, Lin D, et al. Idiopathic right ventricular arrhythmias not arising from the outflow tract: Prevalence, electrocardiographic characteristics, and outcome of catheter ablation. *Heart Rhythm*. 2011;8(4):511–8.

59. Tada H, Tadokoro K, Ito S, et al. Idiopathic ventricular arrhythmias originating from the tricuspid annulus: Prevalence, electrocardiographic characteristics, and results of radiofrequency catheter ablation. *Heart Rhythm*. 2007;4(1):7–16.

60. Sadek MM, Benhayon D, Sureddi R, et al. Idiopathic ventricular arrhythmias originating from the moderator band: Electrocardiographic characteristics and treatment by catheter ablation. *Heart Rhythm*. 2015;12(1):67–75.

61. Doppalapudi H, Yamada T, Ramaswamy K, et al. Idiopathic focal epicardial ventricular tachycardia originating from the crux of the heart. *Heart Rhythm*. 2009;6(1):44–50.

62. Kawamura M, Gerstenfeld EP, Vedantham V, et al. Idiopathic ventricular arrhythmia originating from the cardiac crux or inferior septum: Epicardial idiopathic ventricular arrhythmia. *Circ Arrhythm Electrophysiol*. 2014;7(6):1152–8.

CATHETER ABLATION OF VENTRICULAR FIBRILLATION AND POLYMORPHIC VENTRICULAR TACHYCARDIA

Amin Al-Ahmad, Carola Gianni, and Andrea Natale

CONTENTS

INTRODUCTION

Ventricular fibrillation (VF) and sustained polymorphic ventricular tachycardia (PMVT) are malignant arrhythmias resulting in sudden cardiac death (SCD). SCD is a leading cause of death in the industrialized world, with VF and PMVT accounting for up to one-third of all cases.[1] VF and PMVT are usually associated with structural heart disease, but can occur in patients with structurally normal, albeit electrophysiologically abnormal hearts (Table 24.1). Implantable cardioverter-defibrillators (ICDs) are the first line therapy for secondary prevention of patients with VF/PMVT.[2] Although effective in terminating life-threatening ventricular arrhythmias when they occur, ICDs have no effect on the underlying disease process and do not prevent those arrhythmias from occurring. Consequently, some patients with ICDs will experience multiple shocks, resulting in psychological distress and increased mortality.[3]

Advances in our understanding of VF and PMVT have led to the development of successful catheter ablation strategies. One of the most widely accepted theories propose that VF could be initiated by a single firing focus, that interacts with fixed (anatomical) or functional (electrophysiological) obstacles giving rise to multiple wavelets thus resulting in VF.[4] In most of the described cases of successful VF/PMVT ablation, a premature ventricular complex (PVC) has been isolated as the triggering mechanism (Figure 24.1, Tables 24.2 and 24.3).[5–23] There are surprisingly few sources of VF/PMVT-triggering PVCs that have been reported, and the Purkinje system appears to be the source of the majority of them (Figure 24.2). Catheter ablation strategies that target those PVCs have been employed as a treatment option in the management of patients with recurrent VF/PMVT, either with or without structural heart disease.

Table 24.1   Causes of ventricular fibrillation/polymorphic ventricular tachycardia

Structural heart disease	Non-structural heart disease
Coronary artery disease	Electrophysiological disease
Atherosclerosis	Long QT syndrome[a]
Anomalous coronary circulation	Short QT syndrome
Coronary spasm	Brugada syndrome[a]
Cardiomyopathies	Catecholaminergic polymorphic
Ischemic cardiomyopathy[a]	ventricular tachycardia
Idiopathic dilated cardiomyopathy	Idiopathic ventricular fibrillation[a]
Hypertrophic cardiomyopathy	Early repolarization syndrome[a]
Takotsubo cardiomyopathy	Metabolic disease
Infiltrative cardiomyopathy (e.g., sarcoid, amyloid)	Dyskalemia
Arrhythmogenic right ventricular cardiomyopathy	Hypomagnesemia
Left ventricular noncompaction	Hypocalcemia
Myocarditis	Acidosis
Congenital heart disease	Drugs
Valvular heart disease	
Other	
Wolff–Parkinson–White syndrome	
Commotio cordis	
After cardiac surgery	

[a] Catheter ablation successfully attempted.

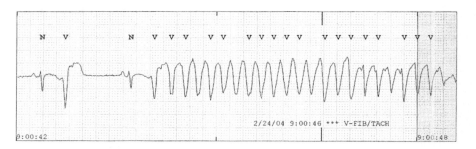

Figure 24.1   PVC triggering VF.

CATHETER ABLATION OF VF/PMVT IN NON-STRUCTURAL HEART DISEASE

Though the majority of VF/PMVT occurs in structurally abnormal hearts, there is a subset of individuals resuscitated from SCD with no structural heart disease. In some of these patients, VF/PMVT is triggered by PVCs that can be mapped and targeted by catheter ablation to prevent subsequent episodes (Table 24.2).

IDIOPATHIC VF

Patients with idiopathic VF are patients with prior history of resuscitated SCD, but without structural heart disease or electrocardiographic abnormalities. Activation mapping identify the area of activation of the initiating PVC, most commonly in the Purkinje network (left or right), as demonstrated by the presence of a sharp potential preceding the QRS by <15 ms

Table 24.2 Catheter ablation of ventricular fibrillation/polymorphic ventricular tachycardia in non-structural heart disease

Author (year)	Etiology	N	Target	Acute success (%)[a]	Follow-up (months)	Long-term success (%)[b]
Haïssaguerre (2002)[5]	Idiopathic VF	16	PVC (PP = 12, RVOT = 4)	81	32	100
Haïssaguerre (2002)[6]	Idiopathic VF	27	PVC (PP = 23, RVOT = 5)	100	24 ± 28	89
Haïssaguerre (2003)[7]	BrS LQTS	7	PVC (PP = 4, RVOT = 3)	100	17 ± 17	100
Noda (2005)[8]	Idiopathic VF/PMVT	16	PVC (RVOT = 16)	100	54 ± 39	75[c]
Haïssaguerre (2008)[9]	ER syndrome	8	PVC (PP or myocardium)	63	NA	NA
Knecht (2009)[10]	Idiopathic VF	38	PVC (PP = 33, RVOT = 4, myocardium = 1)	100	63 (40–80)	82; 95
Nademanee (2011)[11]	BrS	9	Abnormal EGMs (epicardial RVOT)	NA	20 ± 6	89[d]
Van Herendael (2014)[12]	Idiopathic VF	9	PVC (PP = 3, PM = 2, LVOT = 4)	89	14 (5–29)	77
Santoro (2014)[13]	Idiopathic VF	5	PVC (PM = 5)	100	58 ± 11	100

[a] Elimination of triggering PVC, considering only those with PVC at the time of the procedure.

[b] After successful ablation and off-antiarrhythmic drugs; single- and multiple-procedures success rates are reported.

[c] 4 patients on β-blockers at follow-up.

[d] 1 patient on amiodarone at follow-up.

Abbreviations: BrS, Brugada syndrome; EGM, electrogram; ER, early repolarization; LQTS, long QT syndrome; LVOT, left ventricular outflow tract; N, number; NA, not available; PM, papillary muscle; PMVT, polymorphic ventricular tachycardia; PP, Purkinje potentials; PVC, premature ventricular complex; RVOT, right ventricular outflow tract; VF, ventricular fibrillation.

Table 24.3 Catheter ablation of ventricular fibrillation/polymorphic ventricular tachycardia in structural heart disease

Author (year)	Etiology	N	Target	Acute success (%)[a]	Follow-up (months)	Long-term success (%)[b]
Bänsch (2003)[14]	AMI	4	PVC (PP = 4; in the scar)	100	10 (5–28)	100
Szumowski (2004)[15]	AMI	5	PVC (PP = 5; in the scar)	100	20 ± 6	100
Enjoji (2009)[16]	AMI	4	PVC (PP = 4; in the scar)	100	12–48	100
Marrouche (2004)[17]	ICM	8	PVC (PP = 5; in the scar)	100	10 ± 6	87
Peichl (2009)[18]	ICM	9	PVC (PP = 8; in the scar) Abnormal EGMs (scar)	89	13 ± 7	75, 100
Bode (2008)[19]	ICM Myocarditis After AVR	7	PVC (PP = 7; within the scar in ICM)	100	10 (1–27)	100
Kobayashi (2008)[20]	AMI ICM	5	PVC (PP = 7; in the scar)	100	12 (3–24)	100
Hayashi (2014)[21]	AMI ICM	5	PVC (PP = 5)	100	33 ± 22	100
Van Herendael (2014)[12]	AMI ICM IDCM	21	PVC (PP = 6, PM = 6, LVOT = 5; within the scar in 15) Abnormal EGMs (scar)	86	14 (5–29)	90
Sinha (2009)[22]	IDCM	4	PVC (PP = 4)	100	12 ± 5	100
Mlcochova (2006)[23]	Amyloidosis	2	PVC (PP = 2; in the scar)	100	1–8	100

[a] Elimination of triggering PVC, considering only those with PVC at the time of the procedure.
[b] After successful ablation; single- and multiple-procedures success rates are reported.

Abbreviations: AMI, acute myocardial infarction; AVR, aortic valve replacement; EGM, electrogram; ICM, ischemic cardiomyopathy; IDCM, idiopathic dilated cardiomyopathy; PP, Purkinje potentials; PVC, premature ventricular complexes.

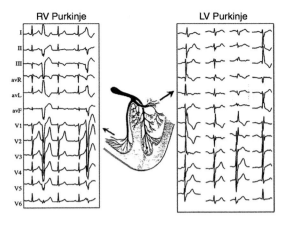

Figure 24.2 Examples of PVC coming from the right and left ventricular Purkinje system.

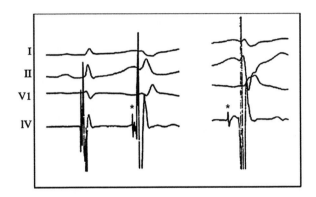

Figure 24.3 Purkinje potential (*) preceding a PVC.

during sinus rhythm (Purkinje potential, PP; Figure 24.3).[5,6,10,12] PVCs originating from the Purkinje network are usually narrow (QRS duration 80–150 ms), they might be polymorphic and their coupling interval is characteristically short (250–270 ms). In some cases, the earliest activation is in the myocardium (right or left ventricular outflow tract—RVOT or LVOT—or papillary muscle—PM), with no pre-systolic PP (Figure 24.4).[5,6,8,10,12,13] Those PVCs are usually wider (QRS duration 130–180 ms), monomorphic with an intermediate coupling interval (320–400 ms). If PVCs are absent at the time of the procedure, pace mapping can be used. Radiofrequency (RF) ablation at these sites eliminates the triggering PVCs and subsequent VF/PMVT in many of these patients.

EARLY REPOLARIZATION SYNDROME

It has been observed that some patients with idiopathic VF have an early repolarization (ER) pattern in the inferior and/or lateral leads, the so-called ER syndrome. Catheter ablation have been successfully employed in this population, with PVCs originating from the Purkinje system or the myocardium.[9] Interestingly, in those with an ER pattern present only in the inferior leads, PVCs originated from the inferior left ventricular wall.

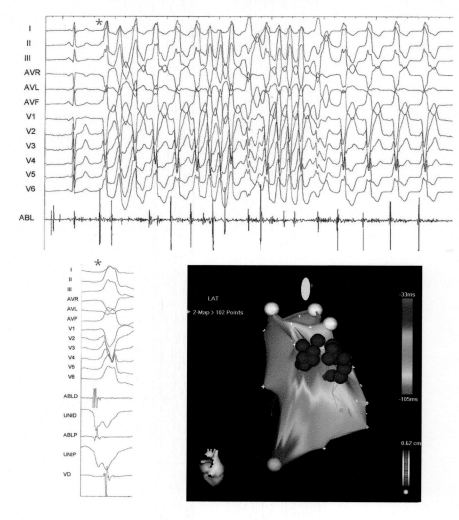

Figure 24.4 PMVT-triggering PVC originating from the RVOT myocardium.

BRUGADA AND CONGENITAL LONG QT SYNDROME

Brugada syndrome and congenital long QT syndrome are arrhythmogenic diseases associated with peculiar ECG repolarization changes secondary to abnormal sodium, potassium, or calcium channel function. Both are associated with an increased risk of SCD and may present with recurrent VF/PMVT often, but not always, initiated by PVCs. As in patients with idiopathic VF, PVC triggers usually arise either from the distal Purkinje network or the RVOT region.[7]

Recently, it has been demonstrated that patients with Brugada syndrome present abnormal voltage areas in the RVOT epicardium.[11] These low-voltage, fragmented potentials can be targeted for ablation, resulting in normalization of the Brugada ECG pattern and in reducing further VF/PMVT episodes at follow-up. This study opens up the possibility of "substrate modification" to treat recurrent VF/PMVT in this population, even if clinical PVCs are not present at the time of the procedure.

VF/PMVT is most commonly associated with structural heart disease. Catheter ablation has been successfully attempted to treat primary VF/PMVT (i.e., not preceded by VT) and electrical storms in patients with structural heart disease of various etiologies. It has been shown that some of these patients also have PVCs triggering those arrhythmias that can be successfully ablated to prevent further arrhythmic episodes (Table 24.3).

ISCHEMIC HEART DISEASE

VF poses a risk in both in the setting of acute myocardial infarction (AMI) and in the natural history of chronic ischemic heart disease, after scar formation. Once again, the Purkinje fibers and their ability to survive transmural myocardial infarction play an important role.[24]

During an AMI, ischemia in the Purkinje system may trigger VF. These arrhythmias are usually managed with recurrent early defibrillation, drugs (β-blockers or amiodarone), and, most importantly, revascularization. In rare cases, incessant VF/PMVT is refractory to medical therapy or successful revascularization. Ablation can be life-saving and has been successfully performed in cases when these arrhythmias are triggered by monomorphic PVCs originating in infarct border zones where PP are present.[12,14–16,20,21]

VF/PMVT in chronic ischemic heart disease is mostly associated with the presence of a myocardial scar. It has been shown that the triggering PVCs usually arise from the scar and are commonly preceded by PP (Figure 24.5).[12,17–21] In some instances, further substrate ablation (isolation of the scar) has been performed at the time of PVC ablation, but it is still unclear if this confers an additional benefit or could be used for primary prevention in ischemic VF/PMVT.

OTHER STRUCTURAL HEART DISEASES

Small case series have shown that successful catheter ablation of VF/PMVT can be achieved in patients with idiopathic dilated cardiomyopathy, amyloidosis, myocarditis, or after cardiac surgery. Again, the triggering PVCs usually originated in areas with PP, but cases in the LVOT and PMs have recently been described.[12,19,22,23]

ABLATION STRATEGY

Before attempting catheter ablation:
- Document that VF/PMVT episodes in a given patient are indeed triggered by a focal PVC trigger:
  - ICD interrogation (far-field electrogram channel)
  - ECG monitoring
- It is important to obtain a 12-lead ECG of the triggering PVC, to plan for the procedure, and to use it in case pace mapping is needed

Catheter ablation procedure:
- To facilitate the presence of the clinical PVC, the procedure should be performed:
  - Following an adequate wash-out period off antiarrhythmic drugs
  - Under conscious or deep sedation in order for the clinical PVC to be present
  - Early after an arrhythmic episode (electrical storm or VF), when PVCs are present, frequent, and easily mappable

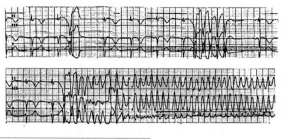
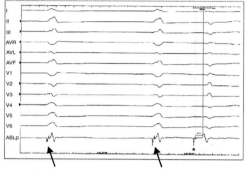
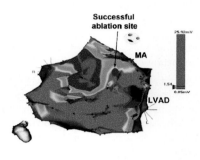

Figure 24.5 PMVT/VF-triggering PVC in a patient with ischemic cardiomyopathy. The PVC was mapped in the border zone of the scar, where Purkinje potentials were seen during sinus rhythm (arrows) and preceding the PVC (*). (Reprinted From *J. Am. Coll. Cardiol.*, 43, Marrouche, N.F. et al., Mode of initiation and ablation of ventricular fibrillation storms in patients with ischemic cardiomyopathy, 1715–1720, Copyright 2004, with permission from Elsevier.)

- Activation mapping of PVCs of identical morphology and coupling interval to the clinical PVC is performed, usually with the aid of 3D electro-anatomical system:
  - A sharp potential before the ventricular electrogram either in sinus rhythm or with a PVC, the origin is identified in the distal Purkinje system (Figure 24.3)
  - In case of polymorphic PVCs, it is advisable to map and target them all.
- If PVCs are not spontaneously present at the time of ablation or too rare to map:
  - Provocative measures can be attempted, such as withdrawing sedation, pacing, or administering drugs (isoproterenol, aminophylline, epinephrine, procainamide, ajmaline, etc.).
  - Pace mapping can be used to identify the putative site of origin (areas with a 12/12 match) – note: this approach is associated with lower clinical success rates.
  - Substrate mapping to look for areas of abnormal voltage or abnormal electrograms can be attempted:
    - Pure substrate-based ablation strategies have been tested only in patients with Brugada syndrome or structural heart disease.
    - Looking for areas with PPs during sinus rhythm or the scar border zone can ease activation mapping if PVCs are infrequent.

- Radiofrequency (RF) ablation is performed at the site of earliest activation to eliminate the VF/PMVT-triggering PVCs or at the chosen putative site with the endpoint of complete local potential abatement.
- The RF lesion set is usually extended to cover a larger area around the focus.

After a successful procedure:
- The patient can be discharged without antiarrhythmic drugs and followed-up to assess freedom from VF/PMVT and PVC recurrence.
  - In case of recurrence, a re-do procedure can be attempted.
- Despite successful ablation, these patients still require an ICD; few to no data is available on long-term follow-up (>5 years) and the published studies were performed in patients with secondary-prevention ICD.

SUMMARY AND CONCLUSIONS

Catheter ablation can be performed in patients with medically refractory VF/PMVT in a variety of arrhythmic substrates, including normal hearts, inherited arrhythmogenic diseases, and cardiomyopathies. It targets PVCs triggering those arrhythmias that usually originate in the Purkinje network. In the studies published to date, acute success rates success rates are near 100%, with long-term success rates ranging from 75% to 100%. Although promising, these are small non-randomized studies conducted in highly specialized centers by expert electrophysiologists and some patients still experiences VF at follow-up. Thus, while reducing the need of anti-arrhythmic medications and the number of shocks, catheter ablation cannot (yet) obviate the need for ICDs.

REFERENCES

1. Zipes DP, Wellens HJ. Sudden cardiac death. *Circulation*. 1998;98(21):2334–2351. doi:10.1161/01.CIR.98.21.2334.
2. Priori SG, Blomström-Lundqvist C, Mazzanti A, et al. 2015 ESC Guidelines for the management of patients with ventricular arrhythmias and the prevention of sudden cardiac death. *Europace*. 2015:euv319. doi:10.1093/europace/euv319.
3. Villacastín J, Almendral J, Arenal A, et al. Incidence and clinical significance of multiple consecutive, appropriate, high-energy discharges in patients with implanted cardioverter-defibrillators. *Circulation*. 1996;93(4):753–762. doi:10.1161/01.CIR.93.4.753.
4. Tabereaux PB, Dosdall DJ, Ideker RE. Mechanisms of VF maintenance: Wandering wavelets, mother rotors, or foci. *Hear Rhythm*. 2009;6(3):405–415. doi:10.1016/j.hrthm.2008.11.005.
5. Haïssaguerre M, Shah DC, Jaïs P, et al. Role of Purkinje conducting system in triggering of idiopathic ventricular fibrillation. *Lancet*. 2002;359(9307):677–678. doi:10.1016/S0140-6736(02)07807-8.
6. Haïssaguerre M, Shoda M, Jaïs P, et al. Mapping and ablation of idiopathic ventricular fibrillation. *Circulation*. 2002;106(8):962–967. doi:10.1161/01.CIR.0000027564.55739.B1.

7. Haïssaguerre M, Extramiana F, Hocini M, et al. Mapping and ablation of ventricular fibrillation associated with long-QT and Brugada syndromes. *Circulation.* 2003;108(8):925–928. doi:10.1161/01.CIR.00000887 81.99943.95.

8. Noda T, Shimizu W, Taguchi A, et al. Malignant entity of idiopathic ventricular fibrillation and polymorphic ventricular tachycardia initiated by premature extrasystoles originating from the right ventricular outflow tract. *J Am Coll Cardiol.* 2005;46(7):1288–1294. doi:10.1016/j.jacc.2005.05.077.

9. Haïssaguerre M, Derval N, Sacher F, et al. Sudden cardiac arrest associated with early repolarization. *N Engl J Med.* 2008;358(19):2016–2023. doi:10.1056/NEJMoa071968.

10. Knecht S, Sacher F, Wright M, et al. Long-term follow-up of idiopathic ventricular fibrillation ablation. A multicenter study. *J Am Coll Cardiol.* 2009;54(6):522–528. doi:10.1016/j.jacc.2009.03.065.

11. Nademanee K, Veerakul G, Chandanamattha P, et al. Prevention of ventricular fibrillation episodes in brugada syndrome by catheter ablation over the anterior right ventricular outflow tract epicardium. *Circulation.* 2011;123(12):1270–1279. doi:10.1161/CIRCULATIONAHA.110.972612.

12. Van Herendael H, Zado ES, Haqqani H, et al. Catheter ablation of ventricular fibrillation: Importance of left ventricular outflow tract and papillary muscle triggers. *Heart Rhythm.* 2014;11(4):566–573. doi:10.1016/j.hrthm.2013.12.030.

13. Santoro F, Di Biase L, Hranitzky P, et al. Ventricular fibrillation triggered by PVCs from papillary muscles: Clinical features and ablation. *J Cardiovasc Electrophysiol.* 2014;25(11):1158–1164. doi:10.1111/jce.12478.

14. Bänsch D, Oyang F, Antz M, et al. Successful catheter ablation of electrical storm after myocardial infarction. *Circulation.* 2003;108(24):3011–3016. doi:10.1161/01.CIR.0000103701.30662.5C.

15. Szumowski L, Sanders P, Walczak F, et al. Mapping and ablation of polymorphic ventricular tachycardia after myocardial infarction. *J Am Coll Cardiol.* 2004;44(8):1700–1706. doi:10.1016/j.jacc.2004.08.034.

16. Enjoji Y, Mizobuchi M, Muranishi H, et al. Catheter ablation of fatal ventricular tachyarrhythmias storm in acute coronary syndrome-role of Purkinje fiber network. *J Interv Card Electrophysiol.* 2009;26(3):207–215. doi:10.1007/s10840-009-9394-7.

17. Marrouche NF, Verma A, Wazni O, et al. Mode of initiation and ablation of ventricular fibrillation storms in patients with ischemic cardiomyopathy. *J Am Coll Cardiol.* 2004;43(9):1715–1720. doi:10.1016/j.jacc.2004.03.004.

18. Peichl P, Čihák R, Koželuhová M, et al. Catheter ablation of arrhythmic storm triggered by monomorphic ectopic beats in patients with coronary artery disease. *J Interv Card Electrophysiol.* 2010;27(1):51–59. doi:10.1007/s10840-009-9443-2.

19. Bode K, Hindricks G, Piorkowski C, et al. Ablation of polymorphic ventricular tachycardias in patients with structural heart disease. *PACE—Pacing Clin Electrophysiol.* 2008;31(12):1585–1591. doi:10.1111/j.1540-8159.2008.01230.x.

20. Kobayashi Y, Iwasaki Y, Miyauchi Y, et al. The role of Purkinje fibers in the emergence of an incessant form of polymorphic ventricular tachycardia or ventricular fibrillation associated with ischemic heart disease. *J Arrhythmia.* 2008;24(4):200–208. doi:10.1016/S1880-4276(08)80029-4.

21. Hayashi M, Miyauchi Y, Murata H, et al. Urgent catheter ablation for sustained ventricular tachyarrhythmias in patients with acute heart failure decompensation. *Europace.* 2014;16(1):9–100. doi:10.1093/europace/eut207.

22. Sinha AM, Schmidt M, Marschang H, et al. Role of left ventricular scar and purkinje-like potentials during mapping and ablation of ventricular fibrillation in dilated cardiomyopathy. *PACE—Pacing Clin Electrophysiol.* 2009;32(3):286–290. doi:10.1111/j.1540-8159.2008.02233.x.

23. Mlcochova H, Saliba WI, Burkhardt DJ, et al. Catheter ablation of ventricular fibrillation storm in patients with infiltrative amyloidosis of the heart. *J Cardiovasc Electrophysiol.* 2006;17(4):426–430. doi:10.1111/j.1540-8167.2005.00321.x.

24. Friedman PL, Stewart JR, Fenoglio JJ, Wit AL. Survival of subendocardial Purkinje fibers after extensive myocardial infarction in dogs. *Circ Res.* 1973;33(5):597–611. doi:10.1161/01.RES.33.5.597.

MAPPING AND CATHETER ABLATION OF POSTMYOCARDIAL INFARCTION VENTRICULAR TACHYCARDIA (VT)
A Substrate-based Approach

Zaid Aziz and Roderick Tung

CONTENTS

Scar-related ventricular tachycardia (VT) is the result of re-entry from fixed or functional unidirectional block, where regions of slow conduction result from viable myocardial interspersed within areas of fibrosis.[1] As the surface morphology represents the exit site of a given VT circuit, the classical construct features slow conduction during diastole within a narrow protected channel, or isthmus, which is the ideal region to target with ablation (Figure 25.1). Mapping during VT remains the most specific method to identify and characterize a critical isthmus, although techniques to approximate and identify surrogates for an isthmus during sinus rhythm have evolved considerably. VT is hemodynamically unstable in the majority (>70%) of cases, which precludes the ability to perform activation mapping to delineate the circuit. Entrainment mapping, which is considered the gold standard for characterizing sites within a circuit, can be performed from candidate sites to assess whether the electrogram of interest is critical to re-entry.

In this chapter, we discuss the most commonly employed techniques used to map and ablate scar-related ventricular tachycardia with an emphasis on sinus rhythm surrogates, high-density electro-anatomic mapping, and ablation strategies.

VT LOCALIZATION

12-LEAD TO PREDICT EXIT SITES

Prior to invasive study, the 12-lead electrocardiogram (ECG) of the clinical tachycardia, when available, can be assessed to localize the site of origin or exit.[2,3] The 12-lead ECG does not predict where the isthmus site is located, but if the exit is in close proximity to the isthmus, a reasonable approximation can be made. VT with a left bundle branch block morphology arises from the right ventricle or left ventricular septum. VT with a right bundle branch block morphology arises from the left ventricle. A superior axis suggests an inferior wall

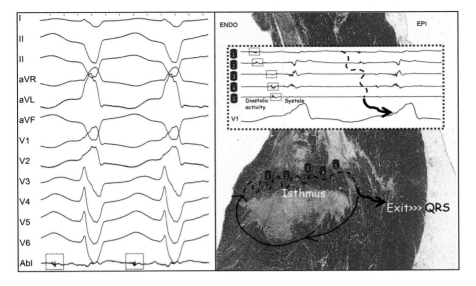

Figure 25.1 Histologic schematic of a reentrant circuit revolving around the region of fibrosis with protected isthmus exhibiting diastolic activation prior to exit, which dictates the QRS morphology. Mid-diastolic electrograms are ideal ablation targets for termination of VT.

location, while an inferior axis suggests a more anterior location. Lead I is typically negative for left free wall sites. The precordial R-wave transition determines how basal or apical the VT circuit exits where positive concordance, or R-wave dominance, suggests a basal location, while a QS pattern throughout suggests an apical location.

EPICARDIAL CRITERIA

Multiple ECG criteria have been proposed and evaluated to suggest epicardial exit sites. In general, the further the site of origin is from the conduction system, the wider the QRS complex. In cases of epicardial VT, wavefront propagation must travel transmyocardially from outside to in before engaging the conduction system endocardially. This results in a wide or slurred initial onset of QRS, which have been quantified as pseudodelta waves or maximum deflection index.[4,5] These predictors perform more optimally in idiopathic VT without structural heart disease. With extensive postmyocardial infarct scar, antiarrhythmic usage, and rapid VTs where QRS onset may be subjective and difficult to discern, these criteria have limited discriminatory value.[6]

VOLTAGE MAPPING: STRUCTURAL DISPLAYS AND ANATOMIC APPROACHES

BORDER ZONE

The original approach to catheter ablation of VT was aimed at mimicking surgical subendocardial resection and encircling ventriculotomy.[7] Marchlinksi et al. were the first to report the feasibility and efficacy of linear lesion sets across scar border zone, as delineated by electro-anatomic mapping and pace mapping.[8] By evaluating the range of normal electrograms, 95% of sampled electrograms of were >1.5 mV, which has since remained the gold standard voltage threshold for low voltage in the left ventricle. Values of <0.5 were chosen arbitrarily for dense scar.

Ablation at the interface between normal and low voltage areas has the potential to close off exits from channels originating deep within scar. Hsia et al. demonstrated by entrainment mapping within different regions of scar that 84% of isthmus sites were localized to dense scar whereas 54% of exit sites were found in border zone tissue (0.5–1.5 mV).[9] In contrast, Verma et al. correlated isthmus sites proven by entrainment mapping within scar and demonstrated that 68% of mappable VTs were successfully ablated at border zone sites.[10] These data suggest that border zone regions can harbor critical isthmuses as well as exit sites.

As a border zone substrate-based approach relies heavily on accurate scar substrate mapping, high mapping density is necessary to delineate the border zone with adequate resolution. Many scars are often too extensive to completely encircle, so localizing the border zone where the circuit exits by pace mapping can guide the operator in the region where more extensive ablation should be performed.

The exact shape of the optimal ablation lesion set is unknown. In addition to encircling a border zone region, a perpendicular line into scar resulting in a "T" shape was implemented in SMASH-VT.[11] Extension of the lesion set into scar increases the likelihood of transecting an isthmus. In EURO-VT, the predominant type of lesion set was linear, aimed to transect the scar.[12] Figure 25.2 shows ablation along the border zone in a patient with basal septal scar and typical lesion sets employed in SMASH-VT and EURO-VT.

RELATIVELY PRESERVED VOLTAGE CHANNELS

Ablation across dense scar can be performed with the goal of transecting a critical isthmus. Arenal at al. first demonstrated that the adjustment of scar voltage thresholds to display dense scar settings can reveal potential macroscopic channels within scar.[13] With a tiered decreasing voltage threshold (0.1–0.5 mV), conducting channels were observed in the majority of patients and related to a clinical or induced VT by pace mapping or entrainment mapping. In a similar

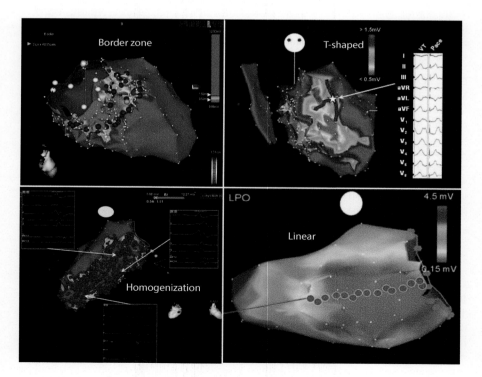

Figure 25.2 Various ablation strategies directed at low-voltage regions defined by electro-anatomic mapping. Circumferential border zone ablation, partial border zone modification, complete homogenization, and linear transection lesions sets are depicted.

fashion, Hsia et al. also performed voltage adjustments for a tiered scar display and found a mean voltage threshold of 0.33 ± 0.15 mV to be the optimal cutpoint for channel detection.

More recently, Mountantonakis et al. correlated critical sites to potential "channels" detected by tiered voltage settings. In contradistinction to previous cohorts, they found a lack of specificity of potential channels for tolerated VT isthmuses in the majority of cases.[14] Although 88% of scar maps revealed channels, only 30% were demonstrated by entrainment to contain the isthmus. The presence of late potentials within a channel increased the specificity to 85%.

HOMOGENIZATION
DiBiase et al. demonstrated that a combined epicardial–endocardial approach aimed to ablate all low-voltage abnormal electrograms in the ventricle resulted in greater freedom from recurrent VT compared to a limited approach in patients with ischemic cardiomyopathy presenting with electrical storm.[15] Such an extensive strategy most closely emulates endocardial resection, as the entire scar is treated (Figure 25.2). Prospective randomized data (VISTA trial)[16] demonstrated that homogenization is superior to limited approaches of ablating only stable clinical VTs. This strategy is practical and pragmatic and aims to modify the entire scar during sinus rhythm, without any targeting of a specific VT morphology.

DECHANNELING
The interconnected nature of channels whereby all LPs are necessarily activated through regions within scar with earlier abnormal activation may allow for achievement of homogenization with less ablation.[17] Importantly, ablation at channel entrances can eliminate remote downstream areas of slow conduction, even modifying electrical activity in regions of scar outside of the known radius of an RF lesion.[18] This technique, which requires detailed mapping with annotation of late electrogram components to track the path of late potential activation has been shown to result in high success rates (>80% freedom) with less ablation.[18,19]

SINUS RHYTHM SURROGATES

PACE MAPPING
Pace mapping can be used to estimate the exit morphology produced from an electrogram of interest. Correlation with the targeted VT exit sites may help localize channels of slow conduction.[14–21] Stimulus latency at matched pacemap sites deeper within scar (>40 ms) has been demonstrated to be more specific for more proximal and isthmus sites[22] (Figure 25.3). However, pace mapping within a reentrant circuit has inherent limitations. In a given scar substrate, there may be numerous pathways for an impulse to exit and this can lead a mismatched pacemap from a common channel. In a cohort of 18 patients with postinfarct monomorphic VT, Stevenson et al. demonstrated a nonmatched pacemap during sinus rhythm in 21% (6/28) of sites where concealed entrainment was demonstrated. Further, pacemap matches were seen in 29% of site where entrainment showed manifest fusion.[22]

Tung et al.[23] demonstrated evidence that multiple exit sites (MES) and pacemapped inductions (PMI) may provide additional functional information for mapping sites critical to re-entry. MES is defined as a pacemap that generates >1 VT exit morphology at a stable site (Figure 25.4); patients who had MES identified and ablated had a significantly higher freedom from VT than those without MES. Sites with access to multiple exits are likely common conducting channels, and this response to pacing may represent an isthmus surrogate. Unintentional induction of VT (pace mapping induction) when burst pacing (400–600 ms), may represent pacing within a slow conduction region with access to the VT exit site. Ablation at these PMI sites, which induce unidirectional block when pacing within a critical channel resulted in a >90% VT termination rate.

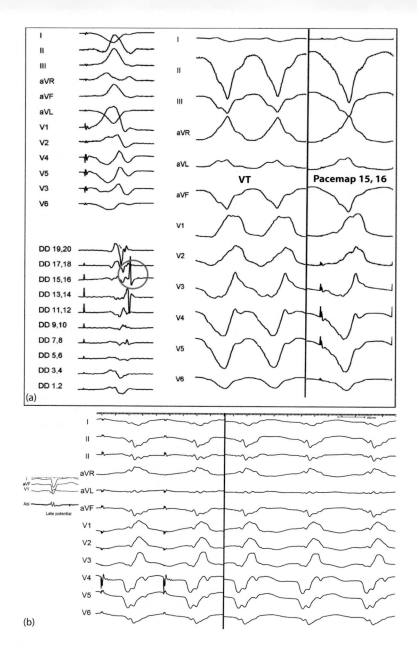

Figure 25.3 Two examples of pace mapping from abnormal electrograms. (a) Pace mapping from split potentials with nearly identical pacemap matches with short S-QRS. (b) Pace mapping from extremely delayed late potential demonstrates long S-QRS, indicating slow conduction from the pacing site out of scar.

"Pacemap mapping" during sinus rhythm, with an automated percentage of concordance to the targeted morphology has been demonstrated to have strong correlation with the reentrant circuit during VT by de Chillou et al.[24] Sites where the pacemap matches abruptly shift from good to poor likely reflect pacing that straddles a line of block or isthmus boundary with capture on either side of it.

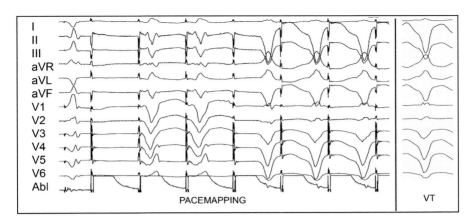

Figure 25.4 Example of multiple exit site, where two pacemap morphologies with different S-QRS latencies are observed. The second morphology matches the targeted VT.

LATE POTENTIALS AND LAVA

Isolated late potentials have been shown to be specific for VT isthmuses, as all critical sites exhibit slow conduction, fixed, or functional. A late potential-based ablation strategy has been shown to be effective in preventing recurrent VT.[25,26] As VT recurrence remained high, newer studies from experienced center had advocated extensive substrate ablation, where elimination of late activity or scar homogenization is the goal. Compared to limited approaches, ablation aimed to eliminate all uncoupled or late activity has been shown to result in improved clinical efficacy.

Jais et al. recently described that critical isthmus sites do not necessarily exhibit fixed conduction with timing after the QRS in sinus rhythm.[27] Rather, isolated potentials that are uncoupled from the local far-field electrogram can be functionally delayed and demonstrated by ventricular ectopics or premature stimuli. Complete elimination of local abnormal ventricular activity was demonstrated to be superior to noninducibility. Similar findings were reported by Vergara et al.,[28] where late potential abolition was used as the procedural endpoint. As the timing of late potentials is dependent on the wavefront of activation, the latest zone of late activation has less specificity for isthmus sites that sites of slow conduction.[29]

ISOCHRONAL LATE ACTIVATION MAPPING

Isochronal late activation mapping (ILAM) is a functional method for electro-anatomical maps to prioritize and distinguish slow conduction regions with delayed late potentials, which merely represent late arrival of the wavefront. Local activation timing of the late potential offset is annotated either manually or via automated mapping methods (Ensite Precision, Last Deflection, Abbott, IL). The propagation map is then displayed as eight equally distributed isochrones of activation (each isochrone are 12.5%). Deceleration zones were defined as slow conducting regions with isochronal crowding with >3 isochrones within 1 cm radius. A functional mapping display can provide complementary information to voltage-based structural displays as wavefront discontinuities are visually evident with isochronal display (Figure 25.5).

Irie et al. demonstrated that the majority of critical sites (90%) resided outside the latest isochrone of activation, implying that the latest late potential may not necessarily participate in the reentrant circuit. All termination sites correlated with areas of crowding of multiple isochronal colors that propagate into the latest isochrones. These data support that deceleration zones with wavefront discontinuities during sinus rhythm are surrogates for isthmus sites (Figure 25.6).[29,30] Studies by Anter et al. in animal models with high-resolution mapping are strongly confirmatory of these findings.[31]

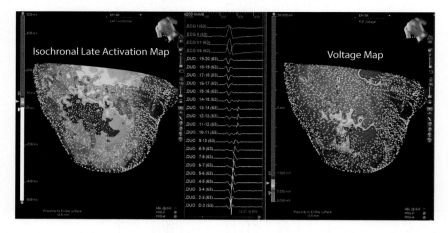

Figure 25.5 Isochronal map reveals a line of block within extensive low-voltage region. Functional propagation (ILAM, left) may be complementary to the structural voltage map (right).

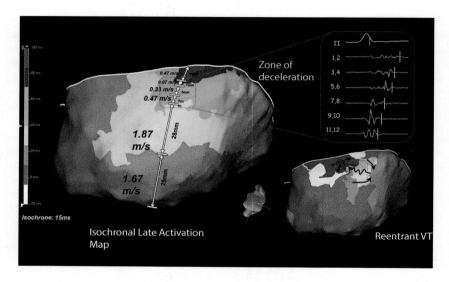

Figure 25.6 Quantification of conduction velocity with deceleration zone (<0.5 m/s) evident as isochronal crowding during sinus rhythm propagation. The deceleration zone correlates with the isthmus site during VT and the latest zone of activation forms the outer loop.

MAPPING DURING VT

ENTRAINMENT MAPPING

Entrainment mapping remains the gold standard methodology to assess the relationship between an electrogram of interest and the reentrant circuit. Entrainment in its simplest terms is continuous resetting (or accelerating the tachycardia to the pacing cycle length) of a circuit with an excitable gap.[32] Pacing typically is performed at a rate slightly faster (~10–30 ms) than the tachycardia cycle length. The tachycardia should not be oscillatory and must continue unchanged after pacing is terminated for interpretation. Overdrive pacing is not sufficient to prove re-entry as a mechanism (compared to focal), as fusion and progressive fusion should be demonstrated.

THREE-POINT CHECKLIST FOR ENTRAINMENT MAPPING OF AN ISTHMUS

When interpreting the response to entrainment, a three-point checklist can be assessed to determine the location of the pacing site in relation to the reentrant circuit: (1) comparison of the postpacing interval (PPI) with the tachycardia cycle length (TCL); (2) presence of overt, or manifest fusion versus concealed fusion; (3) difference between the stimulus to QRS and sensed electrogram to QRS. Most importantly, consistent capture must be confirmed prior to any interpretation. This scar construct developed and popularized by Stevenson et al. demonstrates the various responses to entrainment mapping within a reentrant circuit (Figure 25.7).[33,34]

The PPI is a measure of how close the pacing site is to the tachycardia circuit and is measured from the last pacing stimulus that entrained the tachycardia to the next local electrogram seen at the pacing site. The excess of the PPI compared to the TCL reflects the time required to enter the circuit and exit the circuit back to the pacing electrode. When pacing within the tachycardia circuit, there is no distance required to enter the circuit and return to the pacing electrode (PPI within 30 ms of TCL). Remote bystander sites spatially distinct from the tachycardia circuit have much longer PPI than TCL.

Secondly, the surface QRS morphology should be evaluated for the presence of fusion. When overt surface fusion is seen during pacing, manifest fusion is said to be present whereas concealed fusion is present when no change in surface morphology is seen.[35] Overt or manifest fusion occurs when pacing outside of a protected isthmus as the antidromic wavefront results in myocardial capture distinct from the circuit exit. Remote bystander and outer loop

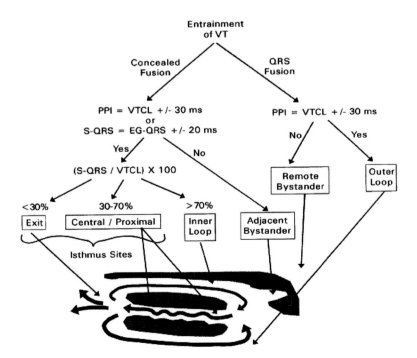

Figure 25.7 Classical construct of scar-reentry with response to entrainment mapping by Stevenson et al.

Mapping and Catheter Ablation of Postmyocardial Infarction Ventricular Tachycardia (VT) 307

sites exhibit manifest fusion. If entrainment is performed within a protected isthmus, the antidromic wavefront collides with the previous orthodromic wavefront within the circuit and only the orthodromic wavefront is seen, which has the same exit morphology. Therefore, fusion is present as collision occurs within the circuit, but it is hidden or concealed because the surface morphology is not altered.[34,36]

The third checkpoint requires the stimulus to QRS latency (S-QRS) to be the same as the timing from the sensed diastolic electrogram to QRS (EGM-QRS). This can help confirm that the site of pacing is the same as the site interpreted for sensing. Bystander sites will exhibit a difference between these two intervals where pacing out of the blind loop will result in a longer S-QRS than the EGM-QRS recorded into the blind loop attached to the isthmus.

At an inner loop site, there concealed fusion is present with a PPI that indicates the site is within the circuit. At an outer loop site, the PPI is within 30 ms of the TCL, although manifest fusion is present. For a bystander site, the PPI exceeds the TCL by the same amount that the S-QRS exceeds the EGM-QRS. When all three parameters on the checklist are fulfilled when targeting diastolic potentials, the rate of VT termination is high (Figure 25.8).[21,37]

ENTRAINMENT LIMITATIONS

Overdrive pacing in an attempt to entrain the reentrant tachycardia may disrupt or perturb the tachycardia. As seen with antitachycardia pacing with ICDs, VT may be overdriven and terminate upon cessation of pacing. Additionally, pacing can be proarrhythmic by accelerating VT, change the morphology, or degenerate into VF. Interpretation of entrainment response may be challenging in cases where the cycle length is not stable, the electrogram component captured is difficult to discern, or the intended electrogram is not captured.

PERCUTANEOUS EPICARDIAL APPROACH

The technique for percutaneous mapping via subxiphoid puncture was first introduced by Sosa et al. using the CARTO system to characterize and target epicardial scar in patients with Chagas disease and ischemic cardiomyopathy refractory to endocardial (Figure 25.9).[38,39] Low voltage regions identified during epicardial mapping may represent epicardial fat (>4 mm) and electrogram characteristics may be useful to differentiate

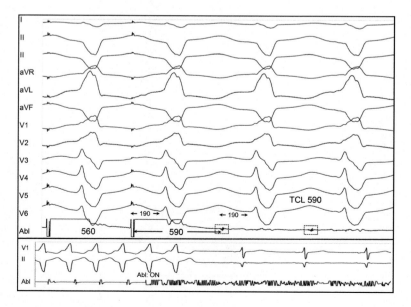

Figure 25.8 Fulfillment of three entrainment criteria with rapid termination of VT from this site.

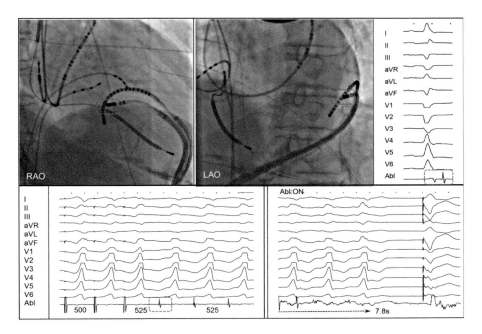

Figure 25.9 Mapping and ablation of VT from percutaneous epicardial approach. Late potential identified on the inferolateral wall is activated during mid-diastole during VT and entrainment fulfills criteria for isthmus.

insulated myocardium from scar.[40] Mapping within the pericardial space is unimpeded by trabeculations (endocardium) and ablation requires a safe distance from coronary arteries and the left phrenic nerve.

The functional contribution of the epicardium in postmyocardial infarct VT has been debated for many decades. In cases of true nonreperfused aneurysms mapping in the operating room, epicardial late potentials are uncommon.[41] Other intraoperative studies demonstrated >32% of circuits involving the epicardium or midmyocardium in postinfarct VT.[42] In clinical practice, epicardial ablation is typically reserved for patients that fail endocardial approach and in those where a paucity of substrate is present endocardially.

TOOLS

ELECTRO-ANATOMIC MAPPING SYSTEMS

Electro-anatomic mapping systems are widely used to delineate scar substrates, allowing for a real-time reproducible precise tool to locate the catheter in three dimensions.[43,44] Three commercially available mapping systems that utilize magnetic emission (CARTO, Biosense-Webster, Diamond Bar, CA and Rhythmia, Boston Scientific, Natick MA) and impedance-based localization (Abbott, Lake Forest, IL) have been validated. Callans and Marchlinski et al. demonstrated excellent correlation between infarct size by pathology low voltage areas that consisted of bipolar electrograms <1.0 mV using CARTO (Biosense Webster, Diamond Bar, CA)[44] and developed the anatomically-based ablation approach of short linear lesions aimed to connect dense scar regions (<0.5 mV) to normal tissue or anatomic boundaries in 2000.[8]

The use of mapping systems reduced the need for fluoroscopy and also allows for recording of ablation history in the virtual chamber created. Scar voltage mapping can be useful prior to induction of ventricular tachycardia to define the area to interrogate, as the critical reentrant sites are found within dense scar (<0.5 mV), and border zone (0.5–1.5 mV) tissue, particularly in regions of heterogeneity.[10,45] Potential channels or isthmuses may be revealed by adjusting voltage settings to more specific settings according to only dense scar (0.1–0.5 mV).[13] The use of multielectrode mapping catheters allows for higher resolution with increased mapping density in a shorter period of time.

Aside from magnetic localization technology, the use of impedance-based electrofield localization (Ensite, Abbott) provides advantages that include the ability to compensate for patient motion and localization of any diagnostic catheter connected to the system. Validation of multielectrode catheter delineation of ventricular substrate was first demonstrated using the Ensite NAVX system in the human right ventricle by Casella et al. (2009) in the left ventricle with combined epicardial–endocardial mapping, a porcine infarct model with a linear duodecapolar catheter (Livewire, 2-2-2) by Tung et al. (2011).[43,46] These studies demonstrated significantly higher density delineation of low-voltage scar in one-third of the mapping of single-point mapping technique, with comparable accuracy (Figure 25.10). In 2013, a fully-automated high-resolution mapping system (Rhythmia, Boston Scientific, Natick, MA) with acquisition from 64 mini-electrodes on a small basket catheter (Orion) was introduced, featuring the highest mapping density (>5000 points) and a noise level of <0.01 mV.

Automated annotation, which has emerged with multielectrode catheter mapping strategies has limitations as the majority of default settings tag the maximum or peak of the local electrogram. This is often a far-field systolic component and in cases where late potentials after

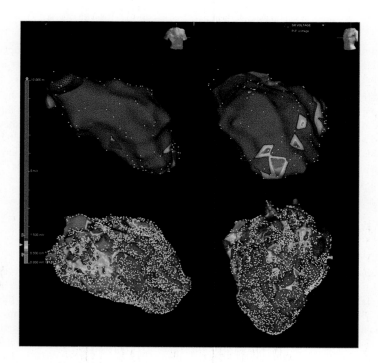

Figure 25.10 Comparison of point-by-point mapping and multielectrode acquisition. Data collection with standard point-by-point collection, with data collection of 300 points over 30 min. Data collection with multipolar catheter results in acquisition of 3000 points in under 30 min.

the QRS may be present, these low-voltage deflections are often not annotated. For fractionated and long-duration electrograms, annotation of a single electrogram component does not capture all of the local information. For these reasons, it is critical that the operator examines electrogram characteristics during map creation as well as postmap review.

MULTIELECTRODE CATHETERS

Multiple shapes and configurations of multielectrode catheters can result in expeditious high-density acquisition. These include multispline (PentaRay, Biosense Webster, Diamond Bar, CA), linear (duodecapolar, Livewire, Abbott or decapolar, DecaNav, Biosense Webster), mini-basket (Orion, Boston Scientific, Natick, MA), and fixed Grid (HF Grid, Abbott, IL). Delineation of border zone and identification of LAVA can be facilitated by multi-electrode mapping relative to point-by-point mapping (Figure 25.11). In addition to pace mapping and entrainment mapping with high density and more candidate electrograms recorded, use of a multipolar catheter allows for mapping of diastolic during hemodynamically unstable, when strategically placed within a region that is suspected to have the highest arrhythmogenicity during sinus rhythm. This strategy provides rapid multisite contact mapping during one beat of VT within scar, which is more efficient than tradition point-by-point mapping (Figure 25.12).

ABLATION CATHETERS AND SETTINGS

Irrigated ablation improves the ability to deliver adequate power into the tissue without temperature limitations from the surface. Ablation is typically performed at 30 W and titrated up to 50 W with a temperature limit of 42°C. Reduction of electrogram amplitude or elimination of late/fractionated is the hallmark of an effective radiofrequency application. Reduction in impedance also demonstrates effective energy delivery and loss of pace capture after ablation can be used to demonstrate tissue inexcitability.[47] Ablation biophysics in scar is different from normal myocardium and dense scar may serve as a barrier

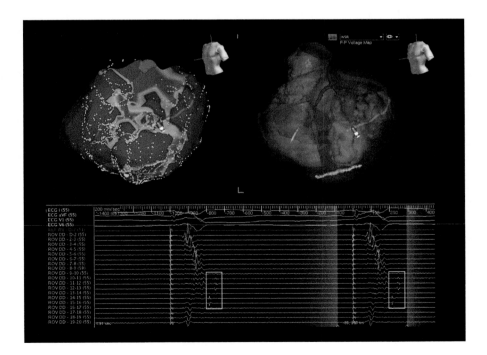

Figure 25.11 Apical infarction mapped with linear multielectrode catheter with late potentials identified on multiple bipoles. Corresponding anatomy of CT scan is shown (right).

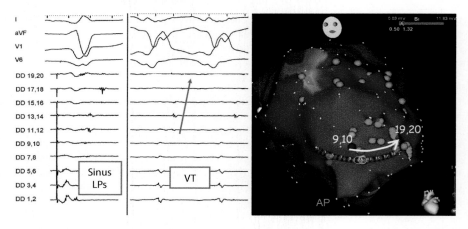

Figure 25.12 Strategic placement of decapolar catheter in anteroapical infarct with sequence of late potentials recorded. The diastolic pathway is mapped with this catheter position in one beat of VT.

for optimal energy delivery. In cases where midmyocardial or epicardial circuitry is suspected (paucity of endocardial substrate or activation gap during VT), epicardial access and ablation can be useful in ICM, where ablation is typically performed at 30–50 W, with a temperature limit of 45°C as the risk of sequelae from char and steam pop is lower in the pericardial space.

CONCLUSIONS

Mapping of low-voltage regions to delineate scar has been greatly facilitated since the advent of electro-anatomic mapping. Pathologic potentials or LAVA that are late, fractionated, or split have been shown to have high sensitivity for critical sites for re-entry.[26] More extensive elimination of the entire substrate results in electrical homogenization, which has been demonstrated to be effective to prevent recurrent VT. Techniques such as dechanneling or targeted ablation of deceleration zones are less reliant on voltage but rather the timing of local electrograms. Regardless of strategy, pace mapping can be employed to approximate the candidate site with the 12-lead VT morphology and entrainment mapping is considered the gold standard for characterizing the circuit response to overdrive pacing. Epicardial ablation and high-density mapping with multielectrode catheters may improve the ability to identify and eliminate arrhythmogenic regions within the scar.

REFERENCES

1. de Bakker JM, van Capelle FJ, Janse MJ et al. Slow conduction in the infarcted human heart. "Zigzag" course of activation. *Circulation.* 1993;88:915–26.
2. Miller JM, Marchlinski FE, Buxton AE, Josephson ME. Relationship between the 12-lead electrocardiogram during ventricular tachycardia and endocardial site of origin in patients with coronary artery disease. *Circulation.* 1988;77:759–66.

3. Josephson ME, Callans DJ. Using the twelve-lead electrocardiogram to localize the site of origin of ventricular tachycardia. *Heart Rhythm.* 2005;2:443–6.

4. Berruezo A, Mont L, Nava S et al. Electrocardiographic recognition of the epicardial origin of ventricular tachycardias. *Circulation.* 2004;109:1842–7.

5. Daniels DV, Lu YY, Morton JB et al. Wilber DJ. Idiopathic epicardial left ventricular tachycardia originating remote from the sinus of Valsalva: Electrophysiological characteristics, catheter ablation, and identification from the 12-lead electrocardiogram. *Circulation.* 2006;113:1659–66.

6. Martinek M, Stevenson WG, Inada K et al. QRS characteristics fail to reliably identify ventricular tachycardias that require epicardial ablation in ischemic heart disease. *J Cardiovasc Electrophysiol.* 2012;23:188–93.

7. Guiraudon G, Fontaine G, Frank R et al. Encircling endocardial ventriculotomy: A new surgical treatment for life-threatening ventricular tachycardias resistant to medical treatment following myocardial infarction. *Ann Thorac Surg.* 1978;26:438–44.

8. Marchlinski FE, Callans DJ, Gottlieb CD, Zado E. Linear ablation lesions for control of unmappable ventricular tachycardia in patients with ischemic and nonischemic cardiomyopathy. *Circulation.* 2000;101:1288–96.

9. Hsia HH, Lin D, Sauer WH et al. Anatomic characterization of endocardial substrate for hemodynamically stable reentrant ventricular tachycardia: Identification of endocardial conducting channels. *Heart Rhythm.* 2006;3:503–12.

10. Verma A, Marrouche NF, Schweikert RA et al. Relationship between successful ablation sites and the scar border zone defined by substrate mapping for ventricular tachycardia post-myocardial infarction. *J Cardiovasc Electrophysiol.* 2005;16:465–71.

11. Reddy VY, Reynolds MR, Neuzil P et al. Prophylactic catheter ablation for the prevention of defibrillator therapy. *N Engl J Med.* 2007;357:2657–65.

12. Tanner H, Hindricks G, Volkmer M et al. Catheter ablation of recurrent scar-related ventricular tachycardia using electroanatomical mapping and irrigated ablation technology: Results of the prospective multicenter Euro-VT-study. *J Cardiovasc Electrophysiol.* 2010;21:47–53.

13. Arenal A, del Castillo S, Gonzalez-Torrecilla E et al. Tachycardia-related channel in the scar tissue in patients with sustained monomorphic ventricular tachycardias: Influence of the voltage scar definition. *Circulation.* 2004;110:2568–74.

14. Mountantonakis SE, Park RE, Frankel DS et al. Relationship between voltage map "channels" and the location of critical isthmus sites in patients with post-infarction cardiomyopathy and ventricular tachycardia. *J Am Coll Cardiol.* 2013;61:2088–95.

15. Di Biase L, Santangeli P, Burkhardt DJ et al. Endo-epicardial homogenization of the scar versus limited substrate ablation for the treatment of electrical storms in patients with ischemic cardiomyopathy. *J Am Coll Cardiol.* 2012;60:132–41.

16. Di Biase L, Burkhardt JD, Lakkireddy D et al. Ablation of stable VTs versus substrate ablation in ischemic cardiomyopathy: The VISTA randomized multicenter trial. *J Am Coll Cardiol* 2015;66:2872–82.

17. Berruezo A, Fernandez-Armenta J, Mont L et al. Combined endocardial and epicardial catheter ablation in arrhythmogenic right ventricular dysplasia incorporating scar dechanneling technique. *Circ Arrhythm Electrophysiol.* 2012;5:111–21.

18. Tung R, Mathuria NS, Nagel R et al. Impact of local ablation on interconnected channels within ventricular scar: Mechanistic implications for substrate modification. *Circ Arrhythm Electrophysiol.* 2013;6:1131–8.

19. Berruezo A, Fernandez-Armenta J, Andreu D et al. Scar dechanneling: New method for scar-related left ventricular tachycardia substrate ablation. *Circ Arrhythm Electrophysiol.* 2015;8:326–36.

20. Brunckhorst CB, Stevenson WG, Soejima K et al. Relationship of slow conduction detected by pace-mapping to ventricular tachycardia re-entry circuit sites after infarction. *J Am Coll Cardiol.* 2003;41:802–9.

21. Bogun F, Bahu M, Knight BP et al. Response to pacing at sites of isolated diastolic potentials during ventricular tachycardia in patients with previous myocardial infarction. *J Am Coll Cardiol.* 1997;30:505–13.

22. Stevenson WG, Sager PT, Natterson PD et al. Relation of pace mapping QRS configuration and conduction delay to ventricular tachycardia reentry circuits in human infarct scars. *J Am Coll Cardiol.* 1995;26:481–8.

23. Tung R, Mathuria N, Michowitz Y et al. Functional pace-mapping responses for identification of targets for catheter ablation of scar-mediated ventricular tachycardia. *Circ Arrhythm Electrophysiol.* 2012;5:264–72.

24. de Chillou C, Groben L, Magnin-Poull I et al. Localizing the critical isthmus of postinfarct ventricular tachycardia: The value of pace-mapping during sinus rhythm. *Heart Rhythm.* 2014;11:175–81.

25. Arenal A, Glez-Torrecilla E, Ortiz M et al. Ablation of electrograms with an isolated, delayed component as treatment of unmappable monomorphic ventricular tachycardias in patients with structural heart disease. *J Am Coll Cardiol.* 2003;41:81–92.

26. Bogun F, Good E, Reich S et al. Isolated potentials during sinus rhythm and pace-mapping within scars as guides for ablation of post-infarction ventricular tachycardia. *J Am Coll Cardiol.* 2006;47:2013–9.

27. Jais P, Maury P, Khairy P et al. Elimination of local abnormal ventricular activities: A new end point for substrate modification in patients with scar-related ventricular tachycardia. *Circulation.* 2012;125:2184–96.

28. Vergara P, Trevisi N, Ricco A et al. Late potentials abolition as an additional technique for reduction of arrhythmia recurrence in scar related ventricular tachycardia ablation. *J Cardiovasc Electrophysiol.* 2012;23:621–7.

29. Irie T, Yu R, Bradfield JS et al. Relationship between sinus rhythm late activation zones and critical sites for scar-related ventricular tachycardia: Systematic analysis of isochronal late activation mapping. *Circ Arrhythm Electrophysiol.* 2015;8:390–9.

30. Raiman M, Tung R. Automated isochronal late activation mapping to identify deceleration zones: Rationale and methodology of a practical electroanatomic mapping approach for ventricular tachycardia ablation. *Comput Biol Med.* 2018.

31. Anter E, Kleber AG, Rottmann M et al. Infarct-related ventricular tachycardia: Redefining the electrophysiological substrate of the isthmus during sinus rhythm. *JACC Clin Electrophysiol.* 2018;4:1033–1048.

32. Waldo AL, Henthorn RW. Use of transient entrainment during ventricular tachycardia to localize a critical area in the reentry circuit for ablation. *Pacing Clin Electrophysiol.* 1989;12:231–44.

33. Stevenson WG, Khan H, Sager P et al. Identification of reentry circuit sites during catheter mapping and radiofrequency ablation of ventricular tachycardia late after myocardial infarction. *Circulation.* 1993;88:1647–70.

34. Stevenson WG, Friedman PL, Sager PT et al. Exploring postinfarction reentrant ventricular tachycardia with entrainment mapping. *J Am Coll Cardiol.* 1997;29:1180–9.

35. Stevenson WG, Sager PT, Friedman PL. Entrainment techniques for mapping atrial and ventricular tachycardias. *J Cardiovasc Electrophysiol.* 1995;6:201–16.

36. Stevenson WG, Soejima K. Catheter ablation for ventricular tachycardia. *Circulation.* 2007;115:2750–60.

37. Bogun F, Hohnloser SH, Bender B et al. Mechanism of ventricular tachycardia termination by pacing at left ventricular sites in patients with coronary artery disease. *J Interv Card Electrophysiol.* 2002;6:35–41.

38. Sosa E, Scanavacca M, d'Avila A et al. Nonsurgical transthoracic epicardial catheter ablation to treat recurrent ventricular tachycardia occurring late after myocardial infarction. *J Am Coll Cardiol.* 2000;35:1442–9.

39. Sosa E, Scanavacca M, D'Avila A et al. Endocardial and epicardial ablation guided by nonsurgical transthoracic epicardial mapping to treat recurrent ventricular tachycardia. *J Cardiovasc Electrophysiol.* 1998;9:229–39.

40. Tung R, Nakahara S, Ramirez R et al. Distinguishing epicardial fat from scar: Analysis of electrograms using high-density electroanatomic mapping in a novel porcine infarct model. *Heart Rhythm.* 2010;7:389–95.

41. Horowitz LN, Josephson ME, Harken AH. Epicardial and endocardial activation during sustained ventricular tachycardia in man. *Circulation.* 1980;61:1227–38.

42. Littmann L, Svenson RH, Gallagher JJ et al. Functional role of the epicardium in postinfarction ventricular tachycardia. Observations derived from computerized epicardial activation mapping, entrainment, and epicardial laser photoablation. *Circulation.* 1991;83:1577–91.

43. Tung R, Nakahara S, Ramirez R et al. Accuracy of combined endocardial and epicardial electroanatomic mapping of a reperfused porcine infarct model: A comparison of electrofield and magnetic systems with histopathologic correlation. *Heart Rhythm.* 2011;8:439–47.

44. Callans DJ, Ren JF, Michele J et al. Electroanatomic left ventricular mapping in the porcine model of healed anterior myocardial infarction. Correlation with intracardiac echocardiography and pathological analysis. *Circulation.* 1999;100:1744–50.

45. Nakahara S, Tung R, Ramirez RJ et al. Distribution of late potentials within infarct scars assessed by ultra high-density mapping. *Heart Rhythm.* 2010.

46. Casella M, Perna F, Dello Russo A et al. Right ventricular substrate mapping using the Ensite navx system: Accuracy of high-density voltage map obtained by automatic point acquisition during geometry reconstruction. *Heart Rhythm.* 2009;6:1598–605.

47. Soejima K, Stevenson WG, Maisel WH et al. Electrically unexcitable scar mapping based on pacing threshold for identification of the reentry circuit isthmus: Feasibility for guiding ventricular tachycardia ablation. *Circulation.* 2002;106:1678–83.

ARRHYTHMOGENIC RIGHT VENTRICULAR CARDIOMYOPATHY

Daniele Muser and Pasquale Santangeli

CONTENTS

INTRODUCTION

Arrhythmogenic right ventricular cardiomyopathy (ARVC) is a genetically determined cardiomyopathy clinically characterized by life-threatening ventricular arrhythmias (VAs) and/or heart failure (HF) predominantly involving the right ventricle (RV).[1] From its initial description in 1977, several progress have been made in the comprehension of the disease etiology, pathogenesis, clinical manifestations, risk stratification, and management.[2] Currently, ARVC is seen as a polygenic-multifactorial disease in which the interaction between a pool of genetic mutations rather than a single gene with other environmental and individual factors such as age, sex, physical activity, infections, and pro-inflammatory conditions leads to the phenotypic manifestation of the disease.[1]

EPIDEMIOLOGY

The prevalence of the disease among the general population has been estimated to range from 1:1000 to 1:5000 with similar distribution in Europe and North America.[3-5]

ARVC is a major cause of sudden cardiac death (SCD) in the young and athletes accounting for 5%–11% and 22% of overall cases, respectively, with a prevalence of male individuals in their second to fourth decade of life.[6-8]

ETIOLOGY AND PATHOGENESIS

ARVC is a genetically determined cardiomyopathy with heterogeneous inheritance and clinical phenotype with variable penetrance and clinical severity of the disease among family trees. In up to 50% of the cases, a definite causal gene mutation cannot be found while desmosomal gene mutations are responsible for the disease in the 70% of cases with a positive genetic test.[9] The first mutations causing the disease were found in 2000 in genes encoding for the desmosomal proteins plakoglobin and desmoplakin among patients with autosomal recessive Naxos and Carvajal cardiocutaneous syndromes, respectively.[10–12] Both present woolly hair, keratoderma and arrhythmogenic cardiomyopathy with a higher incidence of LV involvement in the second one. Other desmosomal genes encoding for plakophilin, desmoglein, and desmocollin have also been discovered and have been associated to both autosomal recessive and dominant forms.[13–15] In a lower proportion of cases, genes encoding for other non-desmosomal proteins like the ryanodine receptor and the transforming growth factor-β3 have been found.[16,17] Mutations in the genes encoding for titin, lamin A/C and phospholamban have also been described and typically lead to arrhythmogenic syndromes characterized by a dilated cardiomyopathy phenotype overlapping with the classical ARVC phenotype.[18–20]

Multiple genes and several exogenous factors interacting with the genetic substrate are probably involved in the pathologic process leading to the clinical expression of the disease.[21–24] Regardless, the underlying genetic mutation, the disease involves the junctions between cardiomyocytes affecting cell to cell mechanical coupling. Therefore, mechanical stretching (especially during effort) can enhance myocyte loss and healing replacement by fibro-fatty tissue.[25] Myocyte loss occurs through an apoptotic mechanism and may be associated with inflammatory infiltrates.[26,27] It starts in early childhood, tends to progress with time, and predominantly affects the RV free wall, usually starting from the epicardium extending to the endocardium. The remodeling process leads to progressive dilation and dysfunction with aneurysm formation especially at the inflow and outflow tract level.[25,28] The resultant disruption of electrical conduction due to preserved islets of myocytes interspersed among fibrofatty tissue serves as the substrate for reentrant VAs.[29]

The disease is not limited to the RV free wall and an LV involvement can be demonstrated in up to 50% of cases. Dominant or isolated LV involvement has also been recognized as a phenotypic variant of the disease characterized by a higher risk of life-threatening VAs and SCD.[30,31]

CLINICAL MANIFESTATIONS AND NATURAL HISTORY

ARVC has a wide spectrum of clinical manifestations ranging from palpitations, syncope, and SCD especially in young males, to congestive heart failure. The clinical onset of the disease usually occurs between the second and fourth decade of life with ventricular arrhythmias of RV origin occurring mostly during effort.

Classically, three stages have been identified in the natural history of the disease:

1   *Subclinical stage:* In this phase, the patient presents no symptoms even if concealed myocardial structural abnormalities mostly represented by healing fibro-fatty replacement may lead to fatal VAs as the only clinical manifestation.[32]

2   *Overt clinical disease:* As the vicious circle of myocardial damage with myocyte loss and scar healing progresses, the disease becomes clinically overt typically presenting with symptomatic VAs of RV origin, which range from premature ventricular complexes

(PVC) to sustained ventricular tachycardia (VT)/ventricular fibrillation (VF). In this phase, the clinical manifestations and the structural changes usually allow to reach a definite diagnosis.[33]

3 *End-stage disease:* The loss of contractile myocardium leads to a progressive RV and LV dilation and dysfunction accounting for severe HF mimicking dilated cardiomyopathy. In this phase, complications like endocavitary thrombosis particularly within aneurysms and polymorphic VAs could be easily seen.

The annual mortality among patients affected by ARVC varies considerably among different cohorts of patients but data from meta-analysis reported an annual rate of cardiac mortality and cardiac transplantation of 0.9%. SCD accounts for one-third of the cases whereas refractory HF is the cause of death in the remaining two-thirds.[34,35]

DIAGNOSIS

Due to the heterogeneous nature of the disease and its clinical manifestations, there is no single criteria allowing a definite diagnosis. Even the structural changes at myocardial biopsy, although suggestive of the disease, can be non-specific as fibro-fatty replacement is the final common pathway of several types of myocardial injury (i.e., ischemia, inflammation). Thus, the diagnosis of the disease should be multi-parametric, based upon several clinical, instrumental, and histological criteria. For these reasons, a pool of diagnostic criteria were established in 1994 and then revised in 2010 to improve sensitivity of the original ones.[33,36] Table 26.1 shows the revised Task Force Criteria for the diagnosis of ARVC: 2 major or 1 major and 2 minor or 4 minor criteria need to be fulfilled for a definite diagnosis, while 1 major and 1 minor or 3 minor are required for a borderline diagnosis and 1 major or 2 minor for a possible diagnosis.

DIAGNOSTIC TOOLS
TWELVE-LEAD ECG AND SIGNAL-AVERAGED ECG
The structural changes involving the myocardium lead to activation delay and repolarization abnormalities that can be visible on the surface ECG particularly on right precordial leads. The classical ECG findings in ARVC comprehend epsilon waves usually visible in leads V_{1-3} and defined as a distinct deflection after the end of the QRS complex. Epsilon waves are more typical of advanced stages of ARVC and can be seen in only 10% of unselected cohorts with definite diagnosis. Activation delay (prolongation of QRS duration >110 ms) specifically in the right precordial leads (V_{1-3}) can also be present. Repolarization abnormalities involve inversion of T waves on precordial leads beyond lead V_1 (usually leads V_{1-3}). In general, the presence of inverted T waves in leads V_{1-3} in the absence of RBBB or beyond V_4 in the presence of RBBB in subjects older than 14 years is the most sensitive ECG abnormality for ARVC (Figure 26.1).

The presence of late potentials as expression conduction delay through areas of scarred myocardium can be unmasked by signal averaged electrocardiogram (SAECG) and currently represents a minor Task Force criterion. There are three parameters commonly evaluated by SAECG: filtered QRS duration (fQRSD), low-amplitude signal duration below 40 μV (LAS), and root mean square voltage in last 40 ms of the QRS (RMS-40). Normal values for fQRSD are <114 ms, for LAS 40 < 38 ms, and for RMS-40 > 20 μV.[37] The SAECG is usually categorized as abnormal if one or more of the above parameters are abnormal.[38] The presence of late potentials detected by SAECG in patients with ARVC can range from 50% to 100% with an higher prevalence among patients presenting with sustained VT.[37,39]

Table 26.1 Revised Task Force Criteria for the diagnosis of ARVC

I. Global or regional dysfunction and structural alterations[a]		
Major		
	By 2D echo:	
	Regional RV akinesia, dyskinesia, or aneurysm and 1 of the following (end diastole):	
		PLAX RVOT $\geq$ 32 mm (corrected for body size $\geq$19 mm/m^2)
		PSAX RVOT $\geq$ 36 mm (corrected for body size $\geq$21 mm/m^2)
		or fractional area change $\leq$33%
	By MRI:	
	Regional RV akinesia or dyskinesia or dyssynchronous RV contraction and 1 of the following:	
		Ratio of RV end-diastolic volume to BSA $\geq$ 110 mL/m^2 (male) or $\geq$100 mL/m^2 (female)
		or RV ejection fraction $\leq$40%
	By RV angiography:	
	Regional RV akinesia, dyskinesia, or aneurysm	
Minor		
	By 2D echo:	
	Regional RV akinesia or dyskinesia	
	and 1 of the following (end diastole):	
		PLAX RVOT $\geq$ 29 to <32 mm (corrected for body size $\geq$16 to <19 mm/m^2)
		PSAX RVOT $\geq$ 32 to <36 mm (corrected for body size $\geq$18 to <21 mm/m^2)
		or fractional area change >33% to $\leq$40%
	By MRI:	
	Regional RV akinesia or dyskinesia or dyssynchronous RV contraction and 1 of the following:	
		Ratio of RV end-diastolic volume to BSA $\geq$ 100 to <110 mL/m^2 (male) or $\geq$90 to <100 mL/m^2 (female)
		or RV ejection fraction >40% to $\leq$45%
II. Tissue characterization of wall		
Major		
	Residual myocytes <60% by morphometric analysis (or <50% if estimated), with fibrous replacement of the RV free wall myocardium in $\geq$1 sample, with or without fatty replacement of tissue on endomyocardial biopsy	
Minor		
	Residual myocytes 60%–75% by morphometric analysis (or 50%–65% if estimated), with fibrous replacement of the RV free wall myocardium in $\geq$1 sample, with or without fatty replacement of tissue on endomyocardial biopsy	

(*Continued*)

Table 26.1 (*Continued*)   Revised Task Force Criteria for the diagnosis of ARVC

III. Repolarization abnormalities	
Major	
	Inverted T waves in right precordial leads (V1, V2, and V3) or beyond in individuals >14 years of age (in the absence of complete right bundle-branch block QRS ≥ 120 ms)
Minor	
	Inverted T waves in leads V1 and V2 in individuals >14 years of age (in the absence of complete right bundle-branch block) or in V4, V5, or V6
	Inverted T waves in leads V1, V2, V3, and V4 in individuals >14 years of age in the presence of complete right bundle-branch block
IV. Depolarization/conduction abnormalities	
Major	
	Epsilon wave (reproducible low-amplitude signals between end of QRS complex to onset of the T wave) in the right precordial leads (V1–V3)
Minor	
	Late potentials by SAECG in ≥1 of 3 parameters in the absence of a QRS duration of ≥110 ms on the standard ECG
	Filtered QRS duration (fQRS) ≥114 ms
	Duration of terminal QRS < 40 µV (low-amplitude signal duration) ≥38 ms
	Root-mean-square voltage of terminal 40 ms <20 µV
	Terminal activation duration of QRS ≥ 55 ms measured from the nadir of the S wave to the end of the QRS, including R', in V1, V2, or V3, in the absence of complete right bundle-branch block
V. Arrhythmias	
Major	
	Non-sustained or sustained ventricular tachycardia of left bundle-branch morphology with superior axis (negative or indeterminate QRS in leads II, III, and aVF and positive in lead aVL)
Minor	
	Non-sustained or sustained ventricular tachycardia of RV outflow configuration, left bundle-branch block morphology with inferior axis (positive QRS in leads II, III, and aVF and negative in lead aVL) or of unknown axis
	>500 PVCs per 24 hours (Holter)
VI. Family history	
Major	
	ARVC/D confirmed in a first-degree relative who meets current Task Force criteria
	ARVC/D confirmed pathologically at autopsy or surgery in a first-degree relative
	Identification of a pathogenic mutation[b] categorized as associated or probably associated with ARVC/D in the patient under evaluation

(*Continued*)

Table 26.1 (*Continued*)   Revised Task Force Criteria for the diagnosis of ARVC

VI. Family history	
Minor	
	History of ARVC/D in a first-degree relative in whom it is not possible or practical to determine whether the family member meets current Task Force criteria
	Premature sudden death (<35 years of age) due to suspected ARVC/D in a first-degree relative
	ARVC/D confirmed pathologically or by current Task Force Criteria in second-degree relative

Notes: Diagnostic terminology: definite diagnosis: 2 major or 1 major and 2 minor criteria or 4 minor from different categories; borderline: 1 major and 1 minor or 3 minor criteria from different categories; possible: 1 major or 2 minor criteria from different categories.

a Hypokinesis is not included in this or subsequent definitions of RV regional wall motion abnormalities for the proposed modified criteria.

b A pathogenic mutation is a DNA alteration associated with ARVC/D that alters or is expected to alter the encoded protein, is unobserved or rare in a large non-ARVC/D control population, and either alters or is predicted to alter the structure or function of the protein or has demonstrated linkage to the disease phenotype in a conclusive pedigree.

Abbreviations: PLAX indicates parasternal long-axis view; RVOT, RV outflow tract; BSA, body surface area; PSAX, parasternal short-axis view.

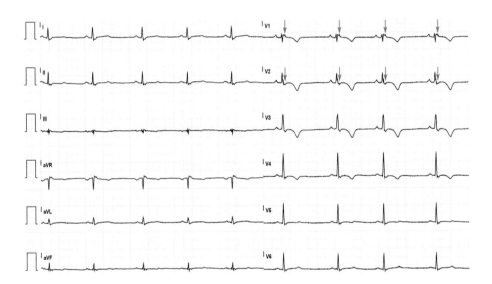

Figure 26.1   ECG of 24 year-old man affected by arrhythmogenic right ventricular cardiomyopathy showing inversion of T waves on precordial leads beyond lead V_1, prolongation of QRS duration >110 ms, and epsilon waves best visible in leads V_{1-2} (red arrows).

ECHOCARDIOGRAPHY

Several structural abnormalities and functional changes of the RV have been described in ARVC with echocardiography. Structural abnormalities include prominent trabeculation, local wall motion abnormalities, focal aneurysms (sometime distributed in sequence along the free wall of the RV in the so-called *"pile d'assiettes"* aspect), and hyperechogenicity of the moderator band. Anterior RV free wall, right ventricular outflow tract (RVOT), and RV apex are the most common regions affected. RV dilatation is common in ARVC particularly for what concerns RVOT (an enlarged RVOT is found in almost all cases) and is often associated with global dysfunction.

None of these elements is per se diagnostic of ARVC but the finding of local wall motion abnormalities (particularly focal aneurysms) in addition to RV dilation and/or dysfunction is highly specific for ARVC and is considered a major diagnostic criterion. The echocardiographic differential diagnosis may be challenging particularly in the early stage of the disease as RV enlargement/dysfunction may be present in several other pathologic conditions and has even been described as adaptation to endurance sports. In this setting, emerging technologic tools like strain analysis by feature tracking may help to quantify subtle functional changes.

VENTRICULAR ANGIOGRAPHY

Ventricular angiography was the first diagnostic tool used to look for structural abnormalities within the RV wall in ARVC but is no long routinely used due to the introduction of several non-invasive imaging modalities (i.e., echocardiography, magnetic resonance, multislice computed tomography). Major findings on ventricular angiography comprehend global RV dilatation and dysfunction, hypertrophic trabeculae visible as a transverse series of deep horizontals fissures, focal aneurysms or bulging, a polycyclic contour of the RV wall ("*cauliflower*" aspect) due to multiple merged sacculations, regionally delayed contrast runoff, and sometimes evidence of thrombotic formations within aneurysms. With the exception of sacculations, most of these findings are not specific for the disease moreover are usually found in advanced stages making ventricular angiography not the imaging modality of choice in early assessment.

CARDIAC MAGNETIC RESONANCE IMAGING (cMRI)

Cardiac MRI has become a fundamental tool in several cardiac conditions over the past decade due to is capability to provide not only a precise quantification of chamber anatomy and function but also an in vivo structural analysis of the myocardium with specific sequences for identification of myocardial edema (T2 imaging), fibro-fatty replacement (T1 imaging), substitutive fibrosis (delayed enhancement imaging), and interstitial fibrosis (T1 mapping). As for other imaging modalities, cMRI findings in ARVC can be grouped into two groups: morphological abnormalities that include intramyocardial fat deposits, focal fibrosis, wall thinning, and RVOT enlargement and functional abnormalities that include RV global dilation and dysfunction and local regional motion abnormalities like aneurysms (Figure 26.2).

Compared to the echo, cMRI has a greater capability to detect and quantify the presence of such abnormalities and moreover can detect fibro-fatty replacement, for these reasons has become the imaging modality of choice for differential diagnosis in patients suspected to be affected by ARVC.

COMPUTED TOMOGRAPHY

The role of multi-detector computed tomography (MDCT) compared to cMRI is relatively limited. Some advantages include a significantly higher spatial resolution (close to 0.5 mm^3) with comparable temporal resolution, its widespread availability, fast acquisition protocol, and relatively low cost. Similar to cMRI, MDCT allows myocardial tissue characterization, however, its lower contrast to noise ratio determines Inferior scar characterization capabilities compared to LGE-cMRI.[40] Quantitative evaluation of RV and LV geometry and function by MDCT have been validated against both TTE and cMRI.[41,42] Due to the widespread use of cMRI and the non-negligible radiation exposure, the use of MDCT is mainly limited to patients in which the cMRI study cannot be performed for safety reasons or due to artifacts related to rhythm abnormalities or ICD-chain. Recently, MDCT has been proposed in patients undergoing catheter ablation (CA) of VT to potentially identify the arrhythmogenic

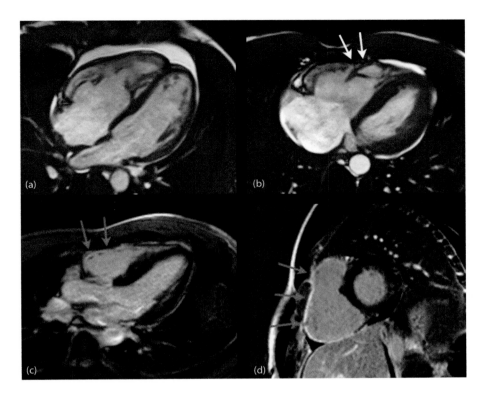

Figure 26.2 Cardiac MRI study of a 24 year-old man affected by arrhythmogenic right ventricular cardiomyopathy showing massive RV dilatation (panel A: four chamber view bright-blood SSFP MR image), RV free wall microaneurysms with the classical "*pile of dishes*" pattern (panel B: white arrows, axial view bright-blood SSFP MR image), and extensive delayed enhancement in the RV free wall (panels C and D: red arrows, contrast-enhanced inversion-recovery gradient-echo MR images).

substrate and guide the procedure. In this regard, a good correlation has been demonstrated between epicardial low-voltage areas on electro-anatomical mapping, presence of abnormal electrograms, and areas of hypodensity on contrast-enhanced MDCT consistent with fibro-fatty infiltration, in 16 patients with ARVC and VT undergoing CA.[43] Identification of intra-myocardial fat by MDCT has also recently been found highly sensitive in identifying LV involvement compared to standard Task Force Criteria.[44]

RISK STRATIFICATION AND ICD-THERAPY

Prevention of SCD is the most important issue in patients with ARVC, unfortunately most of the studies on risk stratification and ICD therapy are retrospective and frequently based on small, high-risk single center cohorts without systematic prospective evaluation of the proposed risk factors. The heterogeneity of the studied populations also explains the wide range of estimated annual risk of life-threatening VAs ranging from less than 0.5% to around 3% among studies.[45,46] In recent meta-analysis, the reported annualized appropriate ICD intervention rate was approximately 10%.[35] Due to these reasons, indications to ICD therapy are challenging especially in the setting of primary prevention.

History of aborted SCD and documented hemodynamically not tolerated sustained ventricular tachycardia (VT) have been demonstrated as the major risk factors for SCD making ICD therapy mandatory in this group of patients.[35] Other reported risk factors include: unexplained syncope, sustained VT without hemodynamic compromise, frequent non-sustained ventricular tachycardia (NSVT) at Holter recording, family history of SCD, extensive RV disease, late gadolinium enhancement (LGE) on cMRI, LV involvement, VT induction at programmed ventricular stimulation (PVS), QRS prolongation (QRS > 125 ms in right precordial leads), and QRS dispersion (>40 ms).[35,47-50] A predictive value of late potentials on signal averaged ECG (SAECG) has never been demonstrated.[51,52] Basing upon the published data, primary prevention ICD implantation should be considered in patients with unexplained syncope.[48] In the Darvin II study, the annual incidence of ICD appropriate therapies among patients with previous unexplained syncope was comparable with that observed in patient with history of cardiac arrest or SVT.[50] For patients that have not experienced syncope, the decision should balance the presence of risk factors like RV and/or LV dysfunction and well-tolerated sustained VT or NSVT on Holter monitoring that place the patient at intermediate risk with the risk of ICD-related complications and his impact on patient's lifestyle.[53] Table 26.2 summarizes indications to ICD implantation based upon currently recognized risk factors.

Even if there are no controlled trials demonstrating the beneficial effect of avoiding sport activity in patients with ARVC, it has been shown that endurance training can increase up to 5-fold the risk of SCD. The mechanism whereby physical training triggers VAs involves volume overload with myocyte stretching and sympathetic stimulation, moreover endurance training may accelerate the degenerative process with progression to RV/LV dysfunction.[6] For these reasons, avoidance of competitive sports is recommended in patients with ARVC.

The selection of a specific device (i.e., single chamber vs. dual chamber vs. subcutaneous ICD) should consider several elements. Endocardial ICD therapy is burdened by an intrinsic risk of lead-related complications reaching 3.7%/year in larger studies, including device-related infections, lead fracture, and loss of ventricular sensing/pacing functions due to myocardium loss with fibrofatty replacement.[35] For these reasons, subcutaneous ICD may be considered especially in young patients. In order to reduce the long-term risk of device-related complications even if its precise in this group of patients needs to be evaluated by larger studies.[54]

Table 26.2 Indications to ICD implantation basing upon patient's recognized risk factors

Life-threatening VAs risk	Risk factors	ICD indication
High	History of aborted SCD	Mandatory
	History of hemodynamically poorly tolerated VT	
	History of unexplained syncope	
Intermediate	History of hemodynamically well tolerated sustained VT	Should be considered
	RV and/or LV dysfunction	
	History of SCD in first-degree family members	
Low	One or more of the other recognized risk factors (QRS prolongation, QRS dispersion, LGE on cMRI, LV involvement, VT induction during PVS)	May be considered taking into account risk of complications and impact of ICD on lifestyle
Very low	Proband fulfilling Task Force Criteria for ARVC without any recognized risk factor	Unjustified

DRUG THERAPY

Most of the data regarding drug therapy in patients with ARVC come from retrospective single center cohorts, moreover the real impact of drug therapy on mortality remains unclear. For these reasons, there are no definite recommendations for medical therapy in asymptomatic patients without RV/LV dysfunction.

In with evidence of arrhythmias, beta-blockers are often used as first-line therapy. Class III antiarrhythmic agents like sotalol have been suggested to be effective in reducing the burden of ventricular arrhythmias in ARVC patients.[55] Amiodarone also has demonstrated to be effective in reducing arrhythmias and prevent ICD interventions but it is usually avoided as long-term therapy due to the high incidence of side effects.[55]

Patients presenting with heart failure should be treated with state-of-the-art heart failure medical regimens including beta-blockers, angiotensin-converting enzyme inhibitors/angiotensin-receptor blockers, and diuretic.

Oral anticoagulation should be taken in account in patients with severe RV/LV dysfunction and ventricular aneurysms well as in patients with supra-ventricular arrhythmias.

CATHETER ABLATION

Owing to the overall limited efficacy of AADs in controlling ventricular arrhythmias in ARVC, CA has been increasingly adopted as an important therapeutic strategy to manage recurrence ventricular arrhythmias in these patients.[56-58] Given the high prevalence of epicardial substrate in ARVC, CA should be performed only in experienced centers and should be considered in patients with frequent PVC/NSVT or recurrent sustained VT in order to avoid ICD shocks.[57,59,60]

As mentioned, due to the more extensive epicardial pathological substrate, endocardial only approaches has led in the past to less satisfactory results with a high VT recurrence rate during an extended follow-up.[29,60,61] Approaches using a combination of endocardial and epicardial ablation and guided by complete VT non-inducibility have shown to significantly improve the long-term VT-free survival with limited need for AADs, particularly amiodarone, in most of the patients.[57,62,63]

The current approach to CA in ARVC comprehends the abolition of all inducible VTs possibly excluding very fast (<250 ms cycle length) ventricular flutter with sine wave morphology, together with a proven comprehensive modification of both the endocardial and epicardial substrate.[56,62] Pre-procedural planning is mandatory and typically comprehend cMRI with LGE imaging in order to characterize the scar amount and location. More recently, contrast-enhanced MDCT has been demonstrated a valuable adjunction in pre-procedural planning.[43] In this setting, MDCT is used to accurately define the anatomy of cardiac chambers, surrounding structures (i.e., coronary vasculature, phrenic nerve), and to identify regions of wall thinning or intramyocardial fat infiltration while LGE-cMRI is used to characterize myocardial scar. The offline 3D reconstruction of the segmented MDCT and cMRI can then be merged with the EAM map by using anatomic landmarks. Overall, imaging-derived substrate has demonstrated to be able to identify up to 90% of abnormal EGMs.[43,64] Moreover, direct visualization of the coronary arteries and phrenic nerve allows to avoid damage during epicardial radiofrequency delivery.[64] This strategy has also demonstrated to reduce arrhythmia recurrence at long-term follow-up.[65]

In our center, the procedure is usually started with conscious sedation due to the possible impact of general anesthesia on VT inducibility. However, it is converted to general anesthesia for cases in which the epicardial approach is necessary. Epicardial procedures under deep sedation with midazolam and remifentanil have been described but we prefer general anesthesia due to a potential for less access-related complications (i.e., avoid patient movement and uncontrolled breathing) and better patient management in case of complications.[66] Whenever possible, antiarrhythmic drugs are stopped at least four half-lives before the procedure.

ENDOCARDIAL VOLTAGE MAPPING

Endocardial RV mapping is typically the first step. In the rarer cases of clinically significant LV involvement with VT arising from the LV (i.e., VT with RBBB morphology), LV mapping is also performed. A sinus or paced rhythm endocardial high-density voltage map of the RV is made with particular care of the perivalvular regions that is more typically involved by the disease. A cut-off of 1.5 and 5.5 mV (8.3 mV for the LV) are widely accepted for the definition of abnormal bipolar and unipolar voltage, respectively.[67,68] A wider extension of the abnormal unipolar voltage area than the abnormal bipolar one is common in ARVC and indicates a wider extension of the scar beyond the endocardium, which can either be midmyocardial or subepicardial.[69] All the areas with abnormal voltage are further evaluated for the presence of abnormal electrograms (i.e., fractionated, multicomponent, or late electrograms), which are carefully tagged.[70] Late or fractionated potentials are usually distributed in clusters within the abnormal voltage area but sometimes they can be found even in areas with higher average voltage beyond established cut-off values.[71]

EPICARDIAL MAPPING

Access to the pericardial space is commonly obtained using the percutaneous subxiphoid approach originally described by Sosa et al.[72] Two different subxiphoid approaches have been described depending on the orientation of the puncture and the resulting site of access:

- *Anterior approach*: The needle is directed superiorly with a shallow trajectory to enter the pericardial space anteriorly over the right ventricle.
- *Inferior access*: The needle is directed towards the left shoulder with a steeper trajectory, entering the pericardial space over the basal-inferior part of the ventricles.

Given the substantial dilatation of the RV and typically high intracavitary pressure in ARVC patients, we currently prefer a posterior approach in these cases to minimize the risk of inadvertent perforation of the thin anterior RV free wall with potential for severe bleeding.

Procedural complications associated with epicardial access have been reported in up to 30% of the cases with effusion/tamponade being the most frequent.[73] In this regard, the use of micropuncture needle has demonstrated to decrease the risk of major complications as well as the need for surgical repair in cases of inadvertent RV puncture.[74] Some complications like effusion, pericarditis, coronary vessels injury, and phrenic nerve injury are common to both approaches while there are some of them almost exclusively seen with a specific approach like injury of the left internal mammary artery with the anterior approach or liver damage, abdominal wall hematoma, and intraperitoneal bleeding with the inferior approach.[73,75]

After the epicardial access is obtained a sinus or paced rhythm epicardial high-density voltage map is performed. The reference value reported for defining abnormal electrograms in the epicardium is <1.0 mV.[62] To further limit the influence of epicardial fat and small-vessel coronary vasculature (i.e., vessels that cannot be directly appreciated by coronary angiogram) on the low-voltage region, the contiguous low-voltage electrograms need to demonstrate not only a low amplitude but also signals with discrete late potentials (recorded after the QRS of the surface ECG) and demonstrate broad multicomponent or split signals within the boundary of the defined contiguous low-voltage abnormality. Signals larger than 1.0 mV that also demonstrate abnormal, multicomponent, split, or late signal should also be tagged.

CATHETER ABLATION

As mentioned, the primary end point of the ablation approach performed in our institution is to eliminate all the mappable clinical and non-clinical VTs. For stable VTs, activation and entrainment mapping are performed at sites showing diastolic activity to identify critical sites of the VT re-entrant circuit.[76] For unstable VTs, a substrate modification approach is performed using established techniques. The site of origin of VT can be approximated using pace mapping to reproduce the VT QRS complex morphology and to identify sites with a long stimulus to QRS interval. These sites together with the adjacent abnormal substrate defined using the above-mentioned electrogram criteria are targeted for CA with the endpoint of local electrogram modification and VT non-inducibility. Other approaches for substrate ablation have been also described and tested in clinical studies.[57,77,78]

Bai et al. described a "scar homogenization" approach in ARVC with catheter ablation of all the abnormal potentials within the substrate without demonstration of critical participation to spontaneous or induced VTs.[63] More recently, Berruezo et al. evaluated the possibility of complete substrate ablation targeting only focal sites typically located at the border of the abnormal substrate that are the earliest breakthrough sites of electrical activation within the scar. This approach is known as "scar dechanneling" and has been suggested to achieve complete scar electrical silence with more focal ablation.[57]

Our approach includes linear and/or cluster lesions that are placed targeting previously identified critical sites by pace mapping, abnormal electrograms, or through channels transecting the abnormal myocardium and extending from the valve annulus to normal myocardium.[56,79] Radiofrequency energy is usually applied with an open irrigated tip catheter using powers up to 50 W with a goal of 12–15 Ω impedance drop or 10% decrease from the baseline impedance. Lesion duration is typically set for 60–90 s but further increases to ≥ 3 min in duration can be applied at sites associated with transient suppression of VT with monitoring to confirm stable impedance drop. Regarding epicardial ablation, coronary artery angiography should be performed before radiofrequency delivery to assess a safe distance of ablation sites from main epicardial coronary vessels. Moreover, sites of phrenic nerve capture during pacing should be marked to avoid the risk of permanent nerve injury during RF delivery. In this regard, in ARVC patients with severely dilated right ventricular outflow tracts, the left phrenic nerve can be adjacent and potentially injured with both endocardial and/or epicardial ablation and caution should be paid to delineate the course of the nerve with high output pacing before ablation (Figure 26.3).

After the procedure end, triamcinolone acetate is usually injected into the pericardial space to prevent post-procedure pericarditis and consequent adhesion formation.[80]

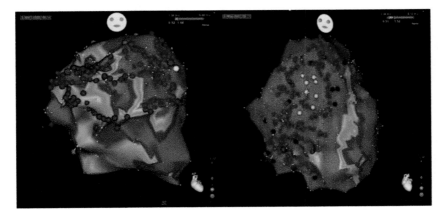

Figure 26.3 Example of endocardial (left) and epicardial (right) substrate ablation radiofrequency lesion set (red circles) in a patient with arrhythmogenic right ventricular cardiomyopathy. Extensive substrate ablation targeting both mappable and unmappable VT rendered VT non-inducible with programmed stimulation. (Reprinted from Santangeli, P. et al., *Circ. Arrhythm. Electrophysiol.*, 8, 1413–1421, 2015. With permission.)

ASSESSMENT OF ACUTE PROCEDURAL OUTCOMES

In our institution, the acute procedural success is assessed by programmed ventricular stimulation at the end of the procedure performed from at least two RV sites with at least two drive cycle lengths and defined as lack of inducibility of any VT with cycle length >250 ms. Non-invasive programmed stimulation is also performed through the ICD in the days following the ablation procedure in patients without spontaneous VT recurrence. A prior study from our group has reported an incremental value of non-invasive programmed stimulation in identifying patients at high risk of recurrence who may need more extensive ablation.[56,81]

LONG-TERM ABLATION OUTCOMES

Table 26.3 summarizes the main studies investigating the role of radiofrequency CA in ARVC. The initial experience with endocardial-only ablation approach failed to achieve an adequate long-term arrhythmia control with recurrence rates up to 70% within 3–5 years follow-up even if acute procedural success was achieved in most of cases.[29] Verma et al. showed a 3-year VT recurrence rate of 47% after endocardial-only ablation while Dalal et al. in their multicenter registry, reported a VT recurrence rate of 91% at 3 years.[60,61] Such unfavorable outcomes were explained by the progressive nature of the disease predisposing to the formation of new arrhythmogenic foci.[60] However, more recently, a progression of endocardial scar has been found only in the minority of patients undergoing serial voltage mapping despite progressive RV dilatation.[82] Moreover, it has been pointed out how most of the critical VT isthmuses in ARVC are located on the epicardial surface due to the propensity of the disease to originate and progress from the epicardium suggesting that an aggressive endo-epi substrate modification may be effective in long-term VT control.[62] Garcia et al. have reported the efficacy of epicardial ablation after previously failed endocardial approach. The authors confirmed a more extensive epicardial involvement in these patients and reported an acute success rate of 85% and a 77% VT-free survival at 18-months follow-up.[62] Similar results have been reported by Bai et al. in a multicenter series of patients undergoing endocardial-only versus endo-epicardial ablatio with a 52% and 85% VT-free survival at 3-years follow-up in the endo-only and endo-epi ablation group, respectively.[63] In the last few years, comprehensive ablation approaches including elimination of clinical VTs as well as endocardial substrate modification with various techniques (i.e., scar dechanneling) with adjuvant epicardial ablation in cases of recurrent VT or persistent inducibility after ENDO-only ablation, have shown to provide excellent long-term outcomes with a VT-free survival up to 75% at 5-years follow-up.[56,77]

Table 26.3 Principal studies investigating the role of catheter ablation in arrhythmogenic right ventricular cardiomyopathy

Study	No. of patients	Epicardial mapping/ ablation	Follow-up (months)	% VT recurrence
Marchlinski et al. (2004)[29]	19	No	27	11
Miljoen et al. (2005)[83]	11	No	20	45
Verma et al. (2005)[61]	22	No	36	47
Satomi et al. (2006)[84]	17	No	26	24
Yao et al. (2007)[85]	32	No	29	19
Dalal et al. (2007)[60]	24	No	32	91
Nogami et al. (2008)[86]	18	No	61	33
Garcia et al. (2009)[62]	13	Yes	18	23
Bai et al. (2011)[63]	49	Yes	40	31
Berruezo et al. (2012)[57]	11	Yes	11	9
Philips et al. (2012)[59]	87	Yes	88	85
Mussigbrodt et al. (2015)[87]	28	Yes	19	47
Santangeli et al. (2015)[56]	62	Yes	56	29

REFERENCES

1. Basso C, Corrado D, Bauce B, Thiene G. Arrhythmogenic right ventricular cardiomyopathy. *Circ Arrhythm Electrophysiol.* 2012;5:1233–1246.

2. Fontaine G, Guiraudon G, Frank R, et al. Arrhythmogenic right ventricular dysplasia and Uhl's disease. *Arch Mal Coeur Vaiss.* 1982;75:361–371.

3. Norman MW, McKenna WJ. Arrhythmogenic right ventricular cardiomyopathy: Perspectives on disease. *Z Für Kardiologie.* 1999;88:550–554.

4. Millar L, Sharma S. Diagnosis and management of inherited cardiomyopathies. *The Practitioner.* 2014;258:21–25, 2–3.

5. Nava A, Thiene G, Canciani B, et al. Familial occurrence of right ventricular dysplasia: A study involving nine families. *J Am Coll Cardiol.* 1988;12:1222–1228.

6. Corrado D, Basso C, Rizzoli G, et al. Does sports activity enhance the risk of sudden death in adolescents and young adults? *J Am Coll Cardiol.* 2003;42:1959–1963.

7. Lopez-Ayala JM, Oliva-Sandoval MJ, Sanchez-Muñoz JJ, Gimeno JR. Arrhythmogenic right ventricular cardiomyopathy. *Lancet Lond Engl.* 2015;385:662.

8. Corrado D, Thiene G, Nava A, et al. Sudden death in young competitive athletes: Clinicopathologic correlations in 22 cases. *Am J Med.* 1990;89(5):588–596.

9. Cox MGPJ, van der Zwaag PA, van der Werf C, et al. Arrhythmogenic right ventricular dysplasia/cardiomyopathy: Pathogenic desmosome mutations in index-patients predict outcome of family screening: Dutch arrhythmogenic right ventricular dysplasia/cardiomyopathy genotype-phenotype follow-up study. *Circulation.* 2011;123:2690–2700.

10. McKoy G, Protonotarios N, Crosby A, et al. Identification of a deletion in plakoglobin in arrhythmogenic right ventricular cardiomyopathy with palmoplantar keratoderma and woolly hair (Naxos disease). *Lancet Lond Engl.* 2000;355:2119–2124.

11. Coonar AS, Protonotarios N, Tsatsopoulou A, et al. Gene for arrhythmogenic right ventricular cardiomyopathy with diffuse nonepidermolytic palmoplantar keratoderma and woolly hair (Naxos disease) maps to 17q21. *Circulation.* 1998;97:2049–2058.

12. Norgett EE, Hatsell SJ, Carvajal-Huerta L, et al. Recessive mutation in desmoplakin disrupts desmoplakin-intermediate filament interactions and causes dilated cardiomyopathy, woolly hair and keratoderma. *Hum Mol Genet.* 2000;9:2761–2766.

13. Gerull B, Heuser A, Wichter T, et al. Mutations in the desmosomal protein plakophilin-2 are common in arrhythmogenic right ventricular cardiomyopathy. *Nat Genet.* 2004;36:1162–1164.

14. Pilichou K, Nava A, Basso C, et al. Mutations in desmoglein-2 gene are associated with arrhythmogenic right ventricular cardiomyopathy. *Circulation.* 2006;113:1171–1179.

15. Syrris P, Ward D, Evans A, et al. Arrhythmogenic right ventricular dysplasia/cardiomyopathy associated with mutations in the desmosomal gene desmocollin-2. *Am J Hum Genet.* 2006;79:978–984.

16. Tiso N, Stephan DA, Nava A, et al. Identification of mutations in the cardiac ryanodine receptor gene in families affected with arrhythmogenic right ventricular cardiomyopathy type 2 (ARVD2). *Hum Mol Genet.* 2001;10:189–194.

17. Beffagna G, Occhi G, Nava A, et al. Regulatory mutations in transforming growth factor-beta3 gene cause arrhythmogenic right ventricular cardiomyopathy type 1. *Cardiovasc Res.* 2005;65:366–373.

18. Taylor M, Graw S, Sinagra G, et al. Genetic variation in titin in arrhythmogenic right ventricular cardiomyopathy-overlap syndromes. *Circulation.* 2011;124:876–885.

19. Quarta G, Syrris P, Ashworth M, et al. Mutations in the Lamin A/C gene mimic arrhythmogenic right ventricular cardiomyopathy. *Eur Heart J*. 2012;33:1128–1136.

20. van der Zwaag PA, van Rijsingen IAW, Asimaki A, et al. Phospholamban R14del mutation in patients diagnosed with dilated cardiomyopathy or arrhythmogenic right ventricular cardiomyopathy: Evidence supporting the concept of arrhythmogenic cardiomyopathy. *Eur J Heart Fail*. 2012;14:1199–1207.

21. Kapplinger JD, Landstrom AP, Salisbury BA, et al. Distinguishing arrhythmogenic right ventricular cardiomyopathy/dysplasia-associated mutations from background genetic noise. *J Am Coll Cardiol*. 2011;57:2317–2327.

22. Bauce B, Nava A, Beffagna G, et al. Multiple mutations in desmosomal proteins encoding genes in arrhythmogenic right ventricular cardiomyopathy/dysplasia. *Heart Rhythm Off J Heart Rhythm Soc*. 2010;7:22–29.

23. Xu T, Yang Z, Vatta M, et al. Multidisciplinary study of right ventricular dysplasia investigators. Compound and digenic heterozygosity contributes to arrhythmogenic right ventricular cardiomyopathy. *J Am Coll Cardiol*. 2010;55:587–597.

24. Protonotarios N, Anastasakis A, Antoniades L, et al. Arrhythmogenic right ventricular cardiomyopathy/dysplasia on the basis of the revised diagnostic criteria in affected families with desmosomal mutations. *Eur Heart J*. 2011;32:1097–1104.

25. Basso C, Thiene G, Corrado D, et al. Arrhythmogenic right ventricular cardiomyopathy. Dysplasia, dystrophy, or myocarditis? *Circulation*. 1996;94:983–991.

26. Thiene G, Corrado D, Nava A, et al. Right ventricular cardiomyopathy: Is there evidence of an inflammatory aetiology? *Eur Heart J*. 1991;12(Suppl D):22–25.

27. Mallat Z, Tedgui A, Fontaliran F, et al. Evidence of apoptosis in arrhythmogenic right ventricular dysplasia. *N Engl J Med*. 1996;335:1190–1196.

28. Corrado D, Basso C, Thiene G, et al. Spectrum of clinicopathologic manifestations of arrhythmogenic right ventricular cardiomyopathy/dysplasia: A multicenter study. *J Am Coll Cardiol*. 1997;30:1512–1520.

29. Marchlinski FE. Electroanatomic substrate and outcome of catheter ablative therapy for ventricular tachycardia in setting of right ventricular cardiomyopathy. *Circulation*. 2004;110:2293–2298.

30. Sen-Chowdhry S, Syrris P, Prasad SK, et al. Left-dominant arrhythmogenic cardiomyopathy: An under-recognized clinical entity. *J Am Coll Cardiol*. 2008;52:2175–2187.

31. Sen-Chowdhry S, Syrris P, Ward D, et al. Clinical and genetic characterization of families with arrhythmogenic right ventricular dysplasia/cardiomyopathy provides novel insights into patterns of disease expression. *Circulation*. 2007;115:1710–1720.

32. Nucifora G, Muser D, Masci PG, et al. Prevalence and prognostic value of concealed structural abnormalities in patients with apparently idiopathic ventricular arrhythmias of left versus right ventricular origin: A magnetic resonance imaging study. *Circ Arrhythm Electrophysiol*. 2014;7:456–462.

33. Marcus FI, McKenna WJ, Sherrill D, et al. Diagnosis of arrhythmogenic right ventricular cardiomyopathy/dysplasia: Proposed modification of the task force criteria. *Circulation*. 2010;121:1533–1541.

34. Hulot J-S, Jouven X, Empana J-P, et al. Natural history and risk stratification of arrhythmogenic right ventricular dysplasia/cardiomyopathy. *Circulation*. 2004;110:1879–1884.

35. Schinkel AFL. Implantable cardioverter defibrillators in arrhythmogenic right ventricular dysplasia/cardiomyopathy: Patient outcomes, incidence of appropriate and inappropriate interventions, and complications. *Circ Arrhythm Electrophysiol*. 2013;6:562–568.

36. McKenna WJ, Thiene G, Nava A, et al. Diagnosis of arrhythmogenic right ventricular dysplasia/cardiomyopathy. Task Force of the Working Group Myocardial and Pericardial Disease of the European Society of Cardiology and of the Scientific Council on Cardiomyopathies of the International Society and Federation of Cardiology. *Br Heart J.* 1994;71:215–218.

37. Nasir K, Bomma C, Tandri H, et al. Electrocardiographic features of arrhythmogenic right ventricular dysplasia/cardiomyopathy according to disease severity: A need to broaden diagnostic criteria. *Circulation.* 2004;110:1527–1534.

38. Marcus FI, Zareba W, Sherrill D. Evaluation of the normal values for signal-averaged electrocardiogram. *J Cardiovasc Electrophysiol.* 2007;18:231–233.

39. Nasir K, Rutberg J, Tandri H, et al. Utility of SAECG in arrhythmogenic right ventricle dysplasia. *Ann Noninvasive Electrocardiol.* 2003;8:112–120.

40. Komatsu Y, Cochet H, Jadidi A, et al. Regional myocardial wall thinning at multidetector computed tomography correlates to arrhythmogenic substrate in postinfarction ventricular tachycardia: Assessment of structural and electrical substrate. *Circ Arrhythm Electrophysiol.* 2013;6:342–350.

41. Doğan H, Kroft LJM, Bax JJ, et al. MDCT assessment of right ventricular systolic function. *AJR Am J Roentgenol.* 2006;186:S366–S370.

42. Raman SV, Cook SC, McCarthy B, Ferketich AK. Usefulness of multidetector row computed tomography to quantify right ventricular size and function in adults with either tetralogy of Fallot or transposition of the great arteries. *Am J Cardiol.* 2005;95:683–686.

43. Komatsu Y, Jadidi A, Sacher F, et al. Relationship between MDCT-imaged myocardial fat and ventricular tachycardia substrate in arrhythmogenic right ventricular cardiomyopathy. *J Am Heart Assoc.* 2014;3(4):e000935.

44. Berte B, Denis A, Amraoui S, et al. Characterization of the left-sided substrate in arrhythmogenic right ventricular cardiomyopathy. *Circ Arrhythm Electrophysiol.* 2015;8:1403–1412.

45. Nava A, Bauce B, Basso C, et al. Clinical profile and long-term follow-up of 37 families with arrhythmogenic right ventricular cardiomyopathy. *J Am Coll Cardiol.* 2000;36:2226–2233.

46. Lemola K, Brunckhorst C, Helfenstein U, et al. Predictors of adverse outcome in patients with arrhythmogenic right ventricular dysplasia/cardiomyopathy: Long term experience of a tertiary care centre. *Heart Br Card Soc.* 2005;91:1167–1172.

47. Roguin A, Bomma CS, Nasir K, et al. Implantable cardioverter-defibrillators in patients with arrhythmogenic right ventricular dysplasia/cardiomyopathy. *J Am Coll Cardiol.* 2004;43:1843–1852.

48. Bhonsale A, James CA, Tichnell C, et al. Incidence and predictors of implantable cardioverter-defibrillator therapy in patients with arrhythmogenic right ventricular dysplasia/cardiomyopathy undergoing implantable cardioverter-defibrillator implantation for primary prevention. *J Am Coll Cardiol.* 2011;58:1485–1496.

49. Corrado D, Leoni L, Link MS, et al. Implantable cardioverter-defibrillator therapy for prevention of sudden death in patients with arrhythmogenic right ventricular cardiomyopathy/dysplasia. *Circulation.* 2003;108:3084–3091.

50. Corrado D, Calkins H, Link MS, et al. Prophylactic implantable defibrillator in patients with arrhythmogenic right ventricular cardiomyopathy/dysplasia and no prior ventricular fibrillation or sustained ventricular tachycardia. *Circulation.* 2010;122:1144–1152.

51. Blomström-Lundqvist C, Olsson SB, Edvardsson N. Follow-up by repeated signal-averaged surface QRS in patients with the syndrome of arrhythmogenic right ventricular dysplasia. *Eur Heart J.* 1989;10(Suppl D):54–60.

52. Leclercq JF, Coumel P. Late potentials in arrhythmogenic right ventricular dysplasia. Prevalence, diagnostic and prognostic values. *Eur Heart J.* 1993;14(Suppl E):80–83.

53. Authors/Task Force Members, Priori SG, Blomström-Lundqvist C, et al. 2015 ESC Guidelines for the management of patients with ventricular arrhythmias and the prevention of sudden cardiac death: The Task Force for the Management of Patients with Ventricular Arrhythmias and the Prevention of Sudden Cardiac Death of the European Society of Cardiology (ESC)Endorsed by: Association for European Paediatric and Congenital Cardiology (AEPC). *Eur Heart J.* 2015;17:1601–1687.

54. Corrado D, Wichter T, Link MS, et al. Treatment of arrhythmogenic right ventricular cardiomyopathy/dysplasia. *Circulation.* 2015;132:441–453.

55. Wichter T, Borggrefe M, Haverkamp W, et al. Efficacy of antiarrhythmic drugs in patients with arrhythmogenic right ventricular disease. Results in patients with inducible and noninducible ventricular tachycardia. *Circulation.* 1992;86:29–37.

56. Santangeli P, Zado ES, Supple GE, et al. Long-term outcome with catheter ablation of ventricular tachycardia in patients with arrhythmogenic right ventricular cardiomyopathy. *Circ Arrhythm Electrophysiol.* 2015;8:1413–1421.

57. Berruezo A, Fernández-Armenta J, Mont L, et al. Combined endocardial and epicardial catheter ablation in arrhythmogenic right ventricular dysplasia incorporating scar dechanneling technique. *Circ Arrhythm Electrophysiol.* 2012;5:111–121.

58. Marcus GM, Glidden DV, Polonsky B, et al. Efficacy of antiarrhythmic drugs in arrhythmogenic right ventricular cardiomyopathy: A report from the North American ARVC registry. *J Am Coll Cardiol.* 2009;54:609–615.

59. Philips B, Madhavan S, James C, et al. Outcomes of catheter ablation of ventricular tachycardia in arrhythmogenic right ventricular dysplasia/cardiomyopathy. *Circ Arrhythm Electrophysiol.* 2012;5:499–505.

60. Dalal D, Jain R, Tandri H, et al. Long-term efficacy of catheter ablation of ventricular tachycardia in patients with arrhythmogenic right ventricular dysplasia/cardiomyopathy. *J Am Coll Cardiol.* 2007;50:432–440.

61. Verma A, Kilicaslan F, Schweikert RA, et al. Short- and long-term success of substrate-based mapping and ablation of ventricular tachycardia in arrhythmogenic right ventricular dysplasia. *Circulation.* 2005;111:3209–3216.

62. Garcia FC, Bazan V, Zado ES, et al. Epicardial substrate and outcome with epicardial ablation of ventricular tachycardia in arrhythmogenic right ventricular cardiomyopathy/dysplasia. *Circulation.* 2009;120:366–375.

63. Bai R, Di Biase L, Shivkumar K, et al. Ablation of ventricular arrhythmias in arrhythmogenic right ventricular dysplasia/cardiomyopathy: Arrhythmia-free survival after endo-epicardial substrate based mapping and ablation. *Circ Arrhythm Electrophysiol.* 2011;4:478–485.

64. Yamashita S, Sacher F, Mahida S, et al. Image integration to guide catheter ablation in scar-related ventricular tachycardia. *J Cardiovasc Electrophysiol.* 2016;27(6):699–708.

65. Yamashita S, Cochet H, Sacher F, et al. Impact of new technologies and approaches for post–myocardial infarction ventricular tachycardia ablation during long-term follow-up. *Circ Arrhythm Electrophysiol.* 2016;9:e003901.

66. Mandel JE, Hutchinson MD, Marchlinski FE. Remifentanil-midazolam sedation provides hemodynamic stability and comfort during epicardial ablation of ventricular tachycardia. *J Cardiovasc Electrophysiol.* 2011;22:464–466.

67. Campos B, Jauregui ME, Park K-M, et al. New unipolar electrogram criteria to identify irreversibility of nonischemic left ventricular cardiomyopathy. *J Am Coll Cardiol.* 2012;60:2194–2204.

68. Hutchinson MD, Gerstenfeld EP, Desjardins B, et al. Endocardial unipolar voltage mapping to detect epicardial ventricular tachycardia substrate in patients with nonischemic left ventricular cardiomyopathy. *Circ Arrhythm Electrophysiol.* 2011;4:49–55.

69. Polin GM, Haqqani H, Tzou W, et al. Endocardial unipolar voltage mapping to identify epicardial substrate in arrhythmogenic right ventricular cardiomyopathy/dysplasia. *Heart Rhythm Off J Heart Rhythm Soc.* 2011;8:76–83.

70. de Bakker JM, van Capelle FJ, Janse MJ, et al. Fractionated electrograms in dilated cardiomyopathy: Origin and relation to abnormal conduction. *J Am Coll Cardiol.* 1996;27:1071–1078.

71. Berte B, Sacher F, Cochet H, et al. Postmyocarditis ventricular tachycardia in patients with epicardial-only scar: A specific entity requiring a specific approach: Epicardial-only VT ablation. *J Cardiovasc Electrophysiol.* 2015;26:42–50.

72. Sosa E, Scanavacca M, d'Avila A, Pilleggi F. A new technique to perform epicardial mapping in the electrophysiology laboratory. *J Cardiovasc Electrophysiol.* 1996;7:531–536.

73. Killu AM, Sugrue A, Munger TM, et al. Impact of sedation vs. general anaesthesia on percutaneous epicardial access safety and procedural outcomes. *Eur Pacing Arrhythm Card Electrophysiol J Work Groups Card Pacing Arrhythm Card Cell Electrophysiol Eur Soc Cardiol.* 2018;20:329–336.

74. Gunda S, Reddy M, Pillarisetti J, et al. Differences in complication rates between large bore needle and a long micropuncture needle during epicardial access: Time to change clinical practice? *Circ Arrhythm Electrophysiol.* 2015;8:890–895.

75. Killu AM, Friedman PA, Mulpuru SK, et al. Atypical complications encountered with epicardial electrophysiological procedures. *Heart Rhythm.* 2013;10:1613–1621.

76. Hsia HH, Lin D, Sauer WH, et al. Relationship of late potentials to the ventricular tachycardia circuit defined by entrainment. *J Interv Card Electrophysiol Int J Arrhythm Pacing.* 2009;26:21–29.

77. Arenal A, del Castillo S, Gonzalez-Torrecilla E, et al. Tachycardia-related channel in the scar tissue in patients with sustained monomorphic ventricular tachycardias influence of the voltage scar definition. *Circulation.* 2004;110:2568–2574.

78. Hsia HH, Lin D, Sauer WH, et al. Anatomic characterization of endocardial substrate for hemodynamically stable reentrant ventricular tachycardia: Identification of endocardial conducting channels. *Heart Rhythm.* 2006;3:503–512.

79. Marchlinski FE, Callans DJ, Gottlieb CD, Zado E. Linear ablation lesions for control of unmappable ventricular tachycardia in patients with ischemic and nonischemic cardiomyopathy. *Circulation.* 2000;101:1288–1296.

80. d'Avila A, Neuzil P, Thiagalingam A, et al. Experimental efficacy of pericardial instillation of anti-inflammatory agents during percutaneous epicardial catheter ablation to prevent postprocedure pericarditis. *J Cardiovasc Electrophysiol.* 2007;18:1178–1183.

81. Frankel DS, Mountantonakis SE, Zado ES, et al. Noninvasive programmed ventricular stimulation early after ventricular tachycardia ablation to predict risk of late recurrence. *J Am Coll Cardiol.* 2012;59:1529–1535.

82. Riley MP, Zado E, Bala R, et al. Lack of uniform progression of endocardial scar in patients with arrhythmogenic right ventricular dysplasia/cardiomyopathy and ventricular tachycardia clinical perspective. *Circ Arrhythm Electrophysiol.* 2010;3:332–338.

83. Miljoen H, State S, de Chillou C, et al. Electroanatomic mapping characteristics of ventricular tachycardia in patients with arrhythmogenic right ventricular cardiomyopathy/dysplasia. *Europace*. 2005;7:516–524.

84. Satomi K, Kurita T, Suyama K, et al. Catheter ablation of stable and unstable ventricular tachycardias in patients with arrhythmogenic right ventricular dysplasia. *J Cardiovasc Electrophysiol*. 2006;17:469–476.

85. Yao Y, Zhang S, He DS, et al. Radiofrequency ablation of the ventricular tachycardia with arrhythmogenic right ventricular cardiomyopathy using non-contact mapping. *Pacing Clin Electrophysiol PACE*. 2007;30:526–533.

86. Nogami A, Sugiyasu A, Tada H, et al. Changes in the isolated delayed component as an endpoint of catheter ablation in arrhythmogenic right ventricular cardiomyopathy: Predictor for long-term success. *J Cardiovasc Electrophysiol*. 2008;19:681–688.

87. Müssigbrodt A, Dinov B, Bertagnoli L, et al. Precordial QRS amplitude ratio predicts long-term outcome after catheter ablation of electrical storm due to ventricular tachycardias in patients with arrhythmogenic right ventricular cardiomyopathy. *J Electrocardiol*. 2015;48:86–92.

NON-ISCHEMIC CARDIOMYOPATHY AND VENTRICULAR ARRHYTHMIAS

Matthew C. Hyman and Gregory E. Supple

CONTENTS

INTRODUCTION

Non-ischemic cardiomyopathy (NICM) is a broad term used to describe a subset of cardiomyopathies characterized by inappropriate ventricular hypertrophy or dilatation in the absence of coronary artery disease.[1] NICM is common comprising 30%–40% of all cardiomyopathy patients.[2] In contrast to ischemic cardiomyopathy, which is mediated by coronary artery disease, non-ischemic myopathies encompass a number of different pathogenic mechanisms that lead to myocardial scarring and fibrosis. This scarring and fibrosis is an essential component of structural heart disease mediated arrhythmias as the resulting admixture of fibrosis and myocytes allows for areas of slow conduction and arrhythmogenic circuits.[3]

Patients with NICM are at an elevated risk of ventricular arrhythmias. This risk of ventricular arrhythmias increases with declining left ventricular function, although ventricular arrhythmias can be present in any heart. Several landmark studies have demonstrated that the risk of arrhythmia-mediated sudden cardiac death is sufficiently elevated in patients with an LVEF below 35% to warrant prophylactic implantable cardioverter-defibrillator (ICD) therapy,[4,5] however the recent Danish Study to Assess the Efficacy of ICDs in Patients with Non-ischemic Systolic Heart Failure on Mortality trial has shown there are many factors that need to be weighed.[6] Many patients with NICM who would have suffered from sudden cardiac death are now presenting for management of their ventricular arrhythmias. For these patients with structural heart disease and demonstrated ventricular arrhythmias, some intervention must be made or up to one-third of patients will present with recurrent ICD therapy.[7]

In the NICM population, ventricular arrhythmias can be managed pharmacologically with anti-arrhythmic medications or through invasive procedures like catheter ablation. For years, anti-arrhythmic drugs were the mainstay of ventricular arrhythmia management though this enthusiasm was always tempered by the associated morbidity of anti-arrhythmic drug therapy.[8] More recently, catheter-based ablation technologies have improved increasing the likelihood of curative therapy with invasive procedures. This has resulted in a shift in clinical practice with a more than three-fold increase in the incidence of ventricular arrhythmia ablation over the last decade.[9] In patients with ischemic cardiomyopathy, randomized-controlled trials have clearly demonstrated that catheter-based ablation leads to a reduction in ICD therapies and longer ventricular arrhythmia free survival when compared to anti-arrhythmic drugs alone.[10,11] In the NICM population, the evidence supporting catheter ablation over anti-arrhythmic drug therapy is less robust. This is further compounded by the fact that the ablation of NICM can be difficult as the arrhythmogenic substrate, electrocardiographic localization, and techniques for ablation differ from other forms of ventricular arrhythmia ablation. Despite those caveats, non-randomized cohorts have shown that catheter ablation leads to a reduction in ventricular tachycardia events in patients who have arrhythmias refractory to anti-arrhythmic medications.[12,13] Further, those patients who undergo ablative therapy are often successfully weaned from anti-arrhythmic medications.[12]

IDENTIFICATION OF ARRHYTHMIC SUBSTRATE IN NON-ISCHEMIC CARDIOMYOPATHY

The scarring and fibrosis of NICMs is distinct from coronary artery disease-mediated scar. While ischemic scar is usually well circumscribed and confined to a vascular territory, non-ischemic scar is often irregular and can cross vascular territories. Within the myocardial wall, ischemic scar localizes to the sub-endocardium. The sub-endocardial predominance of ischemic scar drove the development of VT therapies like surgical sub-endocardial resection and ultimately endocardial catheter-based therapies.[14] By way of contrast, non-ischemic myopathies often involve the mid-myocardial wall and epicardium in a patchy fashion characterized by layers of fibrosis and disordered myocytes.[15,16] While catheter-based therapies for NICM have modeled the same ablation strategies used in ischemic scar, the inherent anatomic differences of non-ischemic myopathies present unique procedural challenges. Substrate identification and subsequent elimination are more challenging when the scar extends (or exists entirely) beyond the sub-endocardium. This is particularly true of traditional endocardial catheter ablation which may not effectively penetrate to the deeper non-ischemic substrate.

One of the first steps in the identification of substrate in a patient with NICM is examination of the surface electrocardiogram. The patient's electrocardiogram can provide information that is useful in identifying or corroborating scar observed in cardiac imaging. Precordial loss of voltage-delayed precordial transitions, late fractionation in QRS complexes all can suggest and localize to areas of underlying myopathic substrate. For this reason, it is important to capture a native conduction ECG in all patients. If a patient is ventricular-paced at baseline with intact conduction, pacing should be inhibited during the pre-procedural planning phase of each patient's evaluation. By examining native conduction in a patient who is otherwise paced, one may "unmask" underlying substrate. While the surface ECG does provide important clues for regionalization of gross myocardial abnormality, its ability to localize to the sub-endocardium, mid-myocardium, or epicardium is more limited.

After the electrocardiogram, cardiac imaging plays a critical role in understanding the layers of myopathic substrate when managing ventricular arrhythmias.[3] Echocardiography can identify scar by demonstrating wall motion abnormalities, thinning, or hyperechoic mid-myocardial scar. Cardiac magnetic resonance imaging (MRI) is often complimentary as myocardial-delayed enhancement following gadolinium injection can be used to visualize areas of scar whether they reside in the endocardium, mid-myocardium, or epicardium.[17,18]

MRI is particularly useful as scars in the mid-myocardium and epicardium may not be appreciable with traditional echocardiography. The presence of myocardial-delayed enhancement on cardiac MRI may be particularly important as it has been associated with elevated risk of sudden cardiac death. Unfortunately, no study to date has been able to clearly define a threshold or scar volume above which a patient's risk of ventricular arrhythmias becomes reliably increased.[18]

When performing cardiac MRIs on patients with implantable cardiac devices, one must consider that such studies historically have been considered "off-label" by the United States Food and Drug Administration.[19] Recent observational cohorts, however, have demonstrated that this practice can be safe and effective and is increasingly being incorporated into routine practice.[20,21]

It is important to recognize that an absence of an appreciable scar on echocardiography or cardiac MRI does not guarantee an absence of scar within a patient's heart. Voltage abnormalities and other signs of myocardial dysfunction during electro-anatomic mapping (EAM) are frequently seen in myopathic patients that lack overt scar with traditional forms of imaging. The resolution of electro-anatomic mapping is currently on the order of tenths of a millimeter and therefore provides a much higher degree of resolution and consequently ability to detect areas of abnormality than more traditional forms of cardiac imaging, however it does rely on detailed mapping with a high density of points sampled in the region of interest to be most effective.[22]

MID-MYOCARDIAL VENTRICULAR ARRHYTHMIAS

Though identification of mid-myocardial scar is challenging, the recognition of this substrate can be critical to the success of a ventricular arrhythmia ablation. Pre-procedural imaging is most useful when scar is observed, but these studies may not always be available and technical limitations may not allow for accurate detection of a scar. Intra-procedure, electro-anatomic endocardial mapping may be used, but the small bipoles used in catheter-based mapping are most sensitive to near-field signals. When the signals of interest are far-field and deeper within the myocardium, a layer of healthy endocardium between that same catheter and a mid-myocardial scar may shield a catheter with a narrow bipole from detecting underlying abnormal and fractionated electrograms. To circumvent the limitations of small bipole spacing, unipolar electrograms (the catheter tip with reference to Wilson's central terminal) have been used to detect areas of deeper scar and myocardial abnormality.[23,24] There are consistent ranges for healthy unipolar and bipolar voltages allowing for the detection of electrical abnormality and scar outside of those ranges.[16,23,25]

Trans-septal conduction time can be used as a specific marker of mid-myocardial septal substrate. The concept of this assessment is that non-ischemic scar tends to be arranged in a layered fashion, which can delay trans-septal conduction and even result in compartmentalization between the left and right ventricles. By pacing from the right ventricular septum and measuring the transit time to another catheter placed along the left ventricular septum, one can get a surrogate evaluation of mid-septal substrate.[26] In one study, mid-myocardial substrate was associated with trans-septal activation times in excess of 40 ms (sensitivity 60%, specificity 100%; $p < 0.001$) and paced local electrocardiogram duration greater than 95 ms (sensitivity 22%, specificity 91%; $p < 0.001$) (Figure 27.1).[26]

While identification of septal substrate can be challenging, ablation of that substrate can be even more difficult. For mid-myocardial ablative therapy, many clinicians have employed long endocardial lesions (usually at lower power but 2–3 times longer than for a ventricular endocardium ablation) with the goal of achieving deeper lesion penetration by allowing

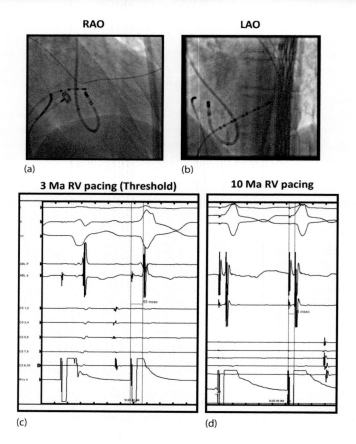

Figure 27.1 Trans-septal conduction: A right ventricular catheter is placed in a basal position and an ablator is placed opposite to it along the left ventricular septum as shown in the RAO (a) and LAO (b) fluoroscopic images. A coronary sinus catheter is present for reference. At threshold pacing, there is an 80 ms delay in conduction across the ventricular septum (c). Note that at higher output, conduction is normal as the mid-myocardial scar is "jumped" by higher pacing outputs (d).

for greater conductive tissue heating.[27] Other techniques for achieving deeper lesion penetration are sequential unipolar ablation (sandwiching the target substrate), simultaneous unipolar ablation (theoretically minimizing conductive cooling from the surface opposite the ablation catheter), and finally bipolar ablation (directing the energy across the target myocardium).[28,29] Others have tried altering the solute mix of the catheter irrigant to optimize current delivery (and thereby resistive heating) to the target tissues.[29] By changing the catheter's irrigant bath, it is possible to achieve larger unipolar ablation lesions (almost twice as large a normal) that are comparable to a bipolar lesion.[29] Beyond changing the lesion duration and irrigant bath, some have attempted to change the site of energy delivery by using a needle-tipped catheter. Energy delivery at the tip of a needle may start the ablative lesion formation below the endocardium closer to the underlying substrate.[30] While each of the aforementioned approaches can create deeper and larger volume lesions, it is worth noting that any technical manipulation that is made to increase energy delivery to the tissue may result in an elevated risk of steam popping. A final, non-catheter based approach to the ablation of non-ischemic tissue is ethanol injection. Both the coronary artery system and the coronary venous system may be used to inject ethanol into the septal myocardium via septal perforators to cause a local infarction.[31] Given the possibility of collateral tissue damage, it is recommended to attempt cold saline injection prior to an irreversible ethanol injection. Cold saline can temporarily render the myocardium electrically in-excitable and thereby provide evidence that targeting the septal perforator will result in termination of the clinical arrhythmia.[32] Balloon occlusion proximal to the venous injection site is also likely needed to better deliver the ethanol to the targeted tissue.

EPICARDIAL VENTRICULAR ARRHYTHMIAS

The epicardium is a common site for arrhythmogenic substrate in non-ischemic cardiomyopathies.[33] When planning an ablative procedure, epicardial substrate may be observed on pre-procedural imaging. This does not mean that the epicardium is the arrhythmic source, however, and the ECG of the clinical arrhythmia must be examined to find additional localization clues. A "Q" wave in lead I is among the most sensitive and specific markers of an epicardial exit (88% for both).[34] Other markers suggestive of an epicardial VT are a "QS" pattern in the inferior leads (although this may also be seen in ischemic patients with inferior MI who should also have inferior Q-waves in their sinus ECG, Figure 27.2), a slurred initial upstroke of the QRS $\geq$ 75 ms and a maximum deflection index ≥ 0.59.[34,35] Even if these ECG criteria are not present, an epicardial focus may be considered when there are no endocardial mid-diastolic or pre-QRS potentials that might explain a re-entrant or automatic ventricular arrhythmia. In these instances, unipolar electrograms can be examined to help identify the possibility of epicardial scar.[23,24] It is worth noting that not all of the epicardium can be mapped as there is a significant amount of peri-valvular and peri-coronary artery fat. This fat can act as an insulator and thereby artificially shielding myocardial electrograms and potentially mimicking scar.[36] This fat is particularly problematic when the critical machinery for the epicardial VT lies under the fat as is often the case in the LV summit. Such VTs are termed "inaccessible" and accordingly have very low rates of arrhythmia termination with epicardial ablation. Success in this site is only seen when a Q-wave ratio of >1.85 in aVL/aVR, a R/S ratio of >2 in V1, and there is no "Q" wave seen in V1; all features that suggest greater distance from the coronary arteries and epicardial fat.[37]

Epicardial access, mapping, and ablation carry an elevated level of risk when compared to traditional endocardial ablation.[38] The coronary arteries are flanked by epicardial fat, but direct ablation on these vessels can result in both spasm and thrombotic occlusion. Care must be taken prior to epicardial ablation to determine the location of the epicardial coronary vasculature to ensure the catheter is a safe distance from nearby arteries. Repeated angiography may be required during a procedure to minimize injury, particularly in cases when ablation is being performed near a coronary arterial branch.

The phrenic nerve also runs along the surface of the heart, though it may be less protected by fat than the coronary vasculature. When ablating along the lateral epicardium, it is recommended to pace at maximum output to "map" the course of the phrenic nerve while noting these sites on the electro-anatomic map. Sites of capture may be too close to the phrenic nerve and therefore at risk of thermal injury from catheter ablation. In such cases where the VT substrate is near the phrenic nerve, pacing the left phrenic nerve from above (from a catheter in the left subclavian vein) can help monitor for any sign of injury during ablation. If the substrate is directly beneath the phrenic nerve, it may be lifted from proximity to the epicardial surface either through infusion of air and fluid into the epicardial space, or through the use of large inflated vascular balloon to physically move the pericardial sac/overlying phrenic nerve.[39]

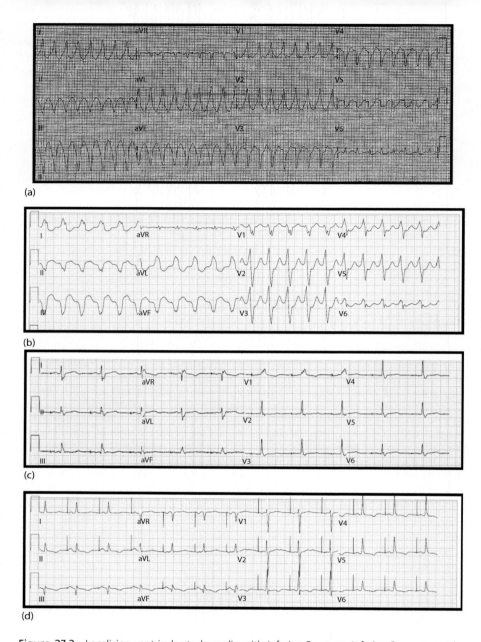

(a)

(b)

(c)

(d)

Figure 27.2 Localizing ventricular tachycardia with inferior Q waves: Inferior Q waves can be seen in both non-ischemic epicardial VT originating from the inferior wall (a) or in ischemic VT with prior inferior wall infarction (b). These two inferior Q wave VTs can often be distinguished pre-procedurally by examining the sinus electrocardiogram. The non-ischemic epicardial VT may not have inferior Q waves at baseline (c), whereas the inferior wall infarction patient often will (d).

PATTERNS OF ARRHYTHMIC SUBSTRATE AND ELECTROCARDIOGRAPHIC CORRELATIONS IN NON-ISCHEMIC CARDIOMYOPATHY

IDIOPATHIC DILATED CARDIOMYOPATHY

Idiopathic dilated cardiomyopathies frequently have scar found near the base of the heart encircling the mitral annulus and extending to the front of the aortic valve. The basal septum and lateral mitral annulus are also sites where focal voltage and myocardial delayed enhancement abnormalities are found.[12,15,40] In terms of myocardial localization, the scar is often sub-epicardial but can extend inward to the endocardial cavity.[16,41] Figure 27.3 shows a patient with a dilated cardiomyopathy with a lateral mitral annular scar. The corresponding intracardiac echocardiography image shows a cross-section of the lateral left ventricle with a prominent stripe of mid-myocardial hyperechoic scar. This scar was recapitulated on pre-procedural contrast-enhanced MRI (Figure 27.3c). The baseline ECG for patients with dilated cardiomyopathy is variable in presentation and dependent on the patient's disease state and extent of myocardial scarring and fibrosis. The baseline ECG may suggest lateral scar if there is a late loss of an "R" wave across the precordium or even Q waves in V6, but these findings are more specific than sensitive. Furthermore, focal peri-annular scar infrequently provides an electro-cardiographic signature on the surface ECG. Ventricular arrhythmias that originate from basal mitral annular regions of the heart are typically right bundle with a late or no precordial transition. The axis is often variable dependent on the arrhythmia's location along the annulus. The inferior mitral annulus yields a superior axis and whereas the superior mitral annulus will have an inferior axis. Peri-aortic valve disease will either have an early precordial transition from left bundle to right or will be right bundle throughout the precordium. The axis is usually a rightward and inferior axis. Ablation outcomes for dilated cardiomyopathy patients are reported to approach VT free survival rates of 70% at 18 months 5 years timepoints.[12,16]

CARDIAC SARCOIDOSIS

Cardiac sarcoidosis is notorious for its variability of presentation and consequently its ability to mimic the presentation of other forms of cardiomyopathies. Scar in patients with cardiac sarcoidosis can be found at any level of the myocardial wall (endocardial, mid-myocardial, or epicardial) and in any manner of regional distributions. In certain circumstances, when the sarcoid-driven scar falls within a vascular territory, this NICM can even masquerade as an ischemic scar. Classically, cardiac sarcoidosis involves the septum and many of the baseline ECG clues reflect this. New conduction abnormalities, prolongation of the PR interval, or even heart block may suggest septal substrate. If the septal scarring is extensive enough, septal Q waves can be seen in leads V1 and V2 (Figure 27.4a). Ventricular arrhythmias arising from the septum are usually left bundle with a precordial transition near V2 or V3. If the VT is exiting from the top of the septum, the ECG has an inferior axis and a superior axis if the septal exit is along the inferoseptum. One clue that suggests septal disease is when a patient has multiple VT or PVC morphologies that appear to exit from the top and bottom of the septum suggesting arrhythmogenic substrate in the mid-septum (Figure 27.4a). In these instances, targeting the mid-septal substrate can be essential to achieving effective ablative therapy. In the largest reported cohort, the effectiveness of VT ablation is limited in the sarcoid population with 50% of patients having VT free survival at 2 years follow-up.[13] The reasons for the recurrence rates in cardiac sarcoid patients are thought to be largely technical as the ventricular arrhythmias are frequently localized to the septum, but are subsequently resistant to termination due to inadequate lesion penetration.

ARRHYTHMOGENIC RIGHT VENTRICULAR DYSPLASIA/CARDIOMYOPATHY

Arrhythmogenic right ventricular cardiomyopathy (ARVC) is unique from most other forms of non-ischemic cardiomyopathy in that the bulk of the arrhythmogenic substrate is found in the right ventricle. ARVC is characterized by fibrofatty replacement of the myocardial wall typically in the epicardial RVOT or the lateral tricuspid annulus.[42-44] The fibrofatty

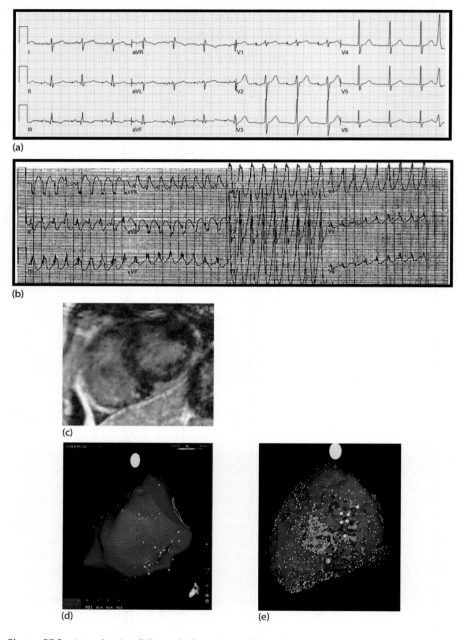

(a)

(b)

(c)

(d)

(e)

Figure 27.3 Lateral epicardial ventricular tachycardia: In this patient with dilated cardiomyopathy, there is no overt sign of lateral scar on the surface ECG (a), though the QS pattern seen in ventricular tachycardia (b) is consistent with an epicardial arrhythmia at this site. Cardiac MRI demonstrated a focal area of lateral wall epicardial myocardial delayed enhancement (c). While endocardial voltage mapping showed preserved LV voltage (d), epicardial voltage mapping revealed the arrhythmogenic focus (e).

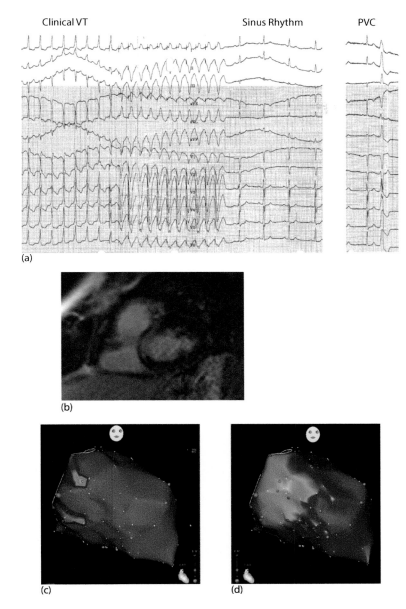

(a)

(b)

(c)   (d)

Figure 27.4   Septal ventricular tachycardia: A rhythm electrocardiogram is shown where a septal VT with an inferior basal exit is overdrive-paced into sinus rhythm (a). A subsequent premature ventricular complex localizes to the basal septum with a more superior exit (a). Cardiac MRI demonstrates a basal stripe of mid-myocardial delayed enhancement (b). Voltage mapping did not show significant endocardial voltage abnormality (c), however unipolar voltage mapping confirmed the presence of mid-myocardial, septal substrate (d).

replacement leads to delayed conduction and repolarization abnormalities that are visible on the surface electrocardiogram and have become incorporated in the diagnostic criteria for this disease.[45] T-wave inversions are often found over the right precordial leads (V1 and V2), but this inversion can extend throughout the precordium. Late fractionation may be present as well in the right precordium and is termed an epsilon wave (Figure 27.5). Ventricular arrhythmias arising from the ARVC population are predominantly found in the free wall of the RVOT where they manifest with a left bundle morphology with late transition (V5 or V6). There will be an inferior axis that frequently shows notching in the inferior leads. Occasionally, the lateral tricuspid annulus will have aneurysmal formation and can be an additional site of arrhythmias. Lateral tricuspid annulus arrhythmias will be left bundle arrhythmias with a late transition (V5 or V6), but the inferior leads will frequently be biphasic in lead II and negative in lead III. One notable aspect of the ARVC population is that while their heart failure course may be progressive, the arrhythmic substrate has been shown to be relatively static over time.[44] This suggests that with a successful initial ablation, ARVC patients can be ventricular arrhythmia free. Achieving successful ablation with endocardial

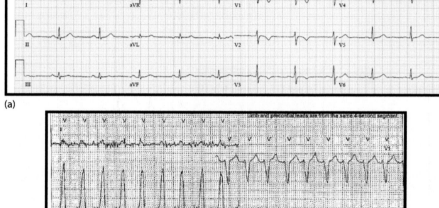

(a)

(b)

Figure 27.5 Ventricular tachycardia in ARVC: At baseline, patients with ARVC may demonstrate early precordial T wave inversions or even late fractionation (a). VT of AVRC is most commonly localized to the RV free wall (b). (*Continued*)

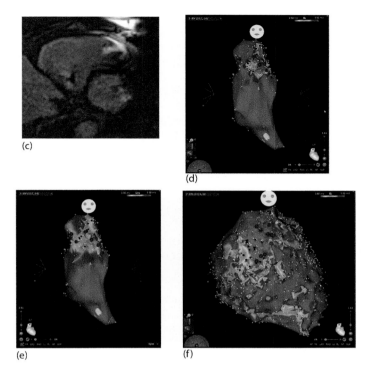

(c)

(d)

(e)

(f)

Figure 27.5 (Continued) Ventricular tachycardia in ARVC: Cardiac MRI will usually show a dilated RV, but myocardial delayed enhancement may be difficult to appreciate due to the thinness of the RV free wall (c). Endocardial bipolar (d) and unipolar (e) and epicardial bipolar (f) voltage maps demonstrate a patch of isolated free wall scar that extends to the tricuspid annulus along the epicardium.

ablation alone can be difficult due to the highly mobile nature of the RV free wall and limited energy delivery to the fibrofatty and epicardial substrate. In a large cohort, 1 year VT free survival is approximately 50% with endocardial ablation alone.[46] When the epicardial substrate is targeted in conjunction with the endocardium, VT free survival is reported to between 64% and 77% at 1 year.[43,46]

HYPERTROPHIC CARDIOMYOPATHY

Hypertrophic cardiomyopathy is characterized by pathologic thickening (non-adaptive) of the ventricular myocardium. This leads to scar development and myofibrillar disarray predisposing this population to ventricular arrhythmias in a manner proportional to wall thickness. Of note, the location of thickening does play some role in arrhythmic risk as aneurysmal formation of the left ventricular apex is associated with higher rates of ventricular arrhythmias than other forms of hypertrophic cardiomyopathy likely due to the formation of apical scarring.[47] Baseline ECG characteristics of patient with hypertrophic cardiomyopathy may demonstrate repolarization abnormalities and precordial T-wave inversions, but the localization will be varied depending on the site of thickening in the ventricle. Similarly, arrhythmias arising in this population can be found wherever the ventricular thickening and scarring occur and consequently there is no pathognomonic ventricular arrhythmia pattern. Ablation in this population is challenging due to small endocardial cavities (leading to limited to catheter manipulation) to inadequate lesion penetration into thickened myocardium; often epicardial ablation is needed in such situations. Despite these limitations, catheter ablation of ventricular arrhythmias in hypertrophic cardiomyopathy can be effective as VT free survival approaches 75% in long-term follow-up.[48,49]

MITRAL VALVE PROLAPSE AND PAPILLARY MUSCLE DISEASE

Another entity on the sudden cardiac death spectrum is the association with mitral valve prolapse and papillary muscle disease.[50] While the exact etiology of this disease is unknown, it is clear that fibrosis and scarring occur within the papillary muscle itself and the adjacent lateral wall myocardium. This scarring is visible both on MRI as well as histopathology.[50] Papillary muscle arrhythmias present with a right bundle branch pattern with a QRS that transitions between leads V3 and V5. There is frequently an rS pattern in V6. While there can be some overlap, the posteromedial papillary muscle is often distinguished from the anterolateral papillary muscle by the axis.[51] The technical aspects of ablating the papillary muscles can be challenging given the highly mobile nature of the structure. Cryoablation may be required to achieve adequate papillary muscle stability when radiofrequency catheter ablation is unsuccessful.[52] The success rate for ablation of papillary muscle ventricular arrhythmias is high with reports up to 80% ventricular arrhythmia free survival.[52,53]

BUNDLE BRANCH RE-ENTRANT VENTRICULAR ARRHYTHMIAS

Bundle branch re-entrant ventricular arrhythmias are a distinct, but important clinical entity found in both ischemic and non-ischemic cardiomyopathies. The majority of bundle branch re-entry ventricular arrhythmias are found in ischemic cardiomyopathies, though they can also be found in NICM as well (40% and 25%, respectively according to a large cohort).[54] The underlying critical substrate for this arrhythmia is the presence of an underlying conduction abnormality. This conduction abnormality can be either a fixed or functional block in the His Purkinje system.[55] In either case, when a patient has differential conduction down the bundle branches, this predisposes the patient to re-entrant arrhythmias using the right and left limbs of the conduction system. This is analogous to the differential conduction seen in the atrioventricular node where slow and fast pathways allow for sustained AV nodal reentrant tachycardias.

The diagnosis of bundle branch reentry should be entertained when a ventricular arrhythmia is induced, which mimics a native bundle branch block. In contrast to a myocardial focus of ventricular arrhythmia, this arrhythmia presents electrocardiographically with a sharp intrinsicoid deflection followed by a "typical" left or right bundle branch pattern that can only be generated by engaging the patient's native right or left bundle branch, respectively (Figure 27.6). Once this diagnosis is suggested by surface electrocardiogram, several additional intracardiac criteria are required for diagnosis: (1) During initiation and maintenance of ventricular arrhythmias, a His recording precedes each QRS complex; (2) changes in the H–H intervals precede changes in the V–V intervals during tachycardia cycle length changes; (3) the recorded HV time is equivalent to or greater than the HV time recorded during sinus rhythm; (4) ablation of the right or left bundle branch renders the arrhythmia non-inducible.[54,56,57]

Given the relatively focal ablative target for bundle branch re-entrant ventricular arrhythmias (the left or right bundle branch), the long-term outcomes of catheter-based therapies for this clinical entity are excellent. Cure rates after a single procedure approach 85%–90%.[54,58] It should be noted that in situations where bundle branch reentrant VT is one of many presenting ventricular arrhythmias, the cure rate for the non-reentrant ventricular arrhythmias can be much lower. The morbidity of bundle branch ablation can be minimized by targeting a retrograde only conducting limb or the right bundle if both have good antegrade conductive properties. Consistent with this, long-term rates of pacemaker requirement do not appear to be elevated in bundle branch re-entry patients who present with a normal baseline HV interval.[54]

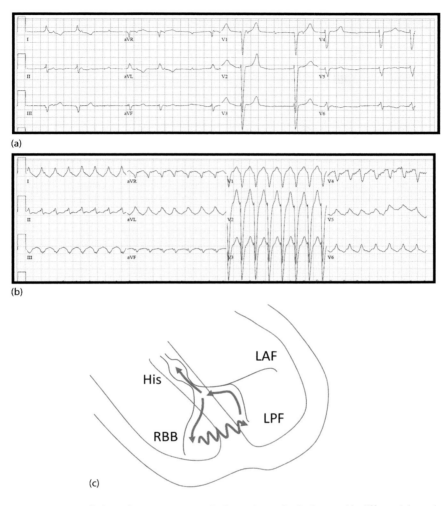

Figure 27.6 Bundle branch re-entrant ventricular tachycardia: Patients with differential conduction between the right and left bundle branches (or true bundle branch block) have the underlying substrate necessary for bundle branch re-entrant tachycardia (a). When present, this form of VT will classically manifest as either a pure right bundle branch or left bundle branch morphology (b). Panel (c) diagrams the re-entrant circuit seen in panel (b). Conduction occurs down the right bundle branch (RBB), across the intraventricular septum and then retrograde up either the left posterior fascicle (LPF) or the left anterior fascicle (LAF) before transiting down the right bundle again.

CONCLUSION

Non-ischemic cardiomyopathies are a unique entity with substrate that varies by myopathy type. The presence of mid-myocardial and epicardial substrate make ablation of arrhythmias in this patient population technically challenging. In spite of these inherent limitation, catheter ablation of non-ischemic ventricular arrhythmias is safe and effective. Future studies will be required to improve on existing ablative therapies to continue to improve overall patient outcomes and arrhythmia free survival.

REFERENCES

1. Maron BJ, Towbin JA, Thiene G, et al. Contemporary definitions and classification of the cardiomyopathies: An American Heart Association scientific statement from the council on clinical cardiology, heart failure and transplantation committee; quality of care and outcomes research and functional genomics and translational biology interdisciplinary working groups; and council on epidemiology and prevention. *Circulation.* 2006;113:1807–1816.

2. Pimentel M, Rohde LE, Zimerman A, Zimerman LI. Sudden cardiac death markers in non-ischemic cardiomyopathy. *J Electrocardiol.* 2016;49:446–451.

3. Aliot EM, Stevenson WG, Almendral-Garrote JM, et al. Ehra/hrs expert consensus on catheter ablation of ventricular arrhythmias: Developed in a partnership with the European Heart Rhythm Association (EHRA), a registered branch of the European Society of Cardiology (ESC), and the Heart Rhythm Society (HRS); in collaboration with the American College of Cardiology (ACC) and the American Heart Association (AHA). *Heart Rhythm.* 2009;6:886–933.

4. Bardy GH, Lee KL, Mark DB, et al. Amiodarone or an implantable cardioverter-defibrillator for congestive heart failure. *N Engl J Med.* 2005;352:225–237.

5. Kadish A, Dyer A, Daubert JP, et al. Prophylactic defibrillator implantation in patients with nonischemic dilated cardiomyopathy. *N Engl J Med.* 2004;350:2151–2158.

6. Kober L, Thune JJ, Nielsen JC, et al. Defibrillator implantation in patients with non-ischemic systolic heart failure. *N Engl J Med.* 2016;375:1221–1230.

7. Reddy VY, Reynolds MR, Neuzil P, et al. Prophylactic catheter ablation for the prevention of defibrillator therapy. *N Engl J Med.* 2007;357:2657–2665.

8. Connolly SJ, Dorian P, Roberts RS, et al. Comparison of beta-blockers, amiodarone plus beta-blockers, or sotalol for prevention of shocks from implantable cardioverter defibrillators: The optic study: A randomized trial. *JAMA.* 2006;295:165–171.

9. Palaniswamy C, Kolte D, Harikrishnan P, et al. Catheter ablation of postinfarction ventricular tachycardia: Ten-year trends in utilization, in-hospital complications, and in-hospital mortality in the United States. *Heart Rhythm.* 2014;11:2056–2063.

10. Kuck KH, Schaumann A, Eckardt L, et al. Catheter ablation of stable ventricular tachycardia before defibrillator implantation in patients with coronary heart disease (vtach): A multicentre randomised controlled trial. *Lancet.* 2010;375:31–40.

11. Sapp JL, Wells GA, Parkash R, et al. Ventricular tachycardia ablation versus escalation of antiarrhythmic drugs. *N Engl J Med.* 2016;375:111–121.

12. Muser D, Santangeli P, Castro SA, et al. Long-term outcome after catheter ablation of ventricular tachycardia in patients with nonischemic dilated cardiomyopathy. *Circ Arrhythm Electrophysiol.* 2016;9.

13. Muser D, Santangeli P, Pathak RK, et al. Long-term outcomes of catheter ablation of ventricular tachycardia in patients with cardiac sarcoidosis. *Circ Arrhythm Electrophysiol.* 2016;9.

14. Miller JM, Kienzle MG, Harken AH, Josephson ME. Subendocardial resection for ventricular tachycardia: Predictors of surgical success. *Circulation.* 1984;70:624–631.

15. Hsia HH, Callans DJ, Marchlinski FE. Characterization of endocardial electrophysiological substrate in patients with nonischemic cardiomyopathy and monomorphic ventricular tachycardia. *Circulation.* 2003;108:704–710.

16. Cano O, Hutchinson M, Lin D, et al. Electroanatomic substrate and ablation outcome for suspected epicardial ventricular tachycardia in left ventricular nonischemic cardiomyopathy. *J Am Coll Cardiol.* 2009;54:799–808.

17. Sasaki T, Miller CF, Hansford R, et al. Impact of nonischemic scar features on local ventricular electrograms and scar-related ventricular tachycardia circuits in patients with nonischemic cardiomyopathy. *Circ Arrhythm Electrophysiol.* 2013;6:1139–1147.

18. Becker MAJ, Cornel JH. The prognostic vale of late gadolinium-enhacned cardiac mgnetic-resonance imagin in nonischemic dilated cardiomyopathy. *JACC: Cardiovascular Imaging.* 2018.

19. Faris OP, Shein M. Food and drug administration perspective: Magnetic resonance imaging of pacemaker and implantable cardioverter-defibrillator patients. *Circulation.* 2006;114:1232–1233.

20. Nazarian S, Hansford R, Rahsepar AA, et al. Safety of magnetic resonance imaging in patients with cardiac devices. *N Engl J Med.* 2017;377:2555–2564.

21. Miller JD, Nazarian S, Halperin HR. Implantable electronic cardiac devices and compatibility with magnetic resonance imaging. *J Am Coll Cardiol.* 2016;68:1590–1598.

22. Ben-Haim SA, Osadchy D, Schuster I, et al. Nonfluoroscopic, in vivo navigation and mapping technology. *Nat Med.* 1996;2:1393–1395.

23. Hutchinson MD, Gerstenfeld EP, Desjardins B, et al. Endocardial unipolar voltage mapping to detect epicardial ventricular tachycardia substrate in patients with nonischemic left ventricular cardiomyopathy. *Circ Arrhythm Electrophysiol.* 2011;4:49–55.

24. Liuba I, Frankel DS, Riley MP, et al. Scar progression in patients with nonischemic cardiomyopathy and ventricular arrhythmias. *Heart Rhythm.* 2014;11:755–762.

25. Polin GM, Haqqani H, Tzou W, et al. Endocardial unipolar voltage mapping to identify epicardial substrate in arrhythmogenic right ventricular cardiomyopathy/dysplasia. *Heart Rhythm.* 2011;8:76–83.

26. Betensky BP, Kapa S, Desjardins B, et al. Characterization of trans-septal activation during septal pacing: Criteria for identification of intramural ventricular tachycardia substrate in nonischemic cardiomyopathy. *Circ Arrhythm Electrophysiol.* 2013;6:1123–1130.

27. Schramm W, Yang D, Wood BJ, et al. Contribution of direct heating, thermal conduction and perfusion during radiofrequency and microwave ablation. *Open Biomed Eng J.* 2007;1:47–52.

28. Koruth JS, Dukkipati S, Miller MA, et al. Bipolar irrigated radiofrequency ablation: A therapeutic option for refractory intramural atrial and ventricular tachycardia circuits. *Heart Rhythm.* 2012;9:1932–1941.

29. Nguyen DT, Gerstenfeld EP, Tzou WS, et al. Radiofrequency ablation using an open irrigated electrode cooled with half-normal saline. *JACC: Electrophysiology.* 2017.

30. Sapp JL, Beeckler C, Pike R, et al. Initial human feasibility of infusion needle catheter ablation for refractory ventricular tachycardia. *Circulation.* 2013;128:2289–2295.

31. Kreidieh B, Rodriguez-Manero M, Schurmann P, et al. Retrograde coronary venous ethanol infusion for ablation of refractory ventricular tachycardia. *Circ Arrhythm Electrophysiol.* 2016;9.

32. Yokokawa M, Morady F, Bogun F. Injection of cold saline for diagnosis of intramural ventricular arrhythmias. *Heart Rhythm.* 2016;13:78–82.

33. Soejima K, Stevenson WG, Sapp JL, et al. Endocardial and epicardial radiofrequency ablation of ventricular tachycardia associated with dilated cardiomyopathy: The importance of low-voltage scars. *J Am Coll Cardiol.* 2004;43:1834–1842.

34. Valles E, Bazan V, Marchlinski FE. ECG criteria to identify epicardial ventricular tachycardia in nonischemic cardiomyopathy. *Circ Arrhythm Electrophysiol.* 2010;3:63–71.

35. Daniels DV, Lu YY, Morton JB, et al. Idiopathic epicardial left ventricular tachycardia originating remote from the sinus of valsalva: Electrophysiological characteristics, catheter ablation, and identification from the 12-lead electrocardiogram. *Circulation*. 2006;113:1659–1666.

36. Dixit S, Narula N, Callans DJ, Marchlinski FE. Electroanatomic mapping of human heart: Epicardial fat can mimic scar. *J Cardiovasc Electrophysiol*. 2003;14:1128.

37. Santangeli P, Marchlinski FE, Zado ES, et al. Percutaneous epicardial ablation of ventricular arrhythmias arising from the left ventricular summit: Outcomes and electrocardiogram correlates of success. *Circ Arrhythm Electrophysiol*. 2015;8:337–343.

38. Della Bella P, Brugada J, Zeppenfeld K, et al. Epicardial ablation for ventricular tachycardia: A European multicenter study. *Circ Arrhythm Electrophysiol*. 2011;4:653–659.

39. Kumar S, Barbhaiya CR, Baldinger SH, et al. Epicardial phrenic nerve displacement during catheter ablation of atrial and ventricular arrhythmias: Procedural experience and outcomes. *Circ Arrhythm Electrophysiol*. 2015;8:896–904.

40. Haqqani HM, Tschabrunn CM, Tzou WS, et al. Isolated septal substrate for ventricular tachycardia in nonischemic dilated cardiomyopathy: Incidence, characterization, and implications. *Heart Rhythm*. 2011;8:1169–1176.

41. Soejima K, Landing BH, Roe TF, Swanson VL. Pathologic studies of the osteoporosis of von Gierke's disease (glycogenosis 1a). *Pediatr Pathol*. 1985;3:307–319.

42. Marchlinski FE, Zado E, Dixit S, et al. Electroanatomic substrate and outcome of catheter ablative therapy for ventricular tachycardia in setting of right ventricular cardiomyopathy. *Circulation*. 2004;110:2293–2298.

43. Garcia FC, Bazan V, Zado ES, et al. Epicardial substrate and outcome with epicardial ablation of ventricular tachycardia in arrhythmogenic right ventricular cardiomyopathy/dysplasia. *Circulation*. 2009;120:366–375.

44. Riley MP, Zado E, Bala R, et al. Lack of uniform progression of endocardial scar in patients with arrhythmogenic right ventricular dysplasia/cardiomyopathy and ventricular tachycardia. *Circ Arrhythm Electrophysiol*. 2010;3:332–338.

45. Marcus FI, McKenna WJ, Sherrill D, et al. Diagnosis of arrhythmogenic right ventricular cardiomyopathy/dysplasia: Proposed modification of the task force criteria. *Circulation*. 2010;121:1533–1541.

46. Philips B, Madhavan S, James C, et al. Outcomes of catheter ablation of ventricular tachycardia in arrhythmogenic right ventricular dysplasia/cardiomyopathy. *Circ Arrhythm Electrophysiol*. 2012;5:499–505.

47. Rowin EJ, Maron BJ, Haas TS, et al. Hypertrophic cardiomyopathy with left ventricular apical aneurysm: Implications for risk stratification and management. *J Am Coll Cardiol*. 2017;69:761–773.

48. Santangeli P, Di Biase L, Lakkireddy D, et al. Radiofrequency catheter ablation of ventricular arrhythmias in patients with hypertrophic cardiomyopathy: Safety and feasibility. *Heart Rhythm*. 2010;7:1036–1042.

49. Santangeli P, Di Biase L, Themistoclakis S, et al. Catheter ablation of atrial fibrillation in hypertrophic cardiomyopathy: Long-term outcomes and mechanisms of arrhythmia recurrence. *Circ Arrhythm Electrophysiol*. 2013;6:1089–1094.

50. Basso C, Perazzolo Marra M, Rizzo S, et al. Arrhythmic mitral valve prolapse and sudden cardiac death. *Circulation*. 2015;132:556–566.

51. Good E, Desjardins B, Jongnarangsin K, et al. Ventricular arrhythmias originating from a papillary muscle in patients without prior infarction: A comparison with fascicular arrhythmias. *Heart Rhythm*. 2008;5:1530–1537.

52. Rivera S, Ricapito Mde L, Tomas L, et al. Results of cryoenergy and radiofrequency-based catheter ablation for treating ventricular arrhythmias arising from the papillary muscles of the left ventricle, guided by intracardiac echocardiography and image integration. *Circ Arrhythm Electrophysiol*. 2016;9:e003874.

53. Yokokawa M, Good E, Desjardins B, et al. Predictors of successful catheter ablation of ventricular arrhythmias arising from the papillary muscles. *Heart Rhythm*. 2010;7:1654–1659.

54. Pathak RK, Fahed J, Santangeli P, Hyman MC. Long-term outcome of catheter ablation for treatment of bundle branch re-entrant tachycardia. *JACC: Clinical Electrophysiology*. 2018.

55. Blanck Z, Jazayeri M, Dhala A, et al. Bundle branch reentry: A mechanism of ventricular tachycardia in the absence of myocardial or valvular dysfunction. *J Am Coll Cardiol*. 1993;22:1718–1722.

56. Tchou P, Jazayeri M, Denker S, et al. Transcatheter electrical ablation of right bundle branch. A method of treating macroreentrant ventricular tachycardia attributed to bundle branch reentry. *Circulation*. 1988;78:246–257.

57. Caceres J, Jazayeri M, McKinnie J, et al. Sustained bundle branch reentry as a mechanism of clinical tachycardia. *Circulation*. 1989;79:256–270.

58. Mehdirad AA, Keim S, Rist K, Tchou P. Long-term clinical outcome of right bundle branch radiofrequency catheter ablation for treatment of bundle branch reentrant ventricular tachycardia. *Pacing Clin Electrophysiol*. 1995;18:2135–2143.

ULTRASOUND IN THE ELECTROPHYSIOLOGY LAB

Carola Gianni, Javier E. Sanchez,
Domenico G. Della Rocca, Amin Al-Ahmad, and Andrea Natale

CONTENTS

INTRODUCTION

Ultrasound (US) is a valuable tool and should be standard of care in any modern electrophysiology (EP) lab. Through real-time imaging of vascular and cardiac anatomy, US is used to obtain central vascular access and to guide EP procedures, reducing complications, procedural times, and increasing success rates.[1] This is a short overview of some of the most important aspects of using real-time US in EP procedures, with the caveat that technical aspects (such as biophysics, ultrasound machine, and knobology, probe manipulation, basic ultrasound anatomy) go beyond the scope of this chapter, but all trained operators should be familiar with them to benefit the most from the use of US.

VASCULAR ULTRASOUND

With a linear, high-frequency (9 to 12 MHz) probe, central vascular access can be obtained safely in both ablation and implant procedures. US-guided vascular access reduces the need for multiple attempts and inadvertent puncture of surrounding structures, thus preventing complications and unsuccessful cannulation.[2-4] To do so, US has to be used real-time, throughout the procedure:

- Establish landmarks (site-specific, e.g., femoral head, lung, ribs, collaterals, and neighboring vessels).
- Identify obstacles (e.g., thrombosis or significant calcification).
- Directly visualize the tip of the needle finding its way into the vessel, thus avoiding surrounding structures and back-walling.
- Confirm correct placement of the wire (Figure 28.1) before advancing the sheath to avoid complications (e.g., hematoma, dissection, pneumothorax).

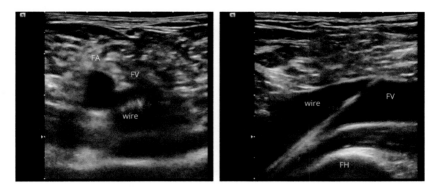

Figure 28.1 Short- and long-axis view of the right FV showing correct intravascular positioning of the metal wire. FA, femoral artery; FH, femoral head; FV, femoral vein.

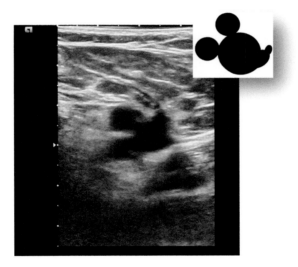

Figure 28.2 Mickey Mouse sign.

Following are some important specific tips for the most common EP-related central vascular access sites:

- Femoral vein:
    - Optimal site is right above the femoral artery bifurcation (Mickey Mouse sign; Figure 28.2) at the level of the saphenofemoral junction, above the femoral head:
        - This prevents going through most of the arterial (e.g., femoral artery, external pudendal artery) and venous (e.g., saphenous vein and collaterals) surrounding vessels.
        - Allows for adequate compression at the time of sheath removal, preventing hematomas and pseudoaneurysm(s).
        - Sometimes the femoral artery bifurcation is high, so it's always important to know where the inguinal ligament/femoral head lies to avoid an intraperitoneal puncture.
    - With below-the-bifurcation access, it is important to carefully scan the target access site looking for all collaterals (best done with probes ≥9 MHz).

- Femoral artery:
    - Optimal site is the common femoral artery, above the femoral artery bifurcation, in the middle of the anterior wall of the vessel, at the level of the femoral head.
        - The needle tip should lie in the center of the vessel, with good blood flow.
            - Sub-intimal intima needle insertion is possible, and advancing the wire when resistance is felt can lead to arterial dissection.
    - To exclude back-walling of the wire, it might be necessary to pull it back and visualize the J-tip freely floating in the lumen.
    - US is also useful when using vascular closure devices, to obtain access in an optimal location and confirm proper epivascular deployment.
- Internal jugular vein:
    - Optimal site is where the vein is more likely to be superficial and lateral to the carotid artery; this is usually in the mid to lower third of the neck.
        - The following are important to avoid lung puncture:
            - The angle of the needle should be as steep as possible (close to 90°); before advancing the wire, the angle can be reduced, making sure to retain access.
            - A sharp (arterial access needle) or smaller gauge needle should be used to minimize tenting and subsequent back-walling.
            - If any doubt of inadvertent lung puncture, lung sliding can be easily assessed using US to prove absence of pneumothorax.
        - Head rotation increases the chance of vein/artery overlap and should be avoided.
- Subclavian/axillary vein:
    - Optimal is where the vein does not lie directly over the lung or artery (e.g., where it overlies the first or second rib; Figure 28.3).
        - A long-axis approach is preferable as it allows to visualize the whole needle, along with the vein, the ribs, and underlying lung.
        - Shrugging the shoulder may help to open up the US window by pulling the clavicle upwards.

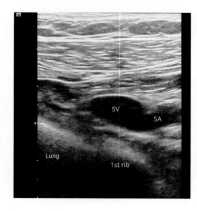

Figure 28.3 Left subclavian vein as it overlies the first rib. SA, subclavian artery; SV, subclavian vein.

Intracardiac ultrasound, usually referred to as intracardiac echocardiography (ICE) with a catheter-based phase array probe allows for real-time imaging of cardiac anatomy, is used to facilitate many EP procedures.[5] ICE is used throughout the procedure with a variety of applications, including (but not limited to):

- Limit radiation exposure to the patient and staff.
- Identify relevant anatomic structures.
- Facilitate trans-septal access.
- Assess accurate placement (including contact) of mapping and ablation catheters.
- Early recognition of complications.

At the beginning of any procedure, a basic cardiac ultrasound survey with ICE should always be performed to identify abnormal/challenging anatomy and quantify baseline for pericardial fluid. The basic views to obtain are the following:

- ICE in the right atrium (RA; Figure 28.4):
  - The probe is positioned at the mid RA, in a neutral position.
  - Initial view ("home view"): Cavotricuspid isthmus (CTI), tricuspid valve (TV).
  - With sequential clock-wise rotation:
    - Right ventricular outflow tract (RVOT), aortic root and valve (with the non-coronary cusp being the closest to the RA), pulmonary valve and artery.
    - Coronary sinus (CS) ostium.
    - Left ventricle (LV), anterior interatrial septum (IAS), mitral valve, left atrial appendage (LAA).
    - Mid IAS, descending aorta/esophagus, left pulmonary veins (PV).
    - Posterior IAS, esophagus.
    - Right PVs, pulmonary artery.
    - Posterior RA, superior vena cava (SVC).
    - Crista terminalis, right atrial appendage (RAA).
- ICE in the right ventricle (RV; Figure 28.5):
  - The probe is positioned in by (i) deflecting the catheter anteriorly when visualizing the RAA, (ii) advancing it past the TV leaflets, (iii) undeflecting the catheter to a neutral position.
    - Do not rely on fluoroscopy, as the heart rotation is variable with a non-negligible risk of perforation when advancing the stiff ICE probe.
  - Initial view: RV, moderator band.
  - With sequential clock-wise rotation:
    - Interventricular septum.
    - LV (inferior and anterior wall), inferoseptal papillary muscle (PM).
    - LV (septal and lateral wall), MV, anterolateral PM, LVOT.
    - Left superior PV, ridge, LAA.
    - Aortic cusps (short axis, with the right coronary cusp closest to the RV and left coronary cusp farthest), left main and proximal left anterior descending/circumflex coronary artery, posterior RVOT.
    - Mid- and anterior RVOT, pulmonary valve, and artery.
    - Aortic root (long axis), right coronary artery.
    - SVC.

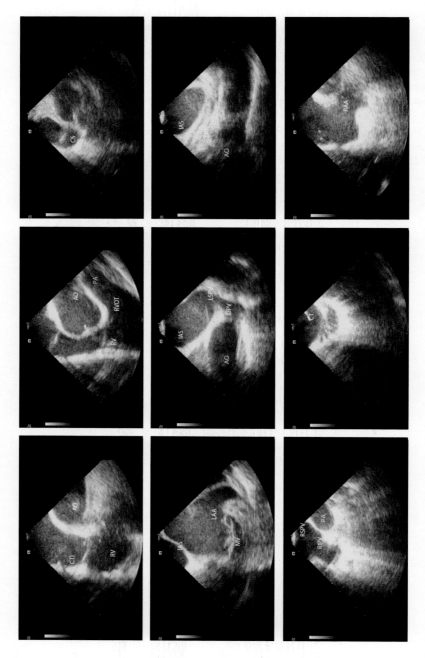

Figure 28.4 Cardiac survey with the ICE probe in the RA (see text). AO, aorta; CS, coronary sinus; CT, crista terminalis; Eso, esophagus; IAS, interatrial septum; ICE, intracardiac echocardiography; LAA, left atrial appendage; LIPV, left inferior pulmonary vein; LSPV, left superior pulmonary vein; MV, mitral valve; RA, right atrium; RAA, right atrial appendage; RIPV, right inferior pulmonary vein; RSPV, right superior pulmonary vein; RV, right ventricle; RVOT, right ventricular outflow tract.

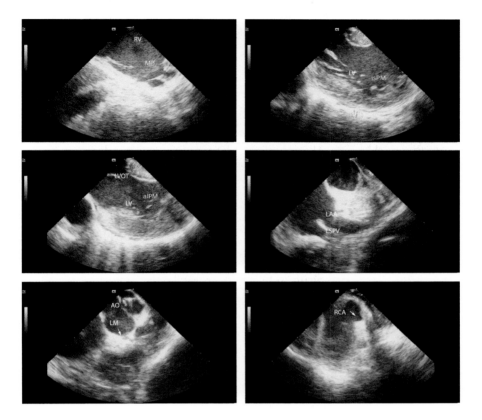

Figure 28.5 Cardiac survey with the ICE probe in the RV (see text). aIPM, antero-lateral papillary muscle; AO, aorta; ICE, intracardiac echocardiography; SPM, septal papillary muscle; LAA, left atrial appendage; LM, left main coronary artery; LSPV, left superior pulmonary vein; MB, moderator band; RCA, right coronary artery; RV, right ventricle.

While the following is not an exhaustive list, the following are some examples of the usefulness of ICE in various EP procedures:

- General applications:
  - Rule out intracardiac thrombosis and baseline pericardial effusion:
    - Perform a complete LAA survey (from the ostium to the tip), best obtained with the probe positioned in the RV (Figure 28.6).
    - LV apex visualization in patients with abnormal LV function.
    - Note any fluid posterior to the RA in the home view and posterior to the LV at the level of the MV.
  - Transseptal access:
    - Uncomplicated LA access is confirmed by real-time visualization of the needle tenting and passing the IAS along with bubbles in the LA when injecting saline through the needle.
      - Pressure monitoring and contrast are superfluous.
    - Access can be performed safely also with otherwise challenging anatomical variants (i.e., lipomatous or aneurysmatic septum) and prior atrial septal defect closure[6] (Figure 28.7).

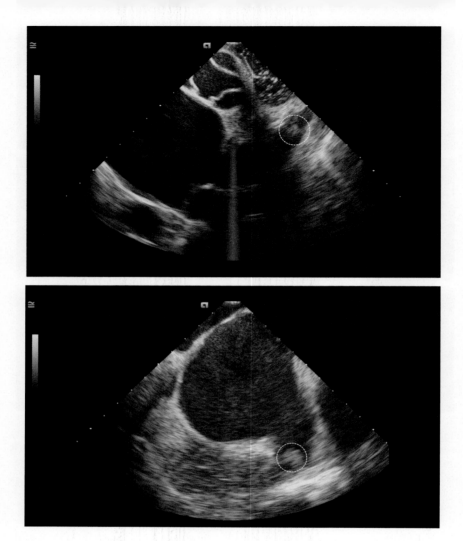

Figure 28.6 Thrombus in the LAA detected with ICE before transseptal access (RV and RA views). ICE, intracardiac echocardiography; LAA, left atrial appendage; RA, right atrium; RV, right ventricle.

- Monitor for complications (Figure 28.8):
  - *Unexpected hypotension*: ICE can quickly rule out devastating vascular complications (aortic dissection, retroperitoneal hematoma) and significant pericardial effusion.
  - *ST segment changes*: It's important to check for thrombus formation or presence of aortic air embolism to guide the proper intervention (i.e., anticoagulation/thrombolysis, air aspiration, PCI).

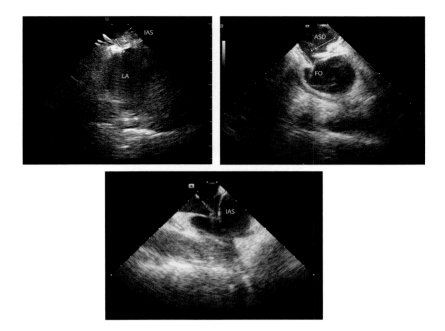

Figure 28.7 Examples of difficult transseptal access, i.e., lipomatous septum (top left), aneurysmatic septum (top right), and ASD closure device (bottom). ASD, atrial septal defect; FO, fossa ovalis; IAS, interatrial septum; LA, left atrium.

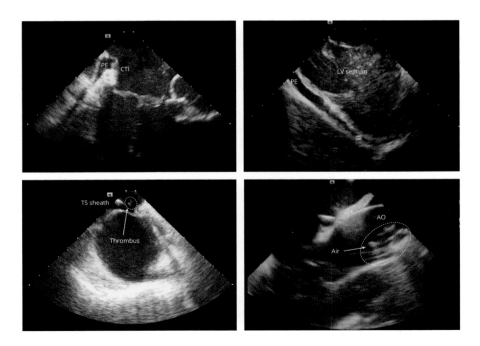

Figure 28.8 Examples of using ICE to monitor for complications. AO, aorta; CTI, cavo-tricuspid isthmus; ICE, intracardiac echocardiography; LV, left ventricle; PE, pericardial effusion; TS, trans-septal.

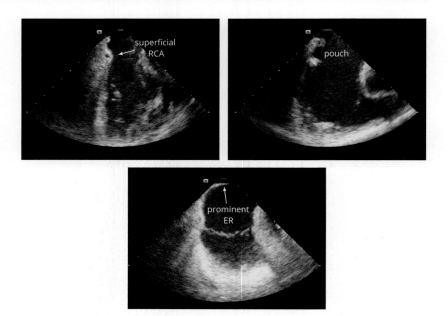

Figure 28.9 CTI anatomical variations. CTI, cavo-tricuspid isthmus; ER, eustachian ridge; RCA, right coronary artery.

- Procedure-specific applications:
  - Atrial fibrillation ablation:
    - To facilitate PV isolation, trans-septal access should be posterior, i.e., through the IAS when the left PVs or posterior wall next to them are in view.
    - Proper antral positioning of the circular mapping and ablation catheters, as well as of cryo- and RF-ablation balloons during PV isolation.
      - The same goes during LAA isolation, where ablation should be performed at the level of the ostium, and not deeper.
    - Real-time visualization of the location of the esophagus.
  - CTI-dependent atrial flutter ablation (Figure 28.9):
    - Delineating the patient's specific CTI anatomy is important, especially in repeat procedures or when bi-directional block is hard to achieve.
      - A prominent Eustachian ridge and pouches are easily visualized and can be navigated with the ablation catheter in real time.
  - LAA occlusion:
    - Transseptal access should be low, and anterior, i.e., through the IAS when the LAA is in view (Figure 28.10).
    - ICE can replace TEE to guide device deployment and proper LAA sealing.
  - Ablation of ventricular arrhythmias:
    - ICE is useful for in all types of access:
      - *LV anterograde*: Trans-septal should be performed anteriorly, where the MV is in view.
      - *LV retrograde access*: Exclude significant aorto-iliac (i.e., atherosclerosis/aneurysm) and aortic valve (i.e., aortic stenosis) disease.
      - *Epicardial access*: Rule out intramyocardial wire course before advancing the sheath; monitor irrigation-related fluid accumulation.

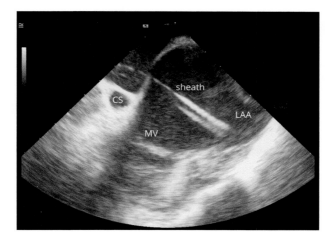

Figure 28.10 Preferable plane for trans-septal access in LAA occlusion procedures. CS, coronary sinus; LAA, left atrial appendage; MV, mitral valve.

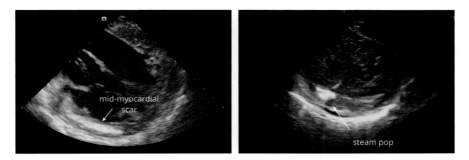

Figure 28.11 Tissue characterization with ICE during ablation of structural VT. ICE, intracardiac echocardiography; VT, ventricular tachycardia.

- Scar-related arrhythmias (Figure 28.11):
  - Identify and delineate the target substrate by real-time visualization of the myocardial scar (presence and location, including endo- vs. mid- vs. epicardial).
  - While ablating in the ventricular trabeculae, ICE can identify tissue overheating (increasing tissue hyperechogenity), even before a steam pop occurs.
  - In patients with significant LV dysfunction, it's useful to monitor the pumping function throughout to exclude further deterioration during the procedure (i.e., due to cardioversions, fluid overload, prolonged hypotension).
- Idiopathic arrhythmias (Figure 28.12):
  - Real-time visualization of right- and left-sided PMs as well as the moderator band.
    - Confirm stability and effective lesion formation during ablation.
  - Easy navigation of the ablation catheter in the RVOT and aortic cusps.
    - Importantly, ICE also allows to locate the coronary arteries ostia and their proximal course on real-time, obviating the need of coronary angiography.

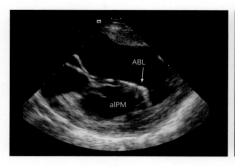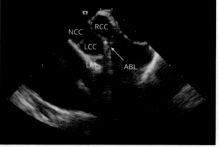

Figure 28.12 Real-time navigation of the ablation catheter with ICE during PM and OT PVC ablation. ABL, ablation catheter; aIPM, anterolateral papillary muscle; ICE, intracardiac echocardiography; LCC, left coronary cusp; LM, left main coronary artery; NCC, non-coronary cusp; OT, outflow tract; PM, papillary muscle; PVC, premature ventricular complex; RCC, right coronary cusp.

- Other procedures:
  - Lead extraction:
    - Identify and assess the extension of lead binding in the SVC, RA, and RV, thus predicting the complexity of the procedure.[7]
  - His bundle pacing:
    - The His area (i.e., anterior RA, right across the bottom of the non-coronary cusp) is easily visualized.
  - Endomyocardial biopsy:
    - As stated above, the scar is easily visualized on ICE thus providing the optimal sampling site for biopsy.[8]

REFERENCES

1. Razminia M, Zei PC, eds. *Fluoroscopy Reduction Techniques for Catheter Ablation of Cardiac Arrhythmias.* Cardiotext Publishing. 2019.

2. Troianos CA, Hartman GS, Glas KE, et al. Guidelines for performing ultrasound guided vascular cannulation: Recommendations of the American Society of Echocardiography and the Society of Cardiovascular Anesthesiologists. *Anesth Analg.* 2012;114(1):46–72. doi:10.1213/ANE.0b013e3182407cd8.

3. AIUM practice guideline for the use of ultrasound to guide vascular access procedures. *J Ultrasound Med.* 2013;32(1):191–215. doi:10.7863/jum.2013.32.1.191.

4. Dietrich CF, Horn R, Morf S, et al. Ultrasound-guided central vascular interventions, comments on the European Federation of Societies for Ultrasound in Medicine and Biology guidelines on interventional ultrasound. *J Thorac Dis.* 2016;8(9):E851–E868. doi:10.21037/jtd.2016.08.49.

5. Enriquez A, Saenz LC, Rosso R, et al. Use of intracardiac echocardiography in interventional cardiology: Working with the anatomy rather than fighting it. *Circulation.* 2018;137(21):2278–2294. doi:10.1161/CIRCULATIONAHA.117.031343.

6. Lakkireddy D, Rangisetty U, Prasad S, et al. Intracardiac echo-guided radiofrequency catheter ablation of atrial fibrillation in patients with atrial septal defect or patent foramen ovale repair: A feasibility, safety, and efficacy study. *J Cardiovasc Electrophysiol.* 2008;19(11):1137–1142. doi:10.1111/j.1540-8167.2008.01249.x.

7. Sadek MM, Cooper JM, Frankel DS, et al. Utility of intracardiac echocardiography during transvenous lead extraction. *Heart Rhythm.* 2017;14(12):1779–1785. doi:10.1016/j.hrthm.2017.08.023.

8. Casella M, Dello Russo A, et al. Electroanatomical mapping systems and intracardiac echo integration for guided endomyocardial biopsy. *Expert Rev Med Devices.* 2017;14(8):609–619. doi:10.1080/17434440.2017.1351875.

LEFT ATRIAL APPENDAGE CLOSURE

Rodney P. Horton, Carola Gianni, and Andrea Natale

CONTENTS

INTRODUCTION

Atrial fibrillation (AF) is the most common arrhythmia in adult humans, affecting 2.4 million patients in the United States alone and represents a major source of rising healthcare costs.[1] While symptoms can range from minor to severe, the most worrisome and ominous consequence of AF remains thromboembolism, most importantly stroke.[2] The left atrial appendage (LAA) remains a focus of thrombus formation in patients with non-valvular AF.[3] Case reports from the 1950s have described surgical amputation of the LAA during open-chest procedures for the explicit purpose of reducing stroke risk in AF patients.[4,5] While this approach was initially sporadic, surgical closure of the LAA has become widely accepted and is now included in the American College of Cardiology (ACC)/American Heart Association (AHA) guidelines for management of patients with valvular heart disease undergoing heart surgery.[6] Moreover, ACC/AHA/Heart Rhythm Society (HRS) guidelines for cardiac surgery patients with a history of AF include surgical LAA closure whenever possible.[7] Historically, stroke prevention has been focused on systemic pharmacologic anti-thrombotic strategies. Aspirin, clopidogrel, warfarin, and various combinations of these agents have been studied. Up until 2005, the oral anticoagulation (OAC) drug warfarin became the agent of choice for reducing stroke risk in patients with higher risk factors based on various risk scores (CHADS$_2$, CHA$_2$DS$_2$-VASc), while aspirin was the recommended agent for the lowest risk patients. Since 2005, newer anti-thrombotic agents (novel oral anticoagulants—NOACs) became available in the form of direct thrombin inhibitors (dabigatran) or factor Xa inhibitors (apixaban, edoxaban, rivaroxaban).[8–11] From an efficacy standpoint, warfarin's primary weakness has been difficulty in maintaining the drug in a therapeutic range. From a patient satisfaction standpoint, the need for regular blood tests to establish efficacy and the drug's impact on diet and other prescribed medications remain common complaints. Because the serum concentration of NAOCs is primarily impacted by renal clearance, the dosing is more predictable thereby avoiding blood testing of efficacy. However, the cost remains a barrier to some patients and they share with warfarin the same issues of major bleeding and non-compliance.

Therefore, non-pharmacologic options have remained attractive alternatives to chronic OAC use for patients with a high stroke risk and contraindications for OAC.[12] In this chapter, the

Table 29.1 FDA-approved devices capable of left atrial appendage closure

Device	Company	Approach	Design	Sizes
Watchman	Boston Scientific	Endocardial occlusion (transcatheter)	Parachute-shaped self-expanding nitinol frame covered by PET membrane	22, 24, 27, 30, and 33 mm
Lariat[a]	SentreHeart	Endo-epicardial ligation (transcatheter)	Non-absorbable suture	40 mm
AtriClip[a]	AtriCure	Epicardial ligation (surgical)	Titanium rods connected by nitinol springs and covered by polyester membrane	35, 40, 45, and 50 mm

[a] FDA approval for tissue approximation only.

author will discuss the three Food and Drug Administration (FDA) approved devices that provide mechanical closure of the LAA: the percutaneous Watchman and Lariat, and AtriClip (Table 29.1).

PATIENT SELECTION

LAA occlusion is indicated in patients with AF and high stroke risk with:

- High risk of bleeding under OAC (i.e., history of bleeding, uncontrolled hypertension, coagulopathy, bleeding disorder).
- Thromboembolic event despite OAC therapy.
- High probability of non-compliance.
- Intolerance/other contraindications for OAC.

Contraindications for LAA closure include:

- Low stroke risk (CHA_2DS_2-VASc = 0).
- Valvular heart disease.
- Other indications for long-term OAC.

WATCHMAN

The Watchman LAA occlusion device consists of the self-expanding nitinol metal frame covered with a porous (160 μm) polyethylene terephthalate (PET) knit fabric (Figure 29.1). The PET membrane covers the proximal surface; the portion which remains in contact with the blood of the left atrial (LA) cavity and promotes healing and endothelialization. Opposite to that, across the nitinol frame perimeter, active fixation hooks are present to anchor to the LAA and ensure stability.

The device is packaged in a pre-loaded containment sheath (delivery system) and is placed in the LAA by means of a 14-F, 75-cm access sheath (Figure 29.2). The device is manufactured in five sizes (21, 24, 27, 30, and 33 mm) to accommodate most LAA dimensions (Figure 29.1). It should be mentioned that the larger devices are also longer: as a result, a LAA with a wider ostial diameter would also need a longer body length to provide adequate sheath position prior to device deployment. The access sheaths are provided in three shapes (Figure 29.2): single-curve, double-curve, and anterior curve. Selection of the access sheath is usually physician reference, although the double-curve and the anterior curve were created to assist in Watchman placement in an LAA with a more superior direction (toward the aortic root).

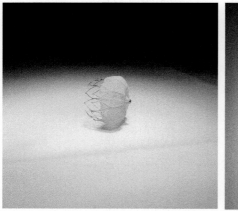
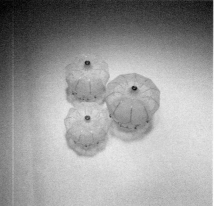

Figure 29.1 Watchman LAA occlusion device.

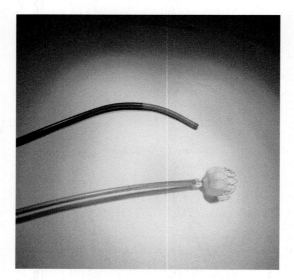

Figure 29.2 Single-curve access sheath (top) and delivery system (bottom).

PRE-PROCEDURE

Pre-procedural imaging, by means of transesophageal echocardiography (TEE) or computed tomography (CT), is essential to exclude LAA thrombus and assess LAA anatomy for suitability for LAA closure and to determine appropriate sizing of the device.

For Watchman, it is important to obtain two LAA dimensions:

- LAA anatomical ostium width (or landing zone), measured from the circumflex artery to the transition between the smooth LA and the trabeculated LAA (usually 1–2 cm distal to the limbus of the LAA-left superior pulmonary vein [LSPV] ridge): Between 17 and 31 mm
- LAA depth, measured from anatomical ostium line to apex of the LAA: Equal or greater than the ostium width

With TEE, the four commonly used views are 0°, 45°, 90°, and 135° (Figure 29.3). In alternative, CT can be employed: it has a superior spatial resolution allowing for 3D reconstructions, and LAA thrombi can be safely ruled out with delayed acquisition imaging.

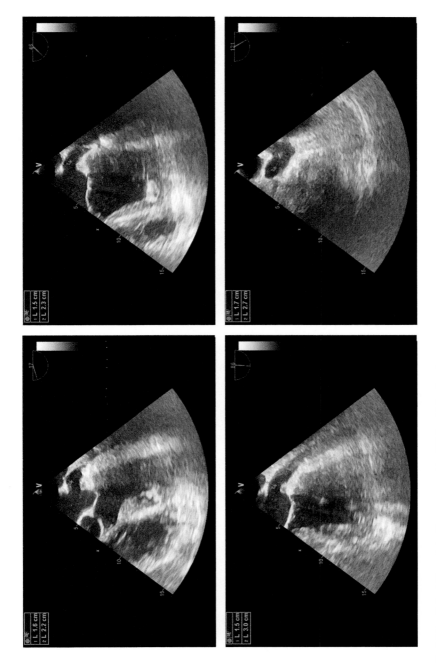

Figure 29.3 LAA ostial width and depth as assessed by TEE (multiple views).

Watchman sizing is based on the maximum LAA ostial width, with oversizing recommended by 10%–20% to ensure stable device positioning. Of note, excessive oversizing may result in compression of the circumflex artery and should be avoided.

PROCEDURE

The procedure is usually under general anesthesia and guided by fluoroscopy and TEE. Anticoagulation is usually stopped before the procedure and antibiotic prophylaxis is administered per protocol.

The following equipment should be available:

- Fluoroscopy and ultrasound (with TEE probe) machine
- Venous introducers
- Trans-septal access: long J-tipped guidewire, 8–8.5 F sheath with dilator, trans-septal needle, pressurized heparinized saline bag
- A long J-tipped 0.035" stiff guidewire
- A 4–6 F pigtail catheter
- Watchman kit: 14 F access sheath with dilator and delivery system (containment sheath with device)
- Iodinated contrast, unfractionated heparin, protamine

The sequence of steps in Watchman deployment are as follows:

- TEE imaging for LAA dimension analysis and device size selection (Figure 29.3).
- Femoral venous access with a skin incision large enough to accommodate a 14-F sheath.
- Heparin administration to a target ACT > 250 s.
- Trans-septal puncture using a standard sheath (crossing low on the septum).
- Sheath exchange to the 14-F access sheath using the stiff exchange guidewire advanced in one of the PVs.
- Removal of guidewire/dilator with care to avoid retained air within the access sheath.
- Placement and advancement of the pigtail catheter to the end of the access sheath.
- Engagement of the LAA using the pigtail catheter (contrast can be used to assess progress).
- Advancement of the access sheath over the pigtail catheter aligning the appropriate radiopaque marker band (corresponding to the device size) at the ostium of the LAA (Figure 29.4).
- Visualization of the LAA in multiple views with angiography (anteroposterior: AP — cranial, right anterior oblique: RAO — 30° cranial 20°, RAO 30°, RAO 30° caudal 20°) and TEE (0°, 45°, 90°, 135°: roughly corresponding to the aforementioned fluoroscopic views) (Figure 29.5).

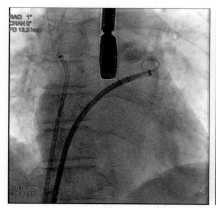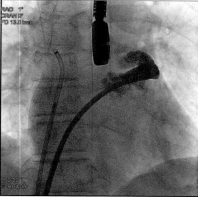

Figure 29.4 Pigtail catheter inside the LAA with the distal radiopaque marker band at the level of the LAA ostium (21 mm device).

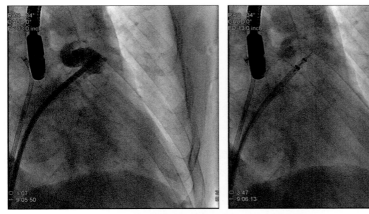

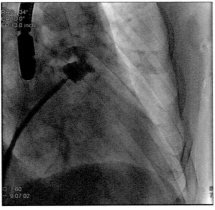

Figure 29.5 Successful deployment of a Watchman device (RAO 30° projection).

- Thoroughly flush the delivery system, making sure the device is aligned to the distal marker band of the containment sheath.
- Removal/exchange of the pigtail catheter with the delivery system (containment sheath/device).
- Advancement of the device until the fluoroscopic marker band located on the containment sheath is aligned to the marker band located distally on the access sheath.
- Retract the access sheath until snapped onto the containment sheath.
- Withdrawal of access/containment sheath assembly while maintaining the device in place until fully deployed (Figure 29.5).
- Before device release, four criteria should be met:
  - *position, assessed with TEE/fluoroscopy*: Device should span the entire LAA ostium, with the maximum device diameter at or distal to the LAA ostium, not protruding too far into the LA (Figures 29.5 and 29.6).
  - If device deployment is too distal, it may be partially recaptured and repositioned:
    - Maintain the device in position while advancing the containment sheath over the device up to (but not beyond) the level of the fixation hooks.
    - Withdraw the containment sheath to the desired position before proceeding to device deployment, as before.

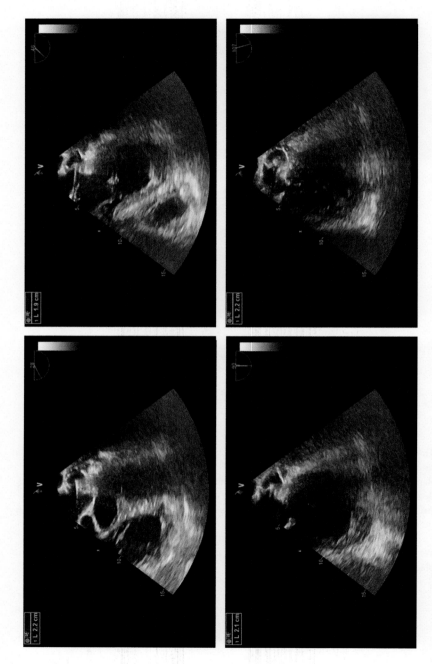

Figure 29.6 Measurement of the maximum WATCHMAN diameter in the LAA (24-mm device).

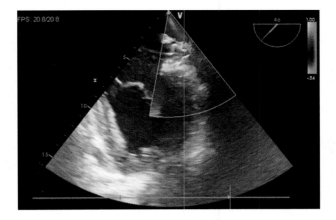

Figure 29.7 Color Doppler showing no peri-device flow.

- If the device is too proximal or sizing/position is suboptimal, it is necessary to fully recapture the device:
  - Advance the containment/delivery sheath assembly beyond the fixation hooks, then withdrawing the device until its distal tines are proximal to the marker band.
  - A new delivery system can be used through the existing 14-F access sheath.
- *stability, assessed with a "tug test"*: Gentle traction on the proximal device post is applied until tactile feedback (sensation of heartbeat) and mild device deformity on TEE and/or fluoroscopy are demonstrated.
- *size, assessed with TEE*: The device widest diameter should be compressed 8%–20% of its original size (e.g., for a 24-mm device, measured width of 19.2–22.1 mm) (Figure 29.6).
- *complete occlusion, assessed with TEE/fluoroscopy*: All LAA lobes should be distal to the proximal face of the device, and with contrast/color Doppler, any peri-device residual flow must be <5 mm (Figure 29.7).
- Once the aforementioned criteria are met, the device can be released by unscrewing the device proximal post with counterclockwise rotation (usually 3–5 rotations).
- Device release is confirmed with angiography and TEE (Figure 29.8).
- Withdrawal of access/containment sheath assembly back into the right atrium.
- Heparin reversal with protamine, as needed.

POST-PROCEDURE

After the procedure, the patient must be placed on acetylsalicylic acid (ASA) 81–100 mg and warfarin with a target INR of 2.0–3.0 for 45 days. A TEE is then required to confirm device placement and adequacy of closure. Any peri-device flow of >5 mm or device thrombus is considered an indication for continued treatment with warfarin. If adequate seal is confirmed, warfarin is discontinued and dual antiplatelet therapy with ASA and clopidogrel 75 mg daily is prescribed for 4.5 months (6 months after the procedure), after which ASA 300–325 mg is usually continued indefinitely.

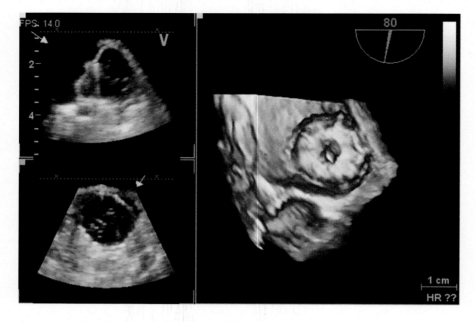

Figure 29.8 3D TEE showing a released Watchman well positioned in the LAA.

LARIAT

LAA closure with the Lariat device is a combined endo-epicardial procedure that allows epicardial LAA ligation with no foreign objects left in the endocardial space. There are five necessary components to perform this procedure: a 12-F Lariat suture delivery device, consisting of a collapsible 40-mm snare with a non-absorbable, size 0 braided polyester pre-tied suture (Figure 29.9); a 15-mm compliant occlusion balloon catheter; two magnet-tipped guidewires (0.025″ and 0.035″) (Figure 29.10); a suture tightener; and a suture cutter.

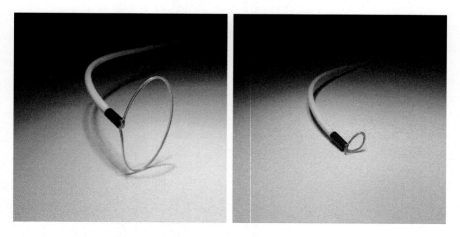

Figure 29.9 Lariat suture delivery device (polyester suture in blue).

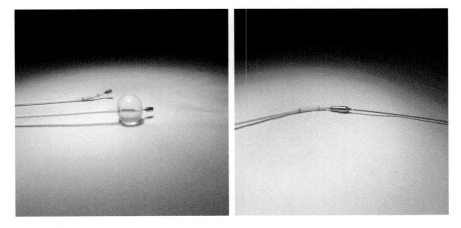

Figure 29.10 Epicardial magnet-tipped wire (top) and endocardial magnet-tipped wire positioned inside the occlusion balloon catheter (bottom); wires magnetically bound.

PRE-PROCEDURE

Because the LAA must be accessed from both the endocardium and epicardium (using an intact pericardium), the patients should be asked about any prior history of heart surgery, pericarditis, or radiation therapy to the chest. These are contraindication to the Lariat procedure, as they render the patient unsuitable for epicardial instrumentation.

For Lariat, LAA imaging with CT is necessary because, besides providing a detailed assessment of LAA morphology, it reveals its relationship with other thoracic structures. More specifically, it is important to evaluate:

- *LAA maximum width*: It should not be >40 mm (exceeding the snare diameter).
- *LAA position*: It should not be oriented posteriorly, with the LAA apex behind to the pulmonary artery (PA).
- *LAA morphology*: It should not consist of multiple lobes oriented in different planes exceeding 40 mm.

On the procedure day, the patient undergoes a TEE to exclude pre-existing thrombus in the LAA.

PROCEDURE

The procedure is usually under general anesthesia and guided by fluoroscopy and TEE. The deployment of the Lariat suture requires three hands; thus, two operators have to be present: the primary operator with either an assistant or an experienced scrub technician. Anticoagulation therapy is stopped before the procedure and antibiotic prophylaxis is administered prior to the procedure.

The following equipment should be available:

- Fluoroscopy and ultrasound (with TEE probe) machine
- Venous introducers
- *Trans-septal access*: Long J-tipped guidewire, 9–9.5-F sheath with dilator, trans-septal needle, pressurized heparinized saline bag
- *Epicardial access*: A 17-gauge blunt-tip epidural needle (Tuohy) or a micropuncture set (21-gauge needle, long J-tipped 0.018" soft guidewire, 4-F sheath/dilator), long J-tipped 0.035" soft guidewire, 14-F sheath with dilator

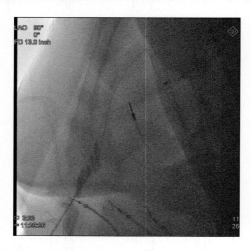

Figure 29.11 Anterior epicardial access with the epicardial wire advancing anterior to the RV (LL projection).

- *Lariat kit*: 15-mm balloon catheter, 0.025" and 0.035" magnet-tipped guidewires, 12-F suture delivery device, suture tightener, suture cutter
- Iodinated contrast, unfractionated heparin, protamine

The steps involved in Lariat closure are as follows:

- Fluoroscopy-guided anterior epicardial access with a sub-xiphoid puncture; a left lateral (LL) view is required to confirm guidewire advancement anterior to the right ventricle (RV) (Figure 29.11).
- Sequential dilation of the puncture site to comfortably place the 14-F epicardial sheath in the pericardial space.
- Femoral venous access.
- Heparin administration with a target ACT > 250 s.
- Trans-septal puncture (preferably low) and advancement of the long sheath into the LA, directed anteriorly toward the LAA.
- Exchange of the guidewire/dilator with the endocardial balloon/0.025" magnet-tipped guidewire assembly.
- Advancement of endocardial magnet-tipped guidewire toward LAA, with the tip placed at the apex (contrast can be used to assess progress) (Figure 29.12).
- Advancement of epicardial 0.035" magnet-tipped guidewire toward the LAA until it magnetically binds to the endocardial guidewire.
- Visualization of the LAA with angiography and/or TEE (preferably with multiple views, i.e., AP, RAO 30° cranial 20°, RAO 30°, RAO 30° caudal 20; a sweep from 0° to 135°).
- Advancement of the 15-mm balloon over the endocardial guidewire at the ostium of the LAA and inflation with a mix of 1:1 saline and contrast for fluoroscopic and/or TEE confirmation of its ostial location.
- Insertion and advancement of the 12-F suture delivery device over the epicardial guidewire until the snare is positioned over the ostium of the LAA (making sure the snare is at the level of the radiopaque marker proximal to the inflated balloon) (Figure 29.13).

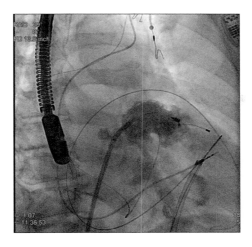

Figure 29.12 Endocardial magnet-tipped wire advanced at the tip of the LAA.

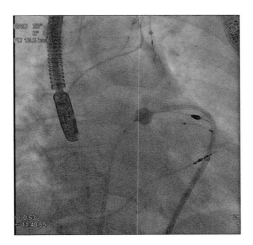

Figure 29.13 Snare at the level of the LAA ostium as evidenced by its position relative to the endocardial balloon.

- Closure of the snare at the LAA ostium.
- Confirmation of proper LAA occlusion by angiography and/or TEE (multiple views) (Figure 29.14).
- Withdrawal of the endocardial balloon/magnet-tipped guidewire assembly out of the LAA.
- Suture deployment from the snare and tightening with the dedicated suture tightener (2 applications, 5 minutes apart).

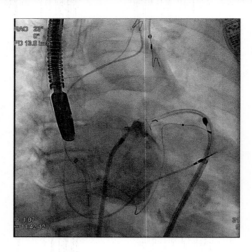

Figure 29.14 Complete LAA occlusion after closure of the snare and suture tightening.

- Final confirmation of proper LAA occlusion by angiography and/or TEE (Figure 29.15).
- Cutting of the red suture-release tab, that is withdrawn from the LAA with the snare completely open.
- Retraction of the suture delivery device and magnet-tipped guidewire from the epicardial space.
- Advancement of the suture cutting device into the epicardial access sheath; cutting of the suture tail near the LAA ostium.
- Exchange of the epicardial sheath with a standard pericardial drain.
- Retraction of the trans-septal catheter to the RA/inferior vena cava.
- Heparin reversal with protamine, as needed.

POST-PROCEDURE

The pericardial drain is kept in place overnight and transthoracic echocardiography is performed to rule out any pericardial effusion before its removal. Colchicine (0.3–0.6 mg twice daily) is recommended for at least 2 weeks following the procedure to mitigate the inflammatory response post-LAA ligation.

There is no consensus on post-procedural antithrombotic regimen (anticoagulation/antiplatelet therapy), thus this is usually left to the operator/patient preference. TEE follow-up by 90 days is highly recommended to assess for residual or de novo leaks, which might require reinitiation of OAC or their closure with other percutaneous approaches.

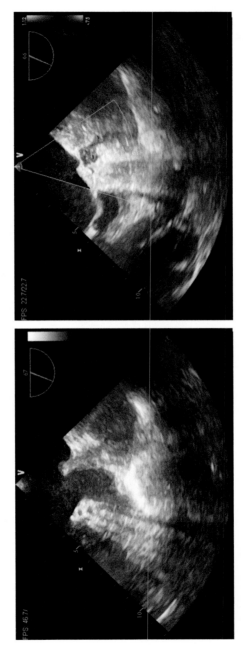

Figure 29.15　Complete LAA occlusion as assessed with TEE.

The AtriClip device is a self-closing clamp that compresses the base of the LAA from the epicardial side (Figure 29.16). It contains two parallel rigid titanium tubes covered by carbothane with a flexible nitinol alloy spring. This frame is covered by a polyester fabric and is manufactured in four sizes (35, 40, 45, and 50 mm). This device is suitable for closure of LAAs between 29 and 50 mm (measured along the mitral valve axis).

Briefly, the device may be applied to the LAA as a concomitant element of an open chest surgical procedure or by means of less invasive approaches such as a limited thoracotomy or thoracoscopy.

With thoracoscopy, the AtripClip device is deployed in the following steps:

- Intubation with dual-lumen endotracheal tube, to allow selective deflation of left bronchus
- Sterile prep of left chest
- Placement of three left thoracoscopic access ports for video imaging and instrument placement; one port must be large enough for insertion of the AtriClip delivery system
- Deflation of left lung

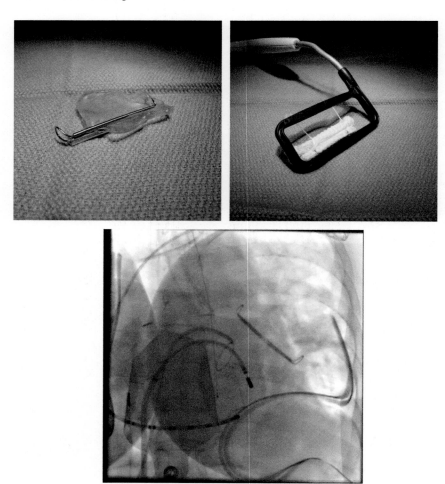

Figure 29.16   AtriClip LAA occlusion device.

- Pericardial access performed under direct videoscopic imaging with care to avoid the left phrenic nerve
- Exposure of the LAA, upon which a measuring device is used to gauge LAA dimension and select the appropriate AtriClip device size
- Insertion of the device through the dedicated chest port
- Placement of the device near the base of the LAA (a maneuver involving gentle prodding/guiding of the LAA into the device)
- Active closure of the device
- TEE confirmation of adequate device positioning/LAA closure
- Release of the restraining sutures on the device
- Removal of the delivery system from the LAA and out of the chest port
- Suture closure of the pericardium
- Re-inflation of the left lung
- Surgical closure of two chest ports, with a chest drain left in one of the ports post-operatively and monitored until any residual thoracic air leak resolves

GENERAL CONSIDERATIONS

While these three LAA closure strategies ultimately close the LAA to prevent cardioembolic events, based on available data (see Table 29.2), several differences should be pointed out between these strategies.

Table 29.2 Major left atrial appendage closure studies[a]

Device	Author, year (study name)	Design	N	Follow-up (average)	Procedure-related complications	Incomplete closure
Watchman	Holmes, 2009[13] Reddy, 2013[14] (PROTECT-AF)	RCT	463	2.3 years	7.4%	32.1% at 1 year[24]
	Reddy, 2011[27] (CAP)	Obs	460	0.4 years	3.7%	NA
	Reddy, 2013[33] (ASAP)	Obs	150	14.4 months	8.7%	NA
	Holmes, 2014[15] (PREVAIL)	RCT	407	18 months	4.7%	NA
Lariat	Bartus, 2014[20]	Obs	89	1 year	3.3%	2%
	Miller, 2014[21]	Obs	41	3.3 months	NA	24%
	Price, 2014[22]	Obs	154	112 days	9.7%	20%
	Pillarisetti, 2015[23]	Obs	259	1 year	NA	13%
	Gianni, 2016[25]	Obs	98	16 months	9%	20% at 1 year
AtriClip	Salzberg, 2010[16]	Obs	34[b]	3 months	8.8%[c]	0%
	Ailawadi, 2011[17]	Obs	71[b]	3 months	48.6%[c]	1.6%
	Emmert, 2014[18]	Obs	40[b]	3.5 years	10%	0%
	Mokraceck, 2015[19]	Obs	30	3 months	0%	0%

[a] Definition varies between studies.
[b] Thoracotomy.
[c] Not device-related.
Obs: observational trial; RCT: randomized clinical trial.

INDICATIONS

In the PROTECT-AF and PREVAIL trials, the Watchman device was studied in patients who were clinically eligible for warfarin therapy and whose clinical history of AF would otherwise warrant long-term OAC therapy.[13-15] The device was studied in comparison to a control group of patients who were instructed to remain on warfarin. In the device group, warfarin was still required for at least 45 days following the procedure, replaced with clopidogrel at if a TEE confirmed adequate closure of the LAA. Therefore, the FDA has approved this device for patients who are eligible to take warfarin therapy but who also possess relative contraindications to chronic OAC use.

In stark contrast, the Lariat device as well as the AtriClip device were developed specifically for LAA closure but were FDA-approved as a general closure device (i.e., a tissue approximation device for structures of ≤40 mm, and 29–50 mm, respectively). These devices demonstrated acceptable safety outcomes.[16-23] However, efficacy in the prevention of strokes was largely inferred from other published LAA closure strategies (primarily from the Watchman data). Despite the current paucity of efficacy data on stroke prevention, the rationale that inspired these devices is likely correct. Furthermore, these devices close the LAA in a fairly predictable fashion without leaving any foreign object in the vascular space. As such, OAC is generally not considered necessary either before or after a Lariat or AtriClip LAA closure. Because of this, most implanters and insurance providers would consider this approach more suitable for patients with absolute contraindication for OAC. Of note, the AtriClip device must be inserted through a trans-thoracic surgical approach: only patients deemed healthy enough for this invasive procedure may be considered.

INCOMPLETE CLOSURE

While each of these LAA closure strategies is intended to completely close the LAA, incomplete closure is seen with all of these approaches. Watchman device leaks have been demonstrated in 41% of patients at the 45-day TEE and 32% of patients at the follow-up TEE at 12 months.[24] Watchman leaks occur along the edge of the device and have been reported when no leak was seen at implant. This may be due to inadequate device contact with a portion of the LAA ostial surface either because of device angulation, LAA shape, and orientation, or both. The Lariat device too has demonstrated residual leaks as well during the postimplantation TEE, with a prevalence as high as 24% at follow-up.[20-23,25] Unlike Watchman, these them are central and usually small (≤5 mm). While no publication describes the impact or treatment strategy for such leaks, some implanters have chosen to close them (for example, with atrial septal defect closure devices or coils) or to leave the patient on OACs.[26] Few data are available on AtriClip positioned via thoracoscopy, however, regardless of the approach, the device appears to be highly successful in complete closure (>95%).[16-19]

COMPLICATIONS

Acute and late complications remain a major source of concern for each of these device strategies. With the Watchman device, acute complications include LAA/cardiac perforation, air or clot emboli, and device embolization. Late complications include thrombus formation on the surface of the device and one report of erosion of the device into the PA. Among early device implants in the PROTECT AF trial, acute bleeding resulting in cardiac tamponade was observed in 10% of procedures.[27] These often required percutaneous drainage or surgical repair. The source of the complication was believed to be related to trans-septal access or mechanical trauma to the LAA from engagement with a guidewire, a deflectable catheter or the access sheath. After procedure modifications prohibiting LAA engagement with any tool other than a pigtail or the delivery sheath, and likely as a learning curve effect, the observed bleeding incidence dropped to 6% range. While embolization has been reported, strict compression criteria prior to device release has resulted in few migrated devices.

With the Lariat device, acute complications have been almost exclusively bleeding in nature. While the endocardial portion of the procedure exposes the same bleeding sources that have been reported with the Watchman procedure, epicardial access exposing to an added risk of bleeding. Percutaneous epicardial access involves needle insertion below the xiphoid process and advancing superiorly and leftward to gain access to the pericardium anterior to the right ventricle. As the needle is advanced, accidental puncture or trauma of the liver, sternal vessels (including the left internal mammary artery), pericardial vessels, and the right ventricle itself can occur. Despite observation of the guidewire in the pericardial space prior to sheath advancement, it remains possible to accidentally puncture the RV in a through and through (mattress stitch) fashion. If this occurs and is unrecognized, advancement of the sheath will result in two holes in the RV, which would likely necessitate surgical repair. Finally, as the needle enters the pericardial space, it remains possible to lacerate the RV free wall with the sharp edge of the needle before the guidewire is inserted. This complication can be minimized by holding ventilation briefly (apnea) until the guidewire can be inserted past the needle into the epicardial space. Late complications of Lariat closure include clinically significant effusions, usually non-hemorrhagic and believed to be the result of intense inflammatory process secondary to LAA necrosis, and thrombosis at the site of ligation, likely due to acute endothelial injury.[21,22,28] For the latter reason, some centers advocate for dual antiplatelet therapy or OAC for 6 weeks, until TEE confirms complete closure and no thrombosis.

In the published AtriClip studies, no complications have been reported that were attributed to the device itself.[16–19] However, procedure-related complications can occur. For stand-alone thoracoscopic procedures, these might include CVA, prolonged thoracic air leak, bleeding requiring conversion to open thoracotomy and refractory heart failure.[29]

ELECTRICAL ISOLATION
The LAA has been shown to be a trigger for AF initiation and maintenance. As a result, ablation and isolation of the structure have been performed as a means of ablating AF.[30] Of the three closure procedures listed, LAA electrical isolation has been demonstrated to occur with the Lariat and AtriClip approaches, but not with the Watchman.[31,32] While further trials are needed to validate the LAA isolation strategy, concomitant electrical isolation during the process of LAA closure may prove to offer the added benefit of surreptitious elimination of one source of AF generation.

CONCLUSION

In summary, there are three mechanical devices available in the US for LAA closure, thereby preventing thrombus formation and/or its embolization from the LAA to the systemic circulation.

The Watchman device has been extensively studied for both safety and efficacy standpoints in comparison to warfarin therapy. Further studies are needed in the OAC contraindicated patient population as well as comparisons of device efficacy with NOAC therapy.

Because the Lariat and AtriClip devices were FDA approved for general tissue approximation, all uses are, by definition, off-label. As such, further prospective efficacy data is needed to provide validation that closure of the LAA with either of these two devices offer comparable stroke reduction as compared to Watchman. Compared to Lariat, the AtriClip device appears to have a higher complete closure rate, but a high incidence of complications associated with the thoracoscopic access limits its use in isolated closure procedures.

REFERENCES

1. Colilla S, Crow A, Petkun W, et al. Estimates of current and future incidence and prevalence of atrial fibrillation in the US adult population. *Am J Cardiol.* 2013;112(8):1142–1147. doi:10.1016/j.amjcard.2013.05.063.

2. Wolf PA, Abbott RD, Kannel WB. Atrial fibrillation as an independent risk factor for stroke: The Framingham Study. *Stroke.* 1991;22(8):983–988. doi:10.1161/01.STR.22.8.983.

3. Johnson WD, Ganjoo AK, Stone CD, et al. The left atrial appendage: Our most lethal human attachment! surgical implications. *Eur J Cardio thoracic Surg.* 2000;17(6):718–722. doi:10.1016/S1010-7940(00)00419-X.

4. Madden JL. Resection of the left auricular appendix: A prophylaxis for recurrent arterial emboli. *J Am Med Assoc.* 1949;140(9):769–772. doi:10.1001/jama.1949.02900440011003.

5. Beal JM, Longmire WP, Leake WH. Resection of the auricular appendages. *Ann Surg.* 1950;132(3):517–527. doi:10.1378/chest.19.3.307.

6. Nishimura RA, Otto CM, Bonow RO, et al. 2014 AHA/ACC guideline for the management of patients with valvular heart disease: Executive summary: A report of the American college of cardiology/American heart association task force on practice guidelines. *J Am Coll Cardiol.* 2014;63(22):2438–2488. doi:10.1016/j.jacc.2014.02.537.

7. January CT, Wann LS, Alpert JS, et al. 2014 AHA/ACC/HRS guideline for the management of patients with atrial fibrillation: A report of the American college of cardiology/American heart association task force on practice guidelines and the heart rhythm society. *Circulation.* 2014;130(23):e199–e267. doi:10.1161/CIR.0000000000000041.

8. Connolly SJ, Ezekowitz MD, Yusuf S, et al. Dabigatran versus warfarin in patients with atrial fibrillation. *N Engl J Med.* 2009;361(12):1139–1151. doi:10.1056/NEJMoa0905561.

9. Patel MR, Mahaffey KW, Garg J, et al. Rivaroxaban versus warfarin in nonvalvular atrial fibrillation. *N Engl J Med.* 2011;365(10):883–891. doi:10.1056/NEJMoa1009638.

10. Granger CB, Alexander JH, McMurray JJ V, et al. Apixaban versus warfarin in patients with atrial fibrillation. *N Engl J Med.* 2011;365(11):981–992. doi:10.1056/NEJMoa1107039.

11. Giugliano RP, Ruff CT, Braunwald E, et al. Edoxaban versus warfarin in patients with atrial fibrillation. *N Engl J Med.* 2013;369(22):2093–2104. doi:10.1056/NEJMoa1310907.

12. Lewalter T, Ibrahim R, Albers B, Camm AJ. An update and current expert opinions on percutaneous left atrial appendage occlusion for stroke prevention in atrial fibrillation. *Europace.* 2013;15(5):652–656. doi:10.1093/europace/eut043.

13. Holmes DR, Reddy VY, Turi ZG, et al. Percutaneous closure of the left atrial appendage versus warfarin therapy for prevention of stroke in patients with atrial fibrillation: A randomised non-inferiority trial. *Lancet.* 2009;374(9689):534–542. doi:10.1016/S0140-6736(09)61343-X.

14. Reddy VY, Doshi SK, Sievert H, et al. Percutaneous left atrial appendage closure for stroke prophylaxis in patients with atrial fibrillation 2.3-year follow-up of the PROTECT AF (Watchman left atrial appendage system for embolic protection in patients with atrial fibrillation) trial. *Circulation.* 2013;127(6):720–729. doi:10.1161/CIRCULATIONAHA.112.114389.

15. Holmes DR, Kar S, Price MJ, et al. Prospective randomized evaluation of the watchman left atrial appendage closure device in patients with atrial fibrillation versus long-term warfarin therapy: The PREVAIL trial. *J Am Coll Cardiol.* 2014;64(1):1–12. doi:10.1016/j.jacc.2014.04.029.

16. Salzberg SP, Plass A, Emmert MY, et al. Left atrial appendage clip occlusion: Early clinical results. *J Thorac Cardiovasc Surg*. 2010;139(5):1269–1274. doi:10.1016/j.jtcvs.2009.06.033.

17. Ailawadi G, Gerdisch MW, Harvey RL, et al. Exclusion of the left atrial appendage with a novel device: Early results of a multicenter trial. *J Thorac Cardiovasc Surg*. 2011;142(5):1002–1009, 1009.e1. doi:10.1016/j.jtcvs.2011.07.052.

18. Emmert MY, Puippe G, Baumüller S, et al. Safe, effective and durable epicardial left atrial appendage clip occlusion in patients with atrial fibrillation undergoing cardiac surgery: First long-term results from a prospective device trial. *Eur J Cardio-Thorac Surg*. 2014;45(1):126–131. doi:10.1093/ejcts/ezt204.

19. Mokracek A, Kurfirst V, Bulava A, et al. Thoracoscopic occlusion of the left atrial appendage. *Innov Technol Tech Cardiothorac Vasc Surg*. 2015;10(3):179–182. doi:10.1097/IMI.0000000000000169.

20. Bartus K, Han FT, Bednarek J, et al. Percutaneous left atrial appendage suture ligation using the Lariat device in patients with atrial fibrillation: Initial clinical experience. *J Am Coll Cardiol*. 2013;62(2):108–118. doi:10.1016/j.jacc.2012.06.046.

21. Miller MA, Gangireddy SR, Doshi SK, et al. Multicenter study on acute and long-term safety and efficacy of percutaneous left atrial appendage closure using an epicardial suture snaring device. *Hear Rhythm*. 2014;11(11):1853–1859. doi:10.1016/j.hrthm.2014.07.032.

22. Price MJ, Gibson DN, Yakubov SJ, et al. Early safety and efficacy of percutaneous left atrial appendage suture ligation. *J Am Coll Cardiol*. 2014;64(6):565–572. doi:10.1016/j.jacc.2014.03.057.

23. Pillarisetti J, Reddy YM, Gunda S, et al. Endocardial (Watchman) vs epicardial (Lariat) left atrial appendage exclusion devices: Understanding the differences in the location and type of leaks and their clinical implications. *Hear Rhythm*. 2015. doi:10.1016/j.hrthm.2015.03.020.

24. Viles-Gonzalez JF, Kar S, Douglas P, et al. The clinical impact of incomplete left atrial appendage closure with the Watchman device in patients with atrial fibrillation. *J Am Coll Cardiol*. 2012;59(10):923–929. doi:10.1016/j.jacc.2011.11.028.

25. Gianni C, Di Biase L, Trivedi C, et al. Clinical implications of leaks following left atrial appendage ligation with the Lariat device. *JACC Cardiovasc Interv*. 2016;9(10):1051–1057. doi:10.1016/j.jcin.2016.01.038.

26. Sahore A, Della Rocca DG, Anannab A, et al. Clinical implications and management strategies for left atrial appendage leaks. *Card Electrophysiol Clin*. 2020;12(1):89–96. doi:10.1016/j.ccep.2019.11.010.

27. Reddy VY, Holmes D, Doshi SK, et al. Safety of percutaneous left atrial appendage closure: Results from the Watchman left atrial appendage system for embolic protection in patients with AF (PROTECT AF) clinical trial and the continued access registry. *Circulation*. 2011;123(4):417–424. doi:10.1161/CIRCULATIONAHA.110.976449.

28. Lakkireddy D, Reddy YM, Di Biase L, et al. Feasibility and safety of uninterrupted rivaroxaban for periprocedural anticoagulation in patients undergoing radiofrequency ablation for atrial fibrillation: Results from a multicenter prospective registry. *J Am Coll Cardiol*. 2014;63(10):982–988. doi:10.1016/j.jacc.2013.11.039.

29. Blackshear JL, Johnson WD, Odell JA, et al. Thoracoscopic extracardiac obliteration of the left atrial appendage for stroke risk reduction in atrial fibrillation. *J Am Coll Cardiol*. 2003;42(7):1249–1252. doi:10.1016/S0735-1097(03)00953-7.

30. Di Biase L, Burkhardt JD, Mohanty P, et al. Left atrial appendage: An underrecognized trigger site of atrial fibrillation. *Circulation*. 2010;122(2):109–118. doi:10.1161/CIRCULATIONAHA.109.928903.

31. Fumoto H, Gillinov AM, Ootaki Y, et al. A novel device for left atrial appendage exclusion: The third-generation atrial exclusion device. *J Thorac Cardiovasc Surg.* 2008;136(4):1019–1027. doi:10.1016/j.jtcvs.2008.06.002.

32. Han FT, Bartus K, Lakkireddy D, et al. The effects of LAA ligation on LAA electrical activity. *Hear Rhythm.* 2014;11(5):864–870. doi:10.1016/j.hrthm.2014.01.019.

33. Reddy VY, Möbius-Winkler S, Miller MA, et al. Left atrial appendage closure with the Watchman device in patients with a contraindication for oral anticoagulation: The ASAP study (ASA plavix feasibility study with Watchman left atrial appendage closure technology). *J Am Coll Cardiol.* 2013;61(25):2551–2556. doi:10.1016/j.jacc.2013.03.035.

ECG FEATURES OF NORMAL HEART PVCs

Robert D. Schaller

CONTENTS

INTRODUCTION

Idiopathic premature ventricular complexes (PVC) are a common phenomenon observed in patients with structurally normal hearts.[1] They are frequently benign and most patients can initially be managed conservatively. If bothersome symptoms persist or the frequent nature of the PVCs has led to a potentially reversible left ventricular (LV) dilatation or a depression in systolic function, suppression with medication or percutaneous catheter ablation is recommended.[2] In the case of the latter, accurate and precise localization of the origin of the PVCs is crucial in order to provide peri-procedural counseling to the patient. The anticipated origin of the PVC may have important implications regarding the likelihood of success, the potential of damage to adjacent structures, and the vascular approach and tools used during the procedure. In patients with normal hearts, the 12-lead electrocardiogram (ECG) is a valuable tool that allows for precise and predictable localization of PVC origin, frequently to within a few millimeters.

ANATOMIC CONSIDERATIONS

There are myriad of factors that may influence PVC morphology other than structural heart disease including patient age, sex, heart rotation and location in the chest, prior cardiac and thoracic surgery, and the position and angle of the ascending aorta.

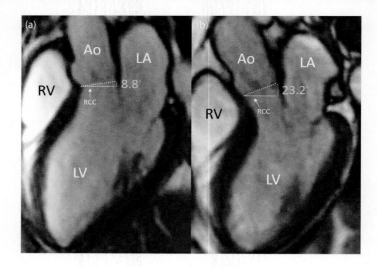

Figure 30.1 Magnetic resonance imaging (MRI) of the left ventricular outflow tract (LVOT) of a 21-year-old woman (a) and 71-year-old woman (b). Note the vertical orientation of the aorta (Ao) in relation to the LVOT in the younger patient as compared to the more horizontal orientation of the older patient. RV: Right ventricle, LA: left atrium, RCC: right coronary cusp, LV: left ventricle. (Courtesy of David Lin, MD.)

Age-related structural changes are common and should be taken into consideration when interpreting PVC morphology. Older patients may have uncoiling of the aortic root with an aortic valve in a vertical position while younger patients frequently have more vertical hearts; both of which can dramatically change the vector of depolarization in relation to the standard 12-lead ECG (Figure 30.1). Maeda et al. have shown that age-related changes in outflow tract anatomy affect pace maps created from the aortic cusp region; specifically, older patients had higher maximal R-wave amplitude in the inferior leads, specifically lead III, when pacing from the left coronary cusp (LCC) versus the right coronary cusp (RCC).[3] 3-Dimensional imaging with cardiac magnetic resonance imaging (MRI), computed tomography (CT), and real-time ultrasound (US) can help to identify variations in patient anatomy that may have implications on PVC origin.

ECG algorithms used for localizing PVCs assume that the limb and precordial leads are in the correct anatomical positions. Small changes in electrocardiographic electrode placement can markedly alter the QRS morphology making proper lead position imperative. Anter et al. have shown that in patients with outflow tract PVCs, superior displacement of leads V1 and V2 can decrease R-wave amplitude while inferior displacement resulted in increased R-wave amplitude and even create a right bundle branch (RBBB) pattern with PVCs from the aortic cusp region. Additionally, anterior displacement of the arm leads from shoulders to chest resulted in the reduction in R-wave amplitude in lead I.[4]

MORPHOLOGICAL CHARACTERISTICS

RIGHT VENTRICULAR OUTFLOW TRACT (RVOT)

RVOT PVCs are the most common type of ventricular ectopy, accounting for approximately 75% of cases and have a characteristic left bundle branch block (LBBB) pattern with an inferior axis and a precordial transition by lead V3 or V4.[5] Jadonath et al. devised a numbering

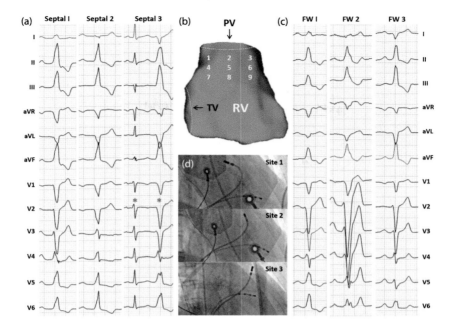

Figure 30.2 (a) PVCs arising from the septal RVOT manifest with a left bundle branch block (LBBB) morphology, inferior axis, and a precordial transition at V3 or V4. Note the earlier transition of the sinus rhythm (asterisk) QRS as compared to the PVC as well as a V2 transition ratio ≤0.60 suggesting origin in the RVOT rather than the left ventricular outflow tract (LVOT). (b) Electro-anatomic map of the right ventricle. Numbers indicate the nine sites in the right ventricular outflow tract (RVOT), which produce distinct characteristic morphologies. (c) PVCs arising from the free wall of the RVOT manifest with a LBBB morphology, inferior axis, and a precordial transition at ≥V4. These PVCs tend to be "notched" and wider than their septal counterparts. (d) Position of the ablation catheter at the most common sites (1–3) in a right anterior oblique (RAO) view. PV: Pulmonic valve, TV: tricuspid valve, FW: free wall, RV: right ventricle.

system, which divided the septal RVOT into nine sites in a right anterior oblique (RAO) fluoroscopic view (Figure 30.2b).[6] Despite close anatomical proximity, each region has discrete morphologic characteristics (Figure 30.2a):

- Lead I is used to differentiate anterior from posterior locations within the RVOT (Figure 30.2d).
  - An R wave in lead I is consistent with a posterior location (site 1).
  - A deep Q wave in lead 1 with a deeper QRS in lead aVL relative to aVR is consistent with an extreme anterior and leftward location (site 3).
    - This morphology is due to the RVOT wrapping anteriorly and leftward of the aortic root.
  - An intermediate location (site 2) typically manifests as multiphasic or flat in lead I.
- A QS pattern in aVR and a monophasic R wave in the inferior leads are seen in almost all patients.
- Sites 4–6 and 7–9 correlate to more caudal locations along the RVOT and manifest with lower amplitude R waves in the inferior leads.

Dixit et al. applied the same numbering system to the free wall of the RVOT in order to delineate these sites from their corresponding septal locations.[7]

R wave amplitude in lead I is still used to predict posterior versus anterior sites along the free wall. As compared to their septal counterparts, free wall sites manifest as such (Figure 30.2c):

- Monophasic R waves in the inferior leads that are smaller and wider.
- "Notching" is frequently present in the inferior leads.
- Precordial transition occurs later, typically in V5 or V6.

While most RVOT PVCs originate from the subvalvular region, myocardial tissue can be found up to 2 cm above the pulmonic valve (PV).[8] Multiple studies have found that PVCs can be successfully mapped and ablated above the PV.[9-13] These PVCs tend to have greater voltage in the inferior leads compared to their RVOT counterparts. Specifically, a cutoff value of more than 18 mV in lead II allows identification of an origin within the PA with 63% sensitivity, 69% specificity.

Other clues as to a supra-valvular origin include[13]:

- Larger R/S ratio in lead V2
- Larger aVL/aVR ratio of Q wave amplitude

Additionally, Tada et al. have also described a dynamic change in morphology after ablation in the RVOT with a significant increase in inferior lead voltage requiring further mapping and ablation above the PV.[11]

TRICUSPID VALVE (TV)

Recent studies have elucidated the differences between RVOT PVCs and ones originating from the TV.[14-18] In one series,[14] Van Herendal et al. demonstrated that 5% of all PVCs from the RV were mapped to the TV annulus with the free wall portion the preferential site of origin.

TV PVCs have a LBBB pattern with an R or r in lead I (Figure 30.3). R wave magnitude in lead I is greater in PVCs arising from the TV than the RVOT due to the location of the RV to the right and basal to the RVOT. Similarly, PVCs from the top of the TV are directed less inferiorly than PVCs arising from the RVOT. While most PVCs from this region are inferiorly directed, there is disparity depending on which segment of the TA it is originating from. PVCs from various locations along the TV manifest as such:

- Anterior/top of the TV (Figure 30.3a):
  - Positive in II, III, and aVF with lead II > III.
  - Deeper Q wave in aVR than aVL.
  - Precordial transition by V3 or V4.
- Posterolateral aspect of the TV (Figure 30.3c):
  - Positive in lead II and negative in lead III with a greater disparity between leads aVR and aVL.
  - Compared to their septal counterparts, PVCs from the free wall tend to be wider, have deeper S waves in leads V1–V3, and are more likely to show "notching" of the mid or late component of the QRS complex.
  - Later transition by V5 or V6.
- Posterior/bottom of the TV (Figure 30.3c):
  - Exhibit negativity in all inferior leads with greater negativity in lead III than lead II.
  - Transition between V4 and V5.

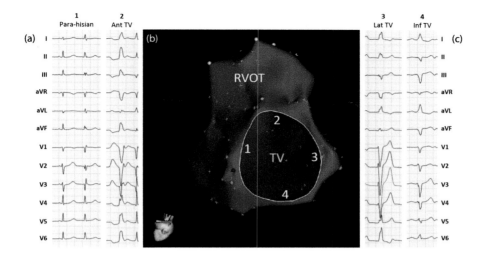

Figure 30.3 (a) Septal para-Hisian and anterior tricuspid valve (TV) PVCs. Note how narrow the para-Hisian PVC is due to its proximity to the conduction system. Lead II > III is characteristic in this region. (b) 3D electro-anatomical voltage map of the right ventricle (RV) pictured in a posterior view. (c) PVCs from the lateral wall of the TV tend to be wider than their septal counterparts frequently with "notching" within the QRS and a precordial transition at ≥V5. Note leads II and aVL (left-sided) are completely positive and leads III and aVR (right-sided) are completely negative. PVCs from the bottom of the TV show a similar R wave in lead I with QR complexes in the inferior leads and a late precordial transition. RVOT: Right ventricular outflow tract, Ant TV: anterior tricuspid valve, Lat TV: lateral tricuspid valve, Inf TV: inferior tricuspid valve.

- Septal para-Hisian region (Figure 30.3a):
    - Relatively narrow (<120 ms) due to close proximity to the central conduction system. They show a LBBB pattern (qS or QS in V1) and usually have an inferior axis. Frequently, lead II is positive and lead III is negative but axis can differ dramatically depending on patient anatomy.
        - In one study of patients with right septal para-Hisian PVCs,[15] the following morphologies were described:
            - LBBB with an inferior axis — 4 patients.
            - LBBB with a superior axis — 3 patients.
            - RBBB with a superior axis — 1 patient.

LEFT VENTRICULAR OUTFLOW TRACT (LVOT)

In general, the LVOT is rightward and posterior to the RVOT and the AV is inferior to the pulmonic valve. A large part of the right and left aortic sinuses of Valsalva overlie the muscular LVOT making for an interesting and convenient place to map PVCs. While the RVOT is a muscular infundibulum circumferentially, the LVOT is part muscular and part fibrous. Because of this and the considerable variability in outflow tract relationships among individuals, the ECG morphology of these PVCs can be somewhat unpredictable. It is important to account for each patient's anatomic differences when approaching a case.

In general, PVCs arising from the LVOT have been shown to manifest two patterns on ECG:[19,20]

- RBBB pattern, inferior axis with a dominant R wave in V1, and a lack of precordial transition with or without a late-appearing S wave in V2 and V6
- LBBB pattern, inferior axis with an early precordial R wave transition (V2 or V3)

Further localization of VT originating from this region can be aided by the QRS morphology in lead I, R wave morphology in lead V1, and the ratio of R waves in limb leads II and III. Due to its posterior location, the precordial transition of LVOT PVCs is usually earlier than that of the RVOT.

Although PVCs have been successfully ablated from the aortic sinuses of Valsalva, it is not clear if the origin of the PVCs represent muscular extensions that course through the valve leaflets or if the aortic root represents a convenient area to access (and ablate) the anterior LV ostium. Regardless of origin, this has become a common location for successful and safe PVC ablation.[21]

The RCC is directly adjacent to the posterior RVOT (Figure 30.4d [asterisk]) and PVCs from here usually manifest[19,20] as:

- LBBB pattern with a leftward and inferior axis.
- Precordial transition at or before V3.

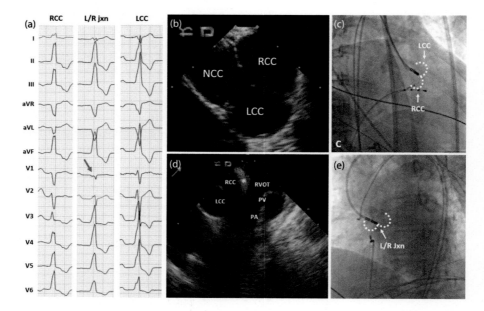

Figure 30.4 (a) PVC morphologies from the right coronary cusp (RCC), left-right coronary cusp junction (L/R jxn), and left coronary cusp (LCC). Note how there is more positivity in lead V1 as the origin of the PVC becomes progressively posterior. There is also greater QRS amplitude in the inferior leads as the origin moves from the RCC to the LCC. PVCs from the L/R jxn have a characteristic notch on the downstroke of V1 (red arrow). (Middle) (b) Intracardiac ultrasound (ICE) imaging of the aortic valve (AV) and (d) AV and right ventricular outflow tract (RVOT) (d) as imaged from the right ventricle (RV). Note that the RCC and Site 1,2 of the RVOT are adjacent to each other accounting for their similar morphology (asterisk). (Right) (c) Right anterior oblique (RAO) and (e) left anterior oblique (LAO) fluoroscopic views of the ablation catheter in the L/R Jxn via a retrograde aortic approach. Dotted lines mark the aortic sinus cusps. PV: Pulmonic valve, PA: pulmonary artery, NCC: non-coronary cusp.

- There is frequently an rS complex in V2 with a wide first component.
- Although the inferior leads are generally all positive, it is common for lead II > III depending on how vertical the heart is in the chest cavity.
  - Similarly, most patients will have a larger S wave in lead aVR compared to aVL.

Due to its position directly posterior to the anterior and mid RVOT, this morphology can be quite similar to that of the RVOT site 1,2 (Figures 30.4d [asterisk] and 30.2a). In general, a PVC that transitions prior to sinus rhythm is suggestive of a more posterior origin within the LVOT rather than the RVOT. In this way, a patient is used as their own "control" in terms of expected precordial QRS transition from negative to positive. When both sinus rhythm and the PVC transition at V3, predicting the closest site of origin is more challenging. Several strategies have been proposed:

- In one study, Ouyang et al. has shown that R wave duration and the R/S wave amplitude ratio in leads V1 and V2 were greater in morphologies originating from the cusp compared with the RVOT.[22]
- An algorithm has been developed comparing the R wave amplitude in V2 for the PVC with that in sinus rhythm. Betensky et al. has shown that in V3 transition PVCs, the R/S wave ratio in V2 compared to the R/S ratio during sinus rhythm is helpful in distinguishing RVOT from LVOT (Figure 30.2a [asterisk]).[23]
  - A ratio of ≥0.6 predicted LVOT origin with a sensitivity of 95% and a specificity of 100%.

Because of its location posterior and leftward to the RCC, PVCs from the LCC usually manifest as such:[19,20,22,24]

- RBBB or intermediate bundle ("m" or "w" pattern) pattern with a more rightward axis.
- Earlier precordial transition ≤V3 (Figure 30.4a).
- Because of its superior location as compared to the RCC, LCC PVCs will frequently manifest with greater R wave amplitude in the inferior leads with lead III > II and a deeper S wave in aVL than aVR (opposite to that of RCC) (Figure 30.4a).

PVCs from the LCC–RCC junction (L/R jxn) can be thought of as a combination of the morphologies from the LCC and RCC.[25,26] V1 is typically LBBB with a characteristic "notching" on the downstroke of the S wave with a precordial transition at V2 or V3 (Figure 30.4a). Lead I is usually multiphasic but is highly dependent on the rotation of the heart within the chest. Figure 4c and 4e show RAO and left anterior oblique (LAO) fluoroscopic views of an ablation catheter within the L/R jxn.

The non-coronary cusp and the posterior aspect of the LCC are continuous with the fibrous aortomitral continuity (AMC), and thus are not characteristically associated with PVCs.

MITRAL VALVE (MV)

PVC morphologies from the basal LV endocardium manifest site-dependent ECG morphologies that can help differentiate medial from lateral locations.

- Dixit et al. have shown that medial sites demonstrate (Figure 30.5)[5]:
  - Narrow QRS complexes (134 ± 28 ms).
  - LBBB morphology.
  - Early precordial transition by V2 or V3.
  - Lead I shows predominantly positive forces (R or Rs morphology).

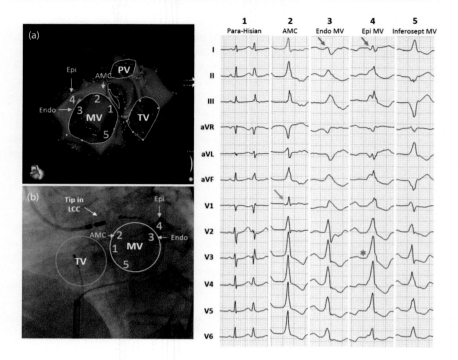

Figure 30.5 (a) Electro-anatomic voltage map of the right and left ventricles viewed posteri-orly. (b) Left anterior oblique (LAO) fluoroscopic view of the heart. Solid lines approximate the mitral valve (MV) and tricuspid valves (TV). Note there is a decapolar catheter within the coronary sinus (CS) with the tip at the great cardiac vein/anteriorly interventricular vein (GCV/AIV) junction. There is an ablation catheter via a retrograde aortic approach with the tip in the left coronary cusp (LCC) adjacent to the GCV/AIV junction. (Right) PVC morphologies from various regions along the mitral valve (MV). (1) Left septal para-Hisian. Note how the PVC QRS is narrow and similar to the sinus beat preceding it. (2) Aortomitral continuity (AMC) with a characteristic qR complex in V1. (3) Endocardial anterolateral MV. Note the initial r wave in lead I (red arrow) indicating endocardial to epicardial activation. (4) Epicardial anterolateral MV. As compared to its endocardial counter-part, there is an initial q wave in lead I (red arrow) indicating epicardial to endocardial activation. (5) Inferoseptal MV with a biphasic pattern in V1 suggesting a more inferoseptal origin rather than along the inferior/bottom portion of the MV. AV: Aortic valve, Epi: epicardial, Endo: endocardial, AMC: aortomitral continuity.

- In comparison, pace maps from lateral basal LV sites (superolateral and lateral MV) demonstrate (Figure 30.5):
  - Wide QRS complexes (182 ± 18 ms).
  - RBBB morphology (R and/or Rs) in lead V1.
  - Absence of precordial transition or late S wave appearance (by V5).
  - rS or qs morphology in lead I (depending on endocardial or epicardial origin — further discussion below).
  - As the origin moves more laterally along the anterolateral wall, lead III becomes more positive than lead II and aVL becomes more negative than aVR.
- Determining whether a PVC has an endocardial or epicardial origin by 12-lead ECG can be challenging. Several clues exist:

- The presence of a "pseudo delta" wave representing early epicardial activation (Figure 30.5 [asterisk]).
  - The degree of initial slurring compared to the total QRS duration has been termed the maximum deflection index (MDI). The initial slurring is indexed by the shortest onset of the QRS to the peak of the R wave in the precordial leads.
  - An MDI $\geq$ 0.55 is highly suggestive of an epicardial origin.[27]
- An initial q wave in lead I (representing epicardial to endocardial activation) suggests an epicardial origin although this has only been validated in patients with nonischemic cardiomyopathy (Figure 30.5 [red arrows]).[28]
- The AMC represents a unique location adjacent to the septal MV with the following features (Figure 30.5)[5,29-34]:
  - RBBB pattern with a leftward axis and no precordial transition.
  - Signature qR morphology in V1 (Figure 30.5 [blue arrow]).
  - R wave ratio >1 in leads II and III.
  - Other studies have found variable morphologies in this region and have been hypothesized to depend on the region of the AMC sampled as well as the involvement of and exit from the His Purkinje system, either actively or passively.[33,34]

LEFT VENTRICULAR SUMMIT

The "LV summit" is the region bounded by the left anterior descending artery (LAD) and the left circumflex artery (LCx) (Figure 30.6). It is broken down into "accessible" and "inaccessible" areas based upon the success rate of catheter-based ablation as it is in the vicinity of pericardial fat and coronary arteries.

LV summit PVCs have distinct characteristics (Figure 30.6):[35,36]

- Depending on whether the exit is endocardial or epicardial, they can contain a "pseudo delta" wave (Figure 30.6 [asterisk]).
- Owing to the proximity to the ventricular septum, PVC morphology can have a RBBB, LBBB, or intermediate bundle branch block pattern in V1.
- PVCs from the "inaccessible" zone uniformly have a LBBB pattern, larger R wave amplitude in the inferior leads, and absence of an S wave in leads V5–V6.
- PVCs from the "accessible" zone may have RBBB or intermediate bundle morphology.
  - Predictors of successful ablation from the epicardium include[36]:
    - Q-wave amplitude ratio in aVL/aVR > 1.85.
    - R/S ratio in V1 > 2.
    - Absence of an initial q wave in lead V1.
- Due to the close proximity of the arterial coronary vessels, ablation from the epicardium is not always prudent. Ablation from adjacent structures such as the left sinus of Valsalva (LSV) and the LV endocardium is common.
  - Predictors of successful ablation from the LSV and endocardium include[37]:
    - Q-wave ratio of <1.45 in aVL/aVR and an anatomical distance of <13.5 mm with a sensitivity and specificity of 89%, 75%, 78%, and 64%, respectively.

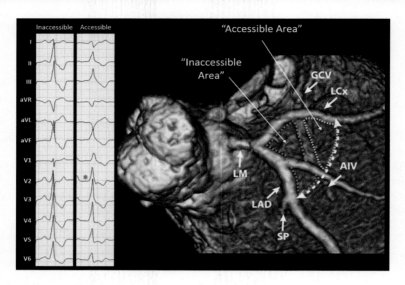

Figure 30.6 (Right) Computed tomography angiogram (CTA) reconstruction of the left ventricular (LV) summit. Blue-dotted line marks the "inaccessible" area medial to the great cardiac vein/anterior interventricular vein (GCV/AIV) bifurcation. Yellow-dotted line marks the "accessible area" lateral to the GCV/AIV bifurcation. (Left) Examples of PVC morphologies from the "inaccessible" and "accessible" regions of the LV summit. The "accessible" PVC has positive predictors of successful ablation including: (1) Q-wave amplitude ratio in aVL/aVR > 1.85. (2) R/S ratio in V1 > 2. (3) Absence of an initial q wave in lead V1. LM: Left main, LCx: left circumflex, LAD: left anterior descending, SP: septal perforator. (Courtesy of Pasquale Santangeli, MD.)

CARDIAC CRUX

- The posterior correlate of the LV summit where the atrioventricular groove and posterior interventricular sulcus intersect is referred to as the basal cardiac crux (BCC) (Figure 30.7). PVCs from this region show:[38–40]
  - LBBB or intermediate morphology.
  - Superior axis (QS pattern).
  - R > S wave in V2.
  - MDI ≥ 0.55.
- PVCs from the BCC are frequently amenable to mapping and ablation within the middle cardiac vein (MCV).
- The apical cardiac crux (ACC) is differentiated from the BCC by a deep S wave in V6, R > S wave in aVR, and occasional RBBB pattern in V1 (Figure 30.7).[39]
  - ACC PVCs can be similar to those from the left posterior fascicle and posteromedial papillary muscle.
  - Useful criteria to distinguish ACC PVCs from endocardial variants include[40]:
    - MDI ≥ 0.55.
    - Monophasic R wave in aVR.
    - QS or r/S ratio <0.15 in V6.
    - Failed endocardial ablation.
- While BCC PVCs are more amenable to ablation from the coronary venous system, apical variants more often require epicardial mapping and ablation.[39]

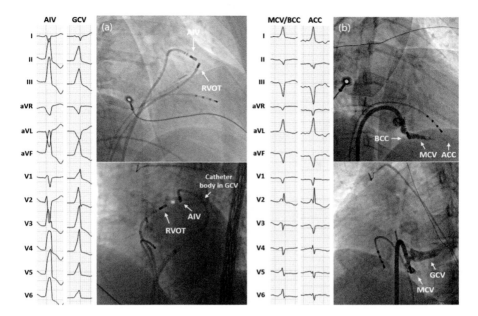

Figure 30.7 (Left) PVCs from the anterior interventricular vein (AIV) and great cardiac vein (GCV). (a) Right anterior oblique and (RAO) left anterior oblique (LAO) fluoroscopic views of ablation catheters within the AIV and the anterior right ventricular outflow tract (RVOT). Note the proximity of the two catheters (asterisk). (Right) PVC morphology from the proximal middle cardiac vein (MCV) or basal cardiac crux (BCC) shows a typical "pattern break" at V2 (asterisk). Contrast is being injected through the sheath. PVC morphology from the apical cardiac crux (ACC) has a similar V2 pattern break but has a later precordial transition due to its more apical location. (b) RAO and LAO fluoroscopic views of an ablation catheter within the proximal MCV.

CORONARY VENOUS SYSTEM

PVCs mapped and ablated in the coronary veins have been described[37,41–46] and in one the largest series[45] represented 9% of all idiopathic arrhythmias.

Whether the branches of the coronary veins represent the origin of these arrhythmias or simply convenient access to the surrounding myocardium is unclear. The great cardiac vein (GCV), anterior interventricular vein (AIV), and MCV represent the most common locations of idiopathic PVCs. Because the coronary venous system is epicardial, signs of epicardial origin that have previously been described ("pseudo delta" wave, MDI $\geq$ 0.55, qS complexes in nearby leads) are typically present.

- GCV PVCs manifest similarly to epicardial MV PVCs (Figure 30.7):
  - RBBB pattern with a rightward axis and no precordial transition.
  - Usually inferiorly-directed but dependent on how anterior the origin is within the GCV.
    - As the origin moves inferiorly, the R wave ratio in III and II increases.
- AIV (Figure 30.7):
  - May have a RBBB, LBBB, or intermediate bundle pattern due to the AIV coursing over the interventricular septum.

- Precordial transition occurs ≤V4 and there is usually no late S wave in V5 or V6.
- Axis is generally rightward but can be highly variable depending on venous anatomy.[45]
- MCV (Figure 30.7):
  - LBBB or intermediate bundle with a late transition by V4 or V5 and a typical pattern break in V2.
  - Lead I shows a large R wave with basal variants which becomes less so as the origin moves more apical.
  - As the MVC is a right-sided structure, S wave in lead III > II.
  - There is usually no r wave in lead II or III representing epicardial to endocardial activation.

LEFT VENTRICULAR PAPILLARY MUSCLES AND FASCICULAR SYSTEM

PVCs from the LV papillary muscles have recently been described.[47–52] Improved tools such as intracardiac ultrasound (ICE) have facilitated more accurate LV mapping and correlation with intracavity structures.

PVCs occur more commonly from the posteromedial papillary muscle (PM Pap) than the anterolateral papillary muscle (AL Pap) as shown in prior studies. Although anatomic variations exist, the PM Pap and AL Pap muscles have distinct morphologic characteristics (Figure 30.8)[50,52]:

- PVCs from the PM Pap share the following features (Figure 30.8):
  - Atypical RBBB frequently with small q wave in V1.
  - Superiorly directed axis.
  - Typically multiphasic in lead I with much variability due to the shape and location of the papillary muscle and whether the PVC exits from a septal or lateral location.
  - Variable precordial transition can range from V3 to V5 depending on how apical the papillary muscle is inserted and which portion the PVC exits from.
- PVCs from the AL Pap share the following features (Figure 30.8):
  - Atypical RBBB
  - Inferior and rightward axis
  - Frequently lead III > II depending on how high the papillary muscle is located on the lateral wall
  - Later transition usually by V5 or V6

PVCs from the left fascicular system are frequently very similar to those from the papillary muscles due to close anatomic proximity (Figure 30.8a–c). Good et al. have described the observed differences in one study of patients with idiopathic ventricular tachycardia from these regions. PVCs from the papillary muscles were described as having the following features in contrast to Purkinje origin (Figure 30.8)[51]:

- Wider QRS (150 ± 15 ms vs. 127 ± 11 ms) due to origin from the terminal aspects of the conduction system
- Lack of discrete Q waves in the lateral or inferior leads
- Typical qR pattern with lack of rsR' pattern in lead V1 that is characteristic for a fascicular etiology

Due to the lack of robust patient cohorts and significant variability in patient anatomy, pre-procedure imaging with a non-invasive imaging modality may facilitate more accurate localization of these important anatomic structures in the EP laboratory.

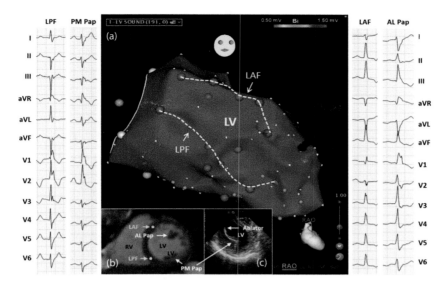

Figure 30.8 (Center) (a) Electro-anatomic map of the left ventricle (LV) in a right anterior oblique (RAO) view. Purple dots and dotted lines indicate the course of the left anterior fascicle (LAF) and the left posterior fascicle (LPF). (b) Magnetic resonance image of the heart in a short-axis view with identification of the anterolateral papillary muscle (AL Pap) and the posterolateral papillary muscle (PM Pap). Yellow dots indicate the presumptive locations of the LAF and LPF. (c) Intracardiac ultrasound (ICE) image of the left ventricle (LV) as imaged from the RV demonstrating the tip of the ablation catheter on the PM Pap. (Left) PVC morphologies from the LPF and PM Pap. The former of which is narrower and contains a typical rSR[I] pattern. (Right) PVC morphologies from the LAF and AL Pap. The former of which is again narrower and less rightward than its AL Pap counterpart.

MODERATOR BAND (MB) AND RV PAPILLARY MUSCLES (RV Pap)

The RV is a highly trabeculated structure with complex anatomy. PVCs from specific intra-cavitary structures in the RV may have been under-recognized in the past due to the inability to directly visualize them with fluoroscopic and computerized mapping systems. The identification and integration of these structures with ICE imaging (Figure 30.9a and b), in particular, has enhanced our knowledge of PVC origin and facilitated targeted ablation procedures. This is particularly true with the moderator band and RV papillary muscles. Due in part to the proximity of these structures to the conduction system, these PVCs have recently been linked with PVC-induced VF in normal hearts.[53-55] Correct interpretation of and localization of these morphologies are crucial to successful ablation.

MB PVCs have a typical LBBB pattern with a leftward and superior axis (Figure 30.9):

- As the MB is a complex structure with insertions on both the RV septum and free wall, the degree of positivity in the inferior leads can be variable.
- Due to the anterior and rightward nature of this structure, the precordial leads usually transition at V5 or V6 and later than the transition in sinus rhythm.
- PVCs have an intermediate QRS duration with a mean duration of 152.7 ± 15.2 ms (range 130–172 ms)[53] due to the proximity to the distal aspects of the right bundle branch.

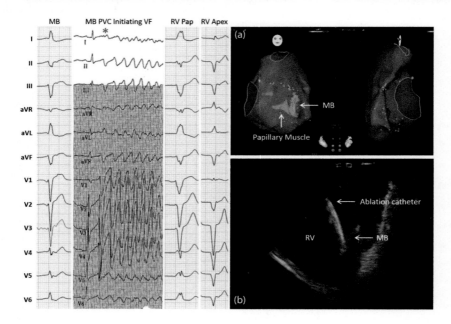

Figure 30.9 (Left) Examples of PVCs from the moderator band (MB) (the second example triggers VF), inferior papillary muscle of the right ventricle (RV Pap), and RV apex. Note the similar morphology of the MB and RV Pap PVCs. As expected, the PVC from the intracavitary structures transitions earlier and have more voltage in lead I due to their more basal locations as compared to the RV apical example. Right (a) electro-anatomic map of the RV with identification and tagging of the MB created with intracardiac ultrasound (ICE) (right anterior oblique [RAO] and posterior views). (b) ICE imaging from within the RV of an ablation catheter on the MB. (Courtesy of Fermin Garcia, MD.)

- Within the RV, the late precordial transition, less positivity in lead I, and more positivity in aVR differentiate them from that of the TV at the level of the RV papillary muscle/moderator band complex.[53]
- Differentiating MB PVCs from RV pap PVCs is challenging. PVCs from the RV Paps have a similar morphology to the MB (Figure 30.9) but have been shown to be slightly wider with a QRS mean duration of 163 ± 21 ms.[56] Crawford et al. have shown that papillary muscle PVCs from the septal RV Pap may manifest with an inferior axis and earlier transition, which is not usual for the MB.[56]
- The degree of positivity in the inferior leads can be variable but axis is typically more superior from the RV pap and may be intermediate from the moderator band with a positive initial component in lead II. Because of the overlap in ECG features, detailed imaging and mapping is required of both the MB and RV pap structure to localize PVCs. Recognition of highly variable anatomy is essential.[53]

CONCLUSION

Normal heart PVCs are common and frequently require treatment with catheter-based ablation. Combined with a basic understanding of normal cardiac anatomy, the 12-lead ECG represents an invaluable tool allowing for precise localization of PVC origin. This knowledge can facilitate patient counseling and procedural planning.

LIST OF ABBREVIATIONS

ACC	apical cardiac crux
AIV	anterior interventricular vein
AL Pap	anterolateral papillary muscle
AMC	aortomitral continuity
BCC	basal cardiac crux
CT	computed tomography
ECG	electrocardiogram
GCV	great cardiac vein
ICE	intracardiac ultrasound
L/R jxn	left/right coronary cusp junction
LAD	left anterior descending
LAO	left anterior oblique
LBBB	left bundle branch block
LCC	left coronary cusp
LCx	left circumflex
LSV	left sinus of Valsalva
LV	left ventricle
LVOT	left ventricular outflow tract
MB	moderator band
MCV	middle cardiac vein
MDI	maximum deflection index
MRI	magnetic resonance imaging
MV	mitral valve
PM	Pap posteromedial papillary muscle
PV	pulmonic valve
PVC	premature ventricular complexes
RAO	right anterior oblique
RBBB	right bundle branch block
RCC	right coronary cusp
RV Pap	right ventricular papillary muscle
RVOT	right ventricular outflow tract
TV	tricuspid valve
US	ultrasound

REFERENCES

1. Kennedy HL, Whitlock JA, Sprague MK, et al. Long-term follow-up of asymptomatic healthy subjects with frequent and complex ventricular ectopy. *N Engl J Med* 1985; 312(4): 193–197.

2. Pedersen CT, Kay GN, Kalman J, et al. EHRA/HRS/APHRS expert consensus on ventricular arrhythmias. *Heart Rhythm* 2014; 11(10): e166–e196.

3. Maeda S, Chik WW, Han Y, et al. Effects of age-related aortic root anatomic changes on left ventricular outflow tract pace-mapping morphologies: A cardiac magnetic resonance imaging validation study. *J Cardiovasc Electrophysiol* 2015; 26: 994–999.

4. Anter E, Frankel DS, Marchlinski FE, et al. Effect of electrocardiographic lead placement on localization of outflow tract tachycardias. *Heart Rhythm* 2012; 9(5): 697–703.

5. Dixit S, Gerstenfeld EP, Lin D, et al. Identification of distinct electrocardiographic patterns from the basal left ventricle: Distinguishing medial and lateral sites of origin in patients with idiopathic ventricular tachycardia. *Heart Rhythm* 2005; 2(5): 485–491.

6. Jadonath RL, Schwartzman DS, Preminger MW, et al. Utility of the 12-lead electrocardiogram in localizing the origin of right ventricular outflow tract tachycardia. *Am Heart J* 1995; 130(5): 1107–1113.

7. Dixit S, Gerstenfeld EP, Callans DJ, et al. Electrocardiographic patterns of superior right ventricular outflow tract tachycardias: Distinguishing septal and free-wall sites of origin. *Cardiovasc Electrophysiol* 2003; 14(1): 1–7.

8. Tada H, Tadokoro K, Miyaji K, et al. Idiopathic ventricular arrhythmias arising from the pulmonary artery: Prevalence, characteristics, and topography of the arrhythmia origin. *Heart Rhythm* 2008; 5(3): 419–426.

9. Timmermans C, Rodriguez LM, Medeiros A, et al. Radiofrequency catheter ablation of idiopathic ventricular tachycardia originating in the main stem of the pulmonary artery. *J Cardiovasc Electrophysiol* 2002; 13(3): 281–284.

10. Timmermans C, Rodriguez LM, Crijns HJ, et al. Idiopathic left bundle-branch block-shaped ventricular tachycardia may originate above the pulmonary valve. *Circulation* 2003; 108(16): 1960–1967.

11. Tada H, Kurosaki K, Ito S, et al. Idiopathic premature ventricular contractions arising from the pulmonary artery: Importance of mapping in the pulmonary artery in left bundle branch block-shaped ventricular arrhythmias. *Circ J* 2005; 69(7): 865–869.

12. Liu CF, Cheung JW, Thomas G, et al. Ubiquitous myocardial extensions into the pulmonary artery demonstrated by integrated intracardiac echocardiography and electroanatomic mapping: changing the paradigm of idiopathic right ventricular outflow tract arrhythmias. *Circ Arrhythm Electrophysiol* 2014; 7(4): 691–700.

13. Sekiguchi Y, Aonuma K, Takahashi A, et al. Electrocardiographic and electrophysiologic characteristics of ventricular tachycardia originating within the pulmonary artery. *J Am Coll Cardiol* 2005; 45(6): 887–895.

14. Van Herendael H, Garcia F, Lin D, et al. Idiopathic right ventricular arrhythmias not arising from the outflow tract: Prevalence, electrocardiographic characteristics, and outcome of catheter ablation. *Heart Rhythm* 2011; 8(4): 511–518.

15. Ban JE, Chen YL, Park HC, et al. Idiopathic ventricular arrhythmia originating from the para-Hisian area: Prevalence, electrocardiographic and electrophysiological characteristics. *J Arrhythmia* 2014; 30(1): 48–54.

16. Tada H, Tadokoro K, Ito S, et al. Idiopathic ventricular arrhythmias originating from the tricuspid annulus: Prevalence, electrocardiographic characteristics, and results of radiofrequency catheter ablation. *Heart Rhythm* 2007; 4(1): 7–16.

17. Yue-Chun L, Wen-Wu Z, Na-Dan Z, et al. Idiopathic premature ventricular contractions and ventricular tachycardias originating from the vicinity of tricuspid annulus: Results of radiofrequency catheter ablation in thirty-five patients. *BMC Cardiovasc Disord* 2012; 12: 32.

18. Satish OS, Yeh KH, Wen MS, et al. Focal right ventricular tachycardia originating from the subtricuspid septum. *Europace* 2005; 7(4): 348–352.

19. Tada H, Nogami A, Naito S, et al. Left ventricular epicardial outflow tract tachycardia: A new distinct subgroup of outflow tract tachycardia. *Jpn Circ J* 2001; 65(8): 723–730.

20. Lin D, Ilkhanoff L, Gerstenfeld E, et al. Twelve-lead electrocardiographic characteristics of the aortic cusp region guided by intracardiac echocardiography and electroanatomic mapping. *Heart Rhythm* 2008; 5(5): 663–669.

21. Hoffmayer KS, Dewland TA, Hsia HH, et al. Safety of radiofrequency catheter ablation without coronary angiography in aortic cusp ventricular arrhythmias. *Heart Rhythm* 2014; 11(7): 1117–1121.

22. Ouyang F, Fotuhi P, Ho SY, et al. Repetitive monomorphic ventricular tachycardia originating from the aortic sinus cusp: Electrocardiographic characterization for guiding catheter ablation. *J Am Coll Cardiol* 2002; 39(3): 500–508.

23. Betensky BP, Park RE, Marchlinski FE, et al. The V(2) transition ratio: A new electrocardiographic criterion for distinguishing left from right ventricular outflow tract tachycardia origin. *J Am Coll Cardiol* 2011; 57(22): 2255–2262.

24. Hutchinson MD, Garcia FC. An organized approach to the localization, mapping, and ablation of outflow tract ventricular arrhythmias. *J Cardiovasc Electrophysiol* 2013; 24(10): 1189–1197.

25. Bala R, Garcia FC, Hutchinson, MD, et al. Electrocardiographic and electrophysiologic features of ventricular arrhythmias originating from the right/left coronary cusp commissure. *Heart Rhythm* 2010; 7(3): 312–322.

26. Yamada T, Yoshida N, Murakami Y, et al. Electrocardiographic characteristics of ventricular arrhythmias originating from the junction of the left and right coronary sinuses of Valsalva in the aorta: The activation pattern as a rationale for the electrocardiographic characteristics. *Heart Rhythm* 2008; 5(2): 184–192.

27. Daniels DV, Lu YY, Morton JB, et al. Idiopathic epicardial left ventricular tachycardia originating remote from the sinus of Valsalva: Electrophysiological characteristics, catheter ablation, and identification from the 12-lead electrocardiogram. *Circulation* 2006; 113(13): 1659–1666.

28. Vallès E, Bazan V, Marchlinski FE. ECG criteria to identify epicardial ventricular tachycardia in nonischemic cardiomyopathy. *Circ Arrhythm Electrophysiol* 2010; 3(1): 63–71.

29. Chen J, Hoff PI, Rossvoll O, et al. Ventricular arrhythmias originating from the aorto-mitral continuity: An uncommon variant of left ventricular outflow tract tachycardia. *Europace* 2012; 14(3): 388–395.

30. Kumagai K, Fukuda K, Wakayama Y, et al. Electrocardiographic characteristics of the variants of idiopathic left ventricular outflow tract ventricular tachyarrhythmias. *J Cardiovasc Electrophysiol* 2008; 19(5): 495–501.

31. Letsas KP, Efremidis M, Kollias G, et al. Electrocardiographic and electrophysiologic characteristics of ventricular extrasystoles arising from the aortomitral continuity. *Cardiol Res Pract* 2011; 2011: 864964.

32. Yamada T, McElderry HT, Okada T, et al. Idiopathic left ventricular arrhythmias originating adjacent to the left aortic sinus of valsalva: Electrophysiological rationale for the surface electrocardiogram. *J Cardiovasc Electrophysiol* 2010; 21(2): 170–176.

33. Mizobuchi M, Enjoji Y. Demonstration of a hidden interaction between the aortomitral continuity and the conduction system in a case of idiopathic left ventricular outflow tract tachycardia. *J Arrhythm* 2015; 31(3): 180–182.

34. Hai JJ, Chahal AA, Friedman PA, et al. Electrophysiologic characteristics of ventricular arrhythmias arising from the aortic mitral continuity-potential role of the conduction system. *J Cardiovasc Electrophysiol* 2015; 26(2): 158–63.

35. Yamada T, McElderry HT, Doppalapudi H, et al. Idiopathic ventricular arrhythmias originating from the left ventricular summit: Anatomic concepts relevant to ablation. *Circ Arrhythmia Electrophysiol* 2010; 3(6): 616–623.

36. Santangeli P, Marchlinski FE, Zado ES, et al. Percutaneous epicardial ablation of ventricular arrhythmias arising from the left ventricular summit: Outcomes and electrocardiogram correlates of success. *Circ Arrhythm Electrophysiol* 2015; 8(2): 337–343.

37. Jaurequi Abularach ME, Campos B, Park KM, et al. Ablation of ventricular arrhythmias arising near the anterior epicardial veins from the left sinus of Valsalva region: ECG features, anatomic distance, and outcome. *Heart Rhythm* 2012; 9(6): 865–873.

38. Doppalapudi H, Yamada T, Ramaswamy K, et al. Idiopathic focal epicardial ventricular tachycardia originating from the crux of the heart *Heart Rhythm* 2009; 6(1): 44–50.

39. Kawamura M, Gerstenfeld EP, Vedantham V, et al. Idiopathic ventricular arrhythmia originating from the cardiac crux or inferior septum: Epicardial idiopathic ventricular arrhythmia. *Circ Arrhythm Electrophysiol* 2014; 7(6): 1152–1158.

40. Kawamura M, Hsu JC, Vedantham V, et al. Clinical and electrocardiographic characteristics of idiopathic ventricular arrhythmias with right bundle branch block and superior axis: Comparison of apical crux area and posterior septal left ventricle. *Heart Rhythm* 2015; 12(6): 1137–1144.

41. Meininger GR, Berger RD. Idiopathic ventricular tachycardia originating in the great cardiac vein. *Heart Rhythm* 2006; 3(4): 464–466.

42. Obel OA, d'Avila A, Neuzil P, et al. Ablation of left ventricular epicardial outflow tract tachycardia from the distal great cardiac vein. *J Am Coll Cardiol* 2006; 48(9): 1813–1817.

43. Baman TS, Ilg KJ, Gupta SK, et al. Mapping and ablation of epicardial idiopathic ventricular arrhythmias from within the coronary venous system. *Circ Arrhythm Electrophysiol* 2010; 3(3): 274–279.

44. Carrigan TP, Patel S, Yokokawa M, et al. Anatomic relationships between the coronary venous system, surrounding structures, and the site of origin of epicardial ventricular arrhythmias. *J Cardiovasc Electrophysiol* 2014; 25(12): 1336–1342.

45. Mountantonakis SE, Frankel DS, Tschabrunn CM, et al. Ventricular arrhythmias from the coronary venous system: Prevalence, mapping, and ablation. *Heart Rhythm* 2015; 12(6): 1145–1153.

46. Steven D, Pott C, Bittner A, et al. Idiopathic ventricular outflow tract arrhythmias from the great cardiac vein: Challenges and risks of catheter ablation. *Int J Cardiol* 2013; 169(5): 366–370.

47. Ablation of ventricular arrhythmias Doppalapudi H, Yamada T, McElderry HT, et al. Ventricular tachycardia originating from the posterior papillary muscle in the left ventricle: A distinct clinical syndrome. *Circ Arrhythm Electrophysiol* 2008; 1(1): 23–29.

48. Yamada T, Doppalapudi H, McElderry HT, et al. Electrocardiographic and electrophysiological characteristics in idiopathic ventricular arrhythmias originating from the papillary muscles in the left ventricle: Relevance for catheter ablation. *Circ Arrhythm Electrophysiol* 2010; 3(4): 324–331.

49. Yamada T, Mcelderry HT, Okada T, et al. Idiopathic focal ventricular arrhythmias originating from the anterior papillary muscle in the left ventricle. *J Cardiovasc Electrophysiol* 2009; 20(8): 866–872.

50. Yokokawa M, Good E, Desjardins B, et al. Predictors of successful catheter ablation of ventricular arrhythmias arising from the papillary muscles. *Heart Rhythm* 2010; 7(11): 1654–1659.

51. Good E, Desjardins B, Jongnarangsin K, et al. Ventricular arrhythmias originating from a papillary muscle in patients without prior infarction: A comparison with fascicular arrhythmias. *Heart Rhythm* 2008; 5(11): 1530–1537.

52. Yamada T, Doppalapudi H, McElderry HT, et al. Idiopathic ventricular arrhythmias originating from the papillary muscles in the left ventricle: Prevalence, electrocardiographic and electrophysiological characteristics, and results of the radiofrequency catheter ablation. *J Cardiovasc Electrophysiol* 2010; 21(1): 62–69.

53. Sadek MM, Benhayon D, Sureddi R, et al. Idiopathic ventricular arrhythmias originating from the moderator band: Electrocardiographic characteristics and treatment by catheter ablation. *Heart Rhythm* 2015; 12(1): 67–75.

54. Santoro F, Di Biase L, Hranitzky P, et al. Ventricular fibrillation triggered by PVCs from papillary muscles: Clinical features and ablation. *J Cardiovasc Electrophysiol* 2014; 25(11): 1158–1164.

55. Anter E, Buxton AE, Silverstein JR, et al. Idiopathic ventricular fibrillation originating from the moderator band. *J Cardiovasc Electrophysiol* 2013; 24(1): 97–100.

56. Crawford T, Mueller G, Good E, et al. Ventricular arrhythmias originating from papillary muscles in the right ventricle. *Heart Rhythm* 2010; 7(6): 725–730.

EPICARDIAL ACCESS AND INDICATIONS

Jason S. Bradfield and Kalyanam Shivkumar

CONTENTS

EPICARDIAL ACCESS INDICATIONS—EPICARDIAL ACCESS TECHNIQUES—EPICARDIAL ACCESS RISKS

Ventricular tachycardia (VT) ablation is the primary treatment modality for medication refractory ventricular arrhythmias. In patients with structural heart disease, these arrhythmias are often re-entrant in nature and can involve complex three-dimensional scars with variable involvement of the endocardium, mid-myocardium, and/or epicardium (Figure 31.1). The complex three-dimensional nature of these substrates[1] is one contributing factor explaining the modest success rates of VT ablation in this patient population.[2]

Techniques that allow a more comprehensive mapping of arrhythmia substrates can potentially improve procedure success rates. Epicardial mapping (percutaneous or surgical), in combination with endocardial mapping, is one such technique. Epicardial access is indicated for mapping of VT when there is thought to be: (1) a critical component of the clinical VT circuit present on the epicardium; (2) a high likelihood of epicardial substrate (fractionated/delayed/late potentials) that may contribute to the current or future VT circuits; and/or (3) mid-myocardial substrates are suspected that might require ablation from both an endocardial and epicardial approach to produce adequate ablation depth.

The current use of epicardial mapping and ablation resulted from the modest acute success rates and long-term freedom from VT seen with endocardial RF ablation alone in patients with various substrates of non-ischemic cardiomyopathy (NICM),[3] including arrhythmogenic right ventricular cardiomyopathy,[4] hypertrophic cardiomyopathy[5,6], and Chagas disease. The initial development of percutaneous epicardial access and mapping came from Sosa and colleagues[7,8] in patients with Chagas disease. Other centers have adopted this technique for NICM patients as first-line approach in combination with endocardial mapping. Experienced centers have also utilized this technique for patients with ischemic cardiomyopathy (ICM) who have recurrences after initial endocardial ablation or even prior to failed procedures if pre-procedure imaging suggests epicardial and/or transmural scar.[9] Epicardial access may also be required in a small percentage of patients with no structural heart disease with premature ventricular complexes or VT that cannot be successfully ablated from an endocardial approach.[10,11] In rare instances, ablation of supraventricular tachycardia may require epicardial access as well.[12]

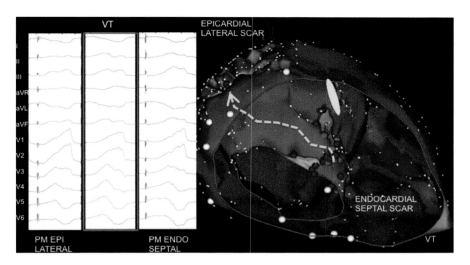

Figure 31.1 Three-dimensional electro-anatomic map (NavX, St. Jude Medical, Minneapolis, MN) with superimposed endocardial and epicardial maps demonstrating the complex anatomic substrates of VT circuits. Pacemaps of the clinical VT are demonstrated on the left panel. The relationship of the endocardial and epicardial sites is demonstrated by the pacemap matches from distant sites with a short stim-QRS latency for the epicardial site and the long stim-QRS latency for the endocardial site. Yellow-dotted arrow indicates direction of activation of the VT circuit from endocardial to epicardial. ENDO = endocardial; EPI = epicardial; PM = pacemap; VT = ventricular tachycardia. (Modified from Bradfield, J. et al., *Indian J. Pacing Electrophysiol.*, 171–180, 2014.)

EPICARDIAL ACCESS INDICATIONS

1   *Substrate considerations*: The probability of an epicardial circuit (area of scar) varies significantly with the underlying cardiac substrate. Patients with NICM have a relatively low ablation success rate with endocardial-only procedures and a combined endocardial/epicardial approach has been suggested either upfront[13] or after assessing endocardial unipolar signals[14,15] that might suggest a distant substrate (mid-myocardial or epicardial). While in most centers epicardial access isn't considered as part of the initial approach for patients with ICM, this technique is frequently utilized in patients who have failed or recurred after an initial procedure, or if pre-procedure imaging suggest an epicardial substrate.[9] Patients with VT related to ARVC,[16,17] Chagas disease,[8] hypertrophic cardiomyopathy,[5,6] myocarditis,[18] and sarcoidosis[19] often require an epicardial approach.

2   *ECG criteria*: ECG criteria[20,21] have been utilized to increase the sensitivity and specificity for predicting an epicardial exit of a given VT. However, recent evidence suggests there are numerous limitations to these criteria including VT rate and utilization of antiarrhythmic drugs.[22,23] Further, while ECG characteristics may predict the exit site of a VT, an epicardial exit does not guarantee the critical component of the circuit is epicardial.

3   *Imaging data*: Transmural or isolated mid-myocardial/epicardial delayed enhancement on cardiac MRI increase the likelihood that epicardial mapping and ablation will be required for control of associated ventricular arrhythmias.[9,24,25]

4   *Prior unsuccessful endocardial ablation(s)*: Previous attempts at endocardial ablation with acute failure or early recurrence suggest the need for more comprehensive mapping

to provide adequate understanding of the VT substrate in a given patient. However, endocardial ablation can fail for a number of reasons including operator inexperience and therefore, epicardial access and ablation while often helpful is not always needed.[26]

EPICARDIAL ACCESS TECHNIQUES

1   A small (1–2 mm) vertical incision is made just left and inferior of the tip of the xiphoid process to avoid resistance with sheath placement later in the procedure.
    (a)   This location increases the likelihood of puncturing an avascular region called the trigonum sternocostal or "Larrey's space."
2   A Tuohy 17G epidural needle can be utilized for access with the needle opening directed toward to left side.
3   Two views should be utilized: either RAO/LAO or AP and lateral.
    (a)   In cases expected to be challenging, a biplane RV angiogram will be useful to use as a roadmap to know the location of the RV free wall (Figure 31.2).
4   The needle is advanced under the rib cage and directed just medial to the patients left shoulder, however, this angle needs to be reassessed in RAO/LAO views based on cardiac chamber enlargement and/or rotation:
    (a)   Fluoroscopically, the ideal site of access should be mid-RV cavity and previously placed pacing/ICD leads or EP catheters can be used as reference points.
5   The initial angle of access should be shallow to avoid liver damage, however, the angle should subsequently be adjusted depending on whether the access will be anterior or posterior:
    (a)   Steeper angle → posterior; shallow angle → anterior (Figure 31.3).
6   A small amount of contrast can be injected as the needle approaches the pericardium to assess location. However, overuse of contrast will impede visualization of access.

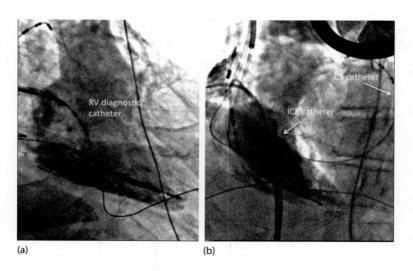

(a)   (b)

Figure 31.2   RAO (a) and LAO (b) RV angiogram images prior to attempted access. CS = coronary sinus; RV = right ventricle.

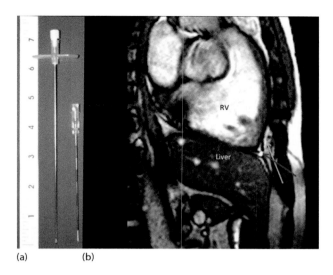

Figure 31.3 Short and long Tuohy needles utilized for percutaneous access (a). Cardiac MRI (b) demonstrating potential access angles for pericardial access. Blue arrow demonstrates a posterior access angle and the orange arrow an anterior angle of access. RV = right ventricle.

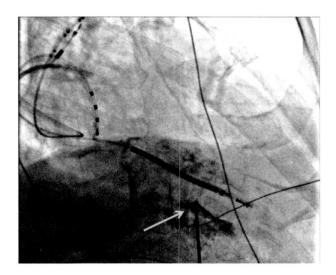

Figure 31.4 RAO view of tenting (yellow arrow) of the pericardium prior to J-wire advancement.

7   When the pericardium is indented, cardiac pulsations can be felt. Pulsations should be initially assessed with inspiration as the heart moves inferiorly.

8   At this point, a small amount of contrast can be injected (via a slip-tip syringe) to demonstrate tenting (Figure 31.4).

9   Puncture of the visceral pericardium may require controlled brisk forward movement of the needle, which leads to release of the resistance:

(a)   At this point, the needle should be withdrawn slightly to avoid RV perforation during ventricular diastole.

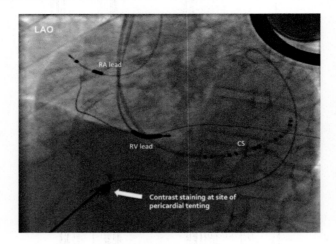

Figure 31.5 LAO view of epicardial access. Residual contrast staining (arrow) is demonstrated and the J-wire advanced along the left heart border ensuring the RV has not been entered. CS = coronary sinus; LAO = left anterior oblique; RA = right atrial; RV = right ventricular.

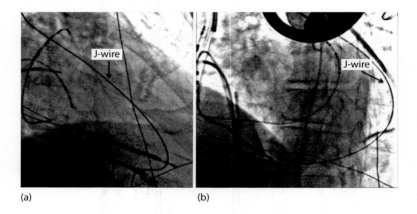

(a) (b)

Figure 31.6 Fluoroscopy demonstrating the importance of verifying wire location in two views. In the RAO image (a), it is not clear whether the J-wire is within the RV or LV chamber. However, in the LAO view (b) the wire takes a course that makes it clear the wire is safely in the pericardial space.

10 The needle should be stabilized and a J-wire can be advanced around the left heart border (in the LAO view) and preferentially across the transverse sinus to the right side (Figure 31.5).

  (a) Understanding wire course to ensure no cardiac chamber access is essential prior to placing a dilator or sheath (Figure 31.6).

  (b) Once the wire position is confirmed, a 4 French soft dilator can then be advanced to perform a pericardiogram (Figure 31.7), to further verify appropriate location within the pericardial space.

11 A long guidewire can then be advanced and a long sheath (SRO/SLO or deflectable Agilis [St. Jude, Minneapolis, MN]) advanced (Figure 31.8). It is essential that an empty sheath not be left in the pericardial space as this may tear or damage a coronary artery; therefore, one should maintain an ablation or balloon-tipped catheter in the sheath with the tip beyond the end of the sheath at all times.

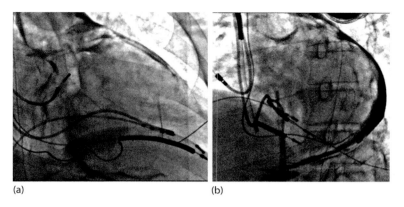

(a)   (b)

Figure 31.7 Pericardiogram demonstrating free-flowing contrast in the pericardial space in the RAO (a) and LAO (b) views.

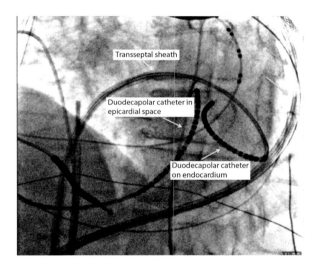

Transseptal sheath

Duodecapolar catheter in epicardial space

Duodecapolar catheter on endocardium

Figure 31.8 LAO view of long sheath advanced safely into the pericardial space (yellow arrow) with a second retained J-wire (orange arrow) after previous double wiring of the long sheath. The additional wire ensures that if access is lost with the long sheath, access does not have to be re-attempted. Two duodecapolar catheters are advanced to opposite surfaces at a critical site for the clinical VT in the LV apex. One mapping catheter is advanced through the long epicardial sheath and another to the endocardial surface via a trans-septal sheath.

An alternative to a Tuohy needle is a micro-puncture needle utilized in some centers. The potential benefit of this needle is its small caliber potentially limiting the size of any inadvertent RV access. One study found that despite similar rates of inadvertent RV puncture, the risk of developing a large pericardial effusion was significantly lower for the micropuncture needle compared to the standard large-bore needle (8.1% vs. 0.9%).[27] The potential downside of such a technique may be some loss of tactile feedback when tenting the pericardium. A needle-in-needle technique has also been reported.[28]

Additional novel techniques have been described to aid access including pericardial pressure transduction,[29] integration of 3D mapping systems,[30] and insufflation of carbon dioxide via intentional right atrial micro-perforation.[31] While these novel concepts provide future promise, the current technique remains the preferred method in most institutions.

After access is obtained and during the procedure, ICE images should be intermittently evaluated for increased fluid collection/bleeding and the pericardial sheath should be suctioned repeatedly to ensure no late bleeding is noted. At the end of the procedure, the pericardium should be drained completely and consideration should be given for injection of steroids[32,33] and repeat pericardiogram to ensure no pockets of fluid remain along with repeat assessment of ICE images for residual fluid or evidence of bleeding.

SURGICAL EPICARDIAL ACCESS

In some cases, percutaneous epicardial access is not feasible and a surgical approach must be considered.[34,35] Patients with previous cardiac surgery (CABG, valve replacement, etc.) are the most common patients encountered that require a surgical approach. These patients may develop epicardial myocardial scar. However, adhesions from the previous cardiac surgery make a percutaneous approach unlikely to succeed, though some centers have reported success in select cases.[36,37]

Even when percutaneous access is successful (Figure 31.9), in a post-surgical patient, complete catheter freedom may still be limited. Therefore, the ability to perform surgical access is essential at high volume VT centers. When surgical access is performed, it is important to choose the access site that will provide the highest yield for epicardial mapping depending on the VT morphology and areas of scar seen on pre-procedure imaging. A subxiphoid approach is best for a VT originating from the inferior wall whereas an anterior or lateral thoracotomy may be best utilized for anterior or lateral VTs.[34]

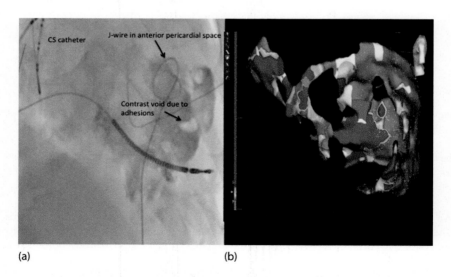

(a)   (b)

Figure 31.9 Fluoroscopy (a) and 3D electro-anatomic mapping image (b) of a patient with significant adhesions limiting wire and catheter movement (a) and 3D mapping density (b).

Percutaneous epicardial access poses numerous risks and potentially serious complications can occur (Figure 31.10). Therefore, adequate training in the procedure itself, as well as a comprehensive understanding of potential complications and the associated treatment is essential.

Initial needle advancement should begin relatively superficial to avoid risk to the liver and abdominal organs and vessels. Liver injury and abdominal bleeding are well-known risks but other complications can occur.[38] The access angle can then be made steeper after the initial advancement if posterior access is preferred.

Right ventricular (RV) perforation is the most common risk[39] given that epicardial access is typically obtained with a "dry" pericardium or with only trace pericardial fluid. Ensuring that the guidewire can be advanced along the left heart border to verify it is outside the heart border and not compatible with intracardiac location is essential to ensure the RV has not been accessed. Given the low-pressure state of the RV, if a sheath is not mistakenly advanced into the RV, the bleeding from RV access is often self-limited and may not preclude further attempts at access or require terminating the procedure. However, this must be monitored closely, especially if anticoagulation is required for a left-sided procedure.

Other more rare complications of epicardial access and procedures have been described[40] including entry into the left pleural space, hemoperitoneum, and abdominal-pericardial fistula.

SUMMARY AND FUTURE DIRECTIONS

VT ablation, particularly in patients with structural heart disease, involves complex substrates that are three-dimensional and may frequently involve the epicardial surface of the heart. When epicardial access and mapping are being considered, careful patient selection is important to optimize patient outcomes and minimize procedure-related risks. However, with appropriate training and technique, epicardial access can be safely obtained, to allow epicardial mapping and ablation as indicated.

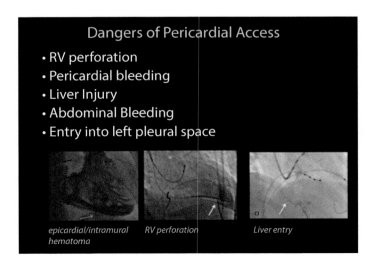

Figure 31.10 Potential risks of pericardial access. RV = right ventricle.

REFERENCES

1. Bradfield JS, Tung R and Shivkumar K. Transmural "Scar-to-Scar" reentrant ventricular tachycardia. *Indian Pacing Electrophysiol J.* 2013;13:212–216.

2. Mathuria N, Tung R and Shivkumar K. Advances in ablation of ventricular tachycardia in nonischemic cardiomyopathy. *Curr Cardiol Rep.* 2012;14:577–583.

3. Cano O, Hutchinson M, Lin D et al. Electroanatomic substrate and ablation outcome for suspected epicardial ventricular tachycardia in left ventricular nonischemic cardiomyopathy. *J Am Coll Cardiol.* 2009;54:799–808.

4. Bai R, Di Biase L, Shivkumar K et al. Ablation of ventricular arrhythmias in arrhythmogenic right ventricular dysplasia/cardiomyopathy: Arrhythmia-free survival after endo-epicardial substrate based mapping and ablation. *Circ Arrhythm Electrophysiol.* 2011;4:478–485.

5. Dukkipati SR, d'Avila A, Soejima K et al. Long-term outcomes of combined epicardial and endocardial ablation of monomorphic ventricular tachycardia related to hypertrophic cardiomyopathy. *Circ Arrhythm Electrophysiol.* 2011;4:185–194.

6. Santangeli P, Di Biase L, Lakkireddy D et al. Radiofrequency catheter ablation of ventricular arrhythmias in patients with hypertrophic cardiomyopathy: Safety and feasibility. *Heart Rhythm.* 2010;7:1036–1042.

7. Sosa E, Scanavacca M, d'Avila A and Pilleggi F. A new technique to perform epicardial mapping in the electrophysiology laboratory. *J Cardiovasc Electrophysiol.* 1996;7:531–536.

8. Sosa E, Scanavacca M, D'Avila A et al. Radiofrequency catheter ablation of ventricular tachycardia guided by nonsurgical epicardial mapping in chronic Chagasic heart disease. *Pacing Clin Electrophysiol.* 1999;22:128–130.

9. Acosta J, Fernandez-Armenta J, Penela D et al. Infarct transmurality as a criterion for first-line endo-epicardial substrate-guided ventricular tachycardia ablation in ischemic cardiomyopathy. *Heart Rhythm.* 2016;13(1):85–95.

10. Lin CY, Chung FP, Lin YJ et al. Radiofrequency catheter ablation of ventricular arrhythmias originating from the continuum between the aortic sinus of Valsalva and the left ventricular summit: Electrocardiographic characteristics and correlative anatomy. *Heart Rhythm.* 2016;13(1):111–121.

11. Santangeli P, Marchlinski FE, Zado ES et al. Percutaneous epicardial ablation of ventricular arrhythmias arising from the left ventricular summit: Outcomes and electrocardiogram correlates of success. *Circ Arrhythm Electrophysiol.* 2015;8:337–43.

12. Scanavacca MI, Sternick EB, Pisani C et al. Accessory atrioventricular pathways refractory to catheter ablation: Role of percutaneous epicardial approach. *Circ Arrhythm Electrophysiol.* 2015;8:128–136.

13. Tung R, Michowitz Y, Yu R et al. Epicardial ablation of ventricular tachycardia: An institutional experience of safety and efficacy. *Heart Rhythm.* 2013;10:490–498.

14. Hutchinson MD, Gerstenfeld EP, Desjardins B et al. Endocardial unipolar voltage mapping to detect epicardial ventricular tachycardia substrate in patients with nonischemic left ventricular cardiomyopathy. *Circ Arrhythm Electrophysiol.* 2011;4:49–55.

15. Polin GM, Haqqani H, Tzou W et al. Endocardial unipolar voltage mapping to identify epicardial substrate in arrhythmogenic right ventricular cardiomyopathy/dysplasia. *Heart Rhythm.* 2011;8:76–83.

16. Philips B, Madhavan S, James C et al. Outcomes of catheter ablation of ventricular tachycardia in arrhythmogenic right ventricular dysplasia/cardiomyopathy. *Circ Arrhythm Electrophysiol.* 2012;5:499–505.

17. Santangeli P, Zado ES, Supple GE et al. Long-term outcome with catheter ablation of ventricular tachycardia in patients with arrhythmogenic right ventricular cardiomyopathy. *Circ Arrhythm Electrophysiol.* 2015;8:1413–1421.

18. Berte B, Sacher F, Cochet H et al. Postmyocarditis ventricular tachycardia in patients with epicardial-only scar: A specific entity requiring a specific approach. *J Cardiovasc Electrophysiol.* 2015;26:42–50.

19. Kumar S, Barbhaiya C, Nagashima K et al. Ventricular tachycardia in cardiac sarcoidosis: Characterization of ventricular substrate and outcomes of catheter ablation. *Circ Arrhythm Electrophysiol.* 2015;8:87–93.

20. Bazan V, Gerstenfeld EP, Garcia FC et al. Site-specific twelve-lead ECG features to identify an epicardial origin for left ventricular tachycardia in the absence of myocardial infarction. *Heart Rhythm.* 2007;4:1403–1410.

21. Berruezo A, Mont L, Nava S et al. Electrocardiographic recognition of the epicardial origin of ventricular tachycardias. *Circulation.* 2004;109:1842–1847.

22. Piers SR, Silva Mde R, Kapel GF et al. Endocardial or epicardial ventricular tachycardia in nonischemic cardiomyopathy? The role of 12-lead ECG criteria in clinical practice. *Heart Rhythm.* 2014;11:1031–1039.

23. Martinek M, Stevenson WG, Inada K et al. QRS characteristics fail to reliably identify ventricular tachycardias that require epicardial ablation in ischemic heart disease. *J Cardiovasc Electrophysiol.* 2012;23:188–193.

24. Andreu D, Ortiz-Perez JT, Boussy T et al. Usefulness of contrast-enhanced cardiac magnetic resonance in identifying the ventricular arrhythmia substrate and the approach needed for ablation. *Eur Heart J.* 2014;35:1316–1326.

25. Piers SR, Tao Q, de Riva Silva M et al. CMR-based identification of critical isthmus sites of ischemic and nonischemic ventricular tachycardia. *JACC Cardiovasc Imaging.* 2014;7:774–784.

26. Schmidt B, Chun KR, Baensch D et al. Catheter ablation for ventricular tachycardia after failed endocardial ablation: Epicardial substrate or inappropriate endocardial ablation? *Heart Rhythm.* 2010;7:1746–1752.

27. Gunda S, Reddy M, Pillarisetti J et al. Differences in complication rates between large bore needle and a long micropuncture needle during epicardial access: Time to change clinical practice? *Circ Arrhythm Electrophysiol.* 2015;8:890–895.

28. Kumar S, Bazaz R, Barbhaiya CR et al. "Needle-in-needle" epicardial access: Preliminary observations with a modified technique for facilitating epicardial interventional procedures. *Heart Rhythm.* 2015;12:1691–1697.

29. Tucker-Schwartz JM, Gillies GT and Mahapatra S. Improved pressure-frequency sensing subxiphoid pericardial access system: Performance characteristics during in vivo testing. *IEEE Trans Biomed Eng.* 2011;58:845–852.

30. Bradfield JS, Tung R, Boyle NG et al. Our approach to minimize risk of epicardial access: Standard techniques with the addition of electroanatomic mapping guidance. *J Cardiovasc Electrophysiol.* 2013;24:723–727.

31. Cronin EM and Zweibel SL. Transatrial pericardial insufflation of carbon dioxide to facilitate percutaneous pericardial access for ablation of ventricular tachycardia. *J Cardiovasc Electrophysiol.* 2016;27(5):615.

32. Dyrda K, Piers SR, van Huls van Taxis CF et al. Influence of steroid therapy on the incidence of pericarditis and atrial fibrillation after percutaneous epicardial mapping and ablation for ventricular tachycardia. *Circ Arrhythm Electrophysiol.* 2014;7:671–676.

33. d'Avila A, Neuzil P, Thiagalingam A et al. Experimental efficacy of pericardial instillation of anti-inflammatory agents during percutaneous epicardial catheter ablation to prevent postprocedure pericarditis. *J Cardiovasc Electrophysiol.* 2007;18:1178–1183.

34. Michowitz Y, Mathuria N, Tung R et al. Hybrid procedures for epicardial catheter ablation of ventricular tachycardia: Value of surgical access. *Heart Rhythm.* 2010;7:1635–1643.

35. Soejima K, Couper G, Cooper JM et al. Subxiphoid surgical approach for epicardial catheter-based mapping and ablation in patients with prior cardiac surgery or difficult pericardial access. *Circulation.* 2004;110:1197–1201.

36. Tschabrunn CM, Haqqani HM, Cooper JM et al. Percutaneous epicardial ventricular tachycardia ablation after noncoronary cardiac surgery or pericarditis. *Heart Rhythm.* 2013;10:165–169.

37. Ebrille E, Killu AM, Anavekar NS et al. Successful percutaneous epicardial access in challenging scenarios. *Pacing Clin Electrophysiol.* 2015;38:84–90.

38. Koruth JS, Aryana A, Dukkipati SR et al. Unusual complications of percutaneous epicardial access and epicardial mapping and ablation of cardiac arrhythmias. *Circ Arrhythm Electrophysiol.* 2011;4:882–888.

39. Sacher F, Roberts-Thomson K, Maury P et al. Epicardial ventricular tachycardia ablation a multicenter safety study. *J Am Coll Cardiol.* 2010;55:2366–2372.

40. Killu AM, Friedman PA, Mulpuru SK et al. Atypical complications encountered with epicardial electrophysiological procedures. *Heart Rhythm.* 2013;10:1613–1621.

41. Bradfield J, Woodbury B, Traina M et al. Repolarization parameters are associated with mortality in chagas disease patients in the United States. *Indian J Pacing Electrophysiol.* 2014;14(4):171–180.

ECG-BASED ORIGIN OF ATRIAL FLUTTER

Decebal Gabriel Laţcu, Nadir Saoudi,
and Francis E. Marchlinski

CONTENTS

INTRODUCTION

For many years, the classification of regular tachycardia at the atrial level has been based exclusively on the ECG. As a historical legacy, the term "flutter" was reserved only for fast rhythms (generally >240 bpm) without an isoelectric line between two atrial deflections. The basis for the current definition[1,2] of atrial tachycardia (AT; including flutter) is the wavefront propagation. Despite the classification, some confusion arose over the recent years as the term "flutter" has often been associated only with macro-re-entrant AT, but not for focal AT, for which atrial activation starts at a small area and spreads centrifugally; in many cases, such AT may also present a flutter-like appearance on the 12-lead ECG.

The expert consensus agreement of 2001 proposed that macro-re-entrant AT may be classified into two categories: "typical (isthmus-dependent) atrial flutter (AFL)" and lesion or disease-dependent macro-re-entrant AFL (or "atypical AFL") (Figure 32.1).

Typical AFL is macro-re-entry around a central obstacle composed of the orifices of the inferior and superior vena cava, posteriorly by the crista terminalis or the sinus venosus and the Eustachian ridge and limited anteriorly by the tricuspid valve. The direction of the propagation around the tricuspid valve yields its two widely known forms: counterclockwise (CCW) and clockwise (CW; or reverse typical).

Atypical AFL is a descriptive term for an AT with an ECG pattern of continuous undulation of the atrial activity, different from typical or reverse typical flutter. Most often, this is an iatrogenic, lesion macro-re-entrant AT, with two types: atriotomy (or incisional) AT and left atrial (LA) macro-re-entrant AT post-LA ablation.

The incidence of these arrhythmias, especially of atypical AFL, has grown with the widespread deployment of atrial fibrillation (AF) ablation. The 12-lead ECG characteristics of all these forms have been the subject of recent review publications[3–5] and will be addressed in this chapter.

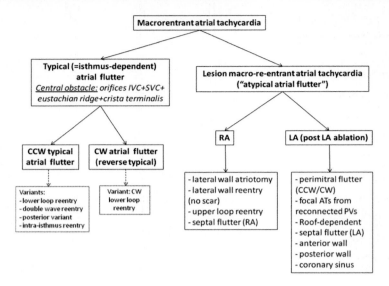

Figure 32.1 Classification of atrial tachycardia, based on wavefront propagation.

DISTINGUISHING RIGHT-SIDED VERSUS LEFT-SIDED FLUTTERS FROM THE ECG

The best lead to distinguish right from left AFL is V_1, especially its initial component. When V_1 has an initial isoelectric (or negative) component (possibly followed by an upright component), this is suggestive of a right AFL. A broad-based upright V_1 is highly predictive of a LA flutter. Conversely, when V_1 is deeply inverted, this is highly suggestive of a right atrium (RA) flutter. However, when V_1 is biphasic or isoelectric (with a terminal positivity), it is not possible to distinguish the chamber of origin based on this criterion alone.[5]

TYPICAL CCW AFL

Typical CCW ECG flutter wave has a well-known "sawtooth" pattern (Figure 32.2a), classically described as a negative deflection in the inferior leads followed by a low-amplitude positive notch preceding a slightly descending plateau. The descending impulse (activation of lateral wall, Figure 32.2c) has shown to be coincident with the nadir of the flutter wave, preceding its ascending part and the plateau.[6,7] Plateau duration in lead III strongly correlates with isthmus conduction time.[8] Moreover, extra isthmus conduction time can be measured on the surface ECG from the beginning of the negative deflection of the flutter wave in lead III to the end of the positive deflection (or beginning of the plateau, Figure 32.2b).[9] Finally, the sharp negative deflection correlates with the wavefront's penetration of the septum.[10]

In the precordial leads, V_1 shows an initial isoelectric component followed by a positive component which falls always later than the negative component of the inferior leads (but biphasic deflections can be seen in some cases). Across the precordium, the initial component rapidly becomes inverted and the second component isoelectric. This produces an "overall impression of an upright flutter wave in V_1 which becomes inverted by V_6"[5] (typically as early as V_3 or V_4). Lead I is low amplitude positive or isoelectric and aVL is usually positive.

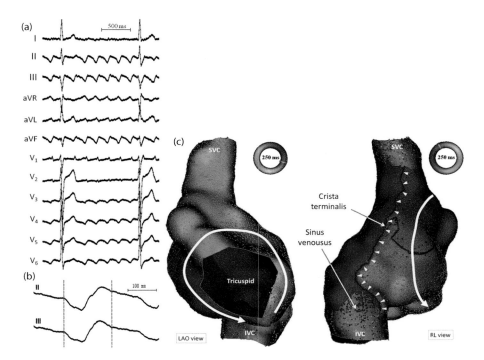

Figure 32.2 Typical CCW flutter. (a) Typical CCW flutter 12-lead ECG pattern. (b) Magnified inferior leads of the typical CCW flutter wave; vertical lines are delineating the beginning of the negative deflection of the P-wave in lead III and the end of the positive deflection (or beginning of the plateau). (c) Ultra-high density mapping (Rhythmia, Boston Scientific) of right atrial (RA) activation during typical CCW flutter. White arrows delineate the crista terminalis location representing a region of functional block (dashed black line) with both SVC and IVC representing the central obstacles for the circuit (see also text). LAO: left anterior oblique; RL: right lateral.

This classic appearance may show morphologic variations, especially in regards to the presence and the amplitude of the terminal positive deflection in the inferior leads. A classification into three subtypes of ECG patterns for CCW cavo-tricuspid isthmus (CTI) dependent flutters was proposed.[11] A terminal positive component of the F-wave in typical CCW flutter seems to identify a patient population with a relatively high likelihood of heart disease, higher incidence of atrial fibrillation (AF) and LA enlargement. It should be stressed that severe atrial disease/ conduction disturbances but also previous AF ablation[12] may yield unusual ECG patterns and the typical circuit may then be difficult to diagnose. Even atypical (e.g., LA flutters, especially in the presence of a pre-existing CTI block[1]) circuits may mimic typical CCW flutter.

VARIANTS OF TYPICAL CCW AFL

CCW LOWER LOOP RE-ENTRY

At times, typical AFL may become irregular and/or accelerates and this led Cheng in 1999[13] to describe a variant of typical flutter: lower loop re-entry (LLR). The circuit is localized in the lower RA, but is also CTI-dependent, has an early breakthrough in the lower anterior RA (due to transversal conduction/shunt through the crista terminalis) and a wavefront collision in the high lateral RA or septum. Alternating LLR (of variable breakthrough sites in the lateral RA) and typical AFL may result in cycle length oscillations. Of note, LA and septum are activated in a similar sequence to CCW typical AFL, producing negative flutter waves in the inferior leads. The morphology of the flutter wave is determined by the site of the breakthrough of the wavefront at the crista terminalis. If the breakthrough occurs at the low lateral RA, the resulting ascending wavefront will collide with the CCW wavefront propagating from the interatrial septum and RA roof, thus abolishing the late descending wavefront seen in typical CCW AFL on the lateral RA wall (the late positive deflection seen on the flutter wave in the inferior leads during CCW typical AFL will be attenuated).[14] A higher breakthrough has been reported as a "posterior variant"[15] of the typical CCW AFL, producing minor changes of the ECG flutter wave (lack of terminal positive deflection in inferior leads in 4/12 instances, and biphasic $\pm$ pattern in V_1 in 5/12 cases).

DOUBLE WAVE RE-ENTRY

Another type of acceleration of typical flutter (with the same ECG morphology) has been reported.[16] This is caused by two successive activation wavefronts circulating in the same direction along the same re-entrant circuit (double-wave re-entry) and was induced by pacing with antidromic block. All of the double-wave re-entry episodes in the initial report were transient. The clinical significance of this rarely observed phenomenon is unknown, but probably limited.

POSTERIOR CTI (POSTERO-EUSTACHIAN) BREAKTHROUGH TO THE SEPTUM

In many cases, the Eustachian valve and ridge form a line of conduction block between the inferior vena cava (IVC) and the coronary sinus (CS) ostium.[17] Conduction through the Eustachian ridge allowing short-circuiting of the CCW circuit posterior to the CS ostium with early activation of the septum has been reported.[14] In this case, a collision at the CTI (anterior to the Eustachian valve) of both the orthodromic CCW wavefront and another front emerging from the CS ostial region may occur. This variant has also been observed with a sudden and sustained cycle length prolongation after radiofrequency (RF) delivery in the anterior portion (sub-Eustachian) of the CTI due to anterior-to-posterior shifting of the septal exit.[18] Concomitant ECG changes of the flutter wave were reported, characterized by a narrower and shallow negative wave in the inferior limb leads, probably due to conduction delay across the isthmus area, resulting in overlap of septal and anterior wall activation.

INTRA-ISTHMUS RE-ENTRY

Intra-isthmus re-entry is a re-entrant tachycardia with a typical CCW ECG pattern in most patients[19] occurring especially in patients with a previous CTI ablation. The circuit seems confined within the CTI itself, and bounded by the medial CTI and the CS ostium. If the term typical is to be applied to re-entrant circuits that are strictly dependent on the CTI, then this is not really the case in the Yang's series of intra-isthmus re-entry, as part of the CTI is frequently out of the circuit and such a flutter can even occur in case of proven complete bidirectional CTI block.[20] Entrainment mapping and recording of fractionated potentials within the CTI (spanning over 34%–71% of the tachycardia cycle length) can facilitate the diagnosis of this unusual variant (Figure 32.3).[21]

TYPICAL CLOCKWISE (REVERSE) AFL

About 10%–30% of typical AFLs have a re-entrant circuit and the anatomical/functional constraints identical within the RA, but rotate in a CW direction around the tricuspid valve from a left anterior oblique perspective[7] (Figure 32.4b). CW AFL may be induced in the EP laboratory; a high percentage of these AFLs occur after ablation of CCW typical flutter.[22]

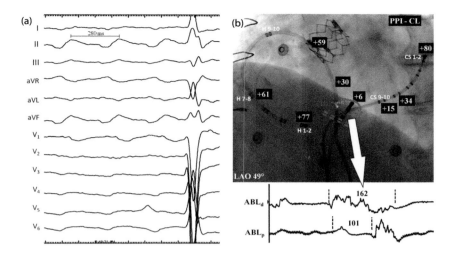

Figure 32.3 Intra-isthmus re-entry. (a) ECG pattern suggesting typical CCW flutter in a patient with previous CTI ablation. (b) Differences between postpacing interval (PPI) and the flutter cycle length (CL) at all the pacing sites are indicated. The maximal duration bipolar electrogram at the septal aspect of the CTI spanned over 58% of the CL (lower panel and large arrow). Based on PPI-CL differences only the septal CTI and possibly the proximal CS were part of the circuit (intra-isthmus re-entry).

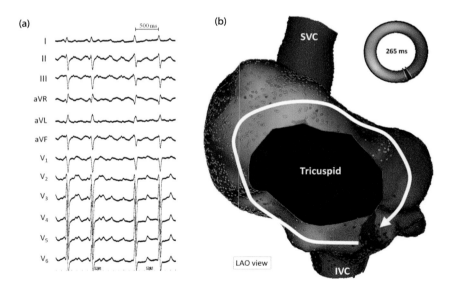

Figure 32.4 Typical CW flutter. (a) Typical CW flutter 12-lead ECG pattern (see text). (b) Ultra-high density mapping (rhythmia) of right atrial (RA) activation during typical CW flutter. LAO: left anterior oblique.

ECG-Based Origin of Atrial Flutter **419**

In the initial series,[7] the classic "sawtooth" pattern was observed in 14 of 18 CW flutters. Although frequently referred to as "positive flutter wave in the inferior leads," in many cases, the appearance can be of continuous undulation without an obviously predominant upright or inverted component. A shorter plateau phase, a widening of the negative component of the F-wave (both possibly suggesting an inconstant impression of positivity), and a negative and frequently bifid F-wave in V_1, are its most consistent findings. In case of CW rotation of the typical flutter, the plateau phase does not correspond solely to the impulse traversing the CTI (end of the plateau in typical CW flutter corresponds to impulse propagation upward in the anterolateral wall).[7] A positive F-wave in V 6 follows in timing the negative deflection in V_1. Lead I is usually upright and aVL is of low amplitude negative and notched (Figure 32.4a).

VARIANT OF TYPICAL CW AFL–CW LOWER LOOP RE-ENTRY

In one study[23] of 12 patients with "positive" flutter waves in the inferior ECG leads suggesting CW typical AFL, it was found with entrainment pacing that the re-entrant circuit involved the lower RA around the IVC in 7 patients; nevertheless, the authors did not report any ECG specificity for this variant.

ATYPICAL RA AFL

RA FREE WALL ATYPICAL AFL

The most common form of atypical RA flutter is macro-re-entry in the RA free wall. The central area of block is a surgical or a spontaneous scar in the posterolateral RA wall.[14,24]

IATROGENIC SCAR-RELATED RA AFL

Atriotomy scar, a septal prosthetic patch, a suture line, or a line of fixed block secondary to prior RF catheter ablation may represent (as standalone or combined with anatomic structures located in the vicinity of the scar—i.e., SVC, IVC) the central obstacle of the macro-re-entrant circuit.

The ECG aspect of scar-related RA AFL is highly variable; it depends on the anatomic location, the direction of the rotation, the coexisting conduction disturbances in the atrium, the existence of a simultaneous peritricuspid circuit or a pre-existing CTI block, as well as the presence of antiarrhythmic drugs. Depending on the predominant direction of septal activation, RA free wall flutter can mimic either CW or CCW flutter morphology. A negative F-wave in lead V_1 will almost certainly identify the RA origin of the arrhythmia (Figure 32.5).

The best characterized atriotomy macro-re-entrant AT is due to activation around a surgical incision scar in the lateral RA wall, with the incision having a superoinferior axis. Low-voltage electrograms characteristic of areas of scar can be observed during both sinus rhythm and AFL. A line of double potentials is recorded in the lateral RA, extending vertically (superoinferior), corresponding to the atriotomy scar. They are widely split in the middle of the incision scar and tend to be narrow as the catheter approaches the scar end only to fuse at its superior and inferior ends. A linear RF lesion extending from the inferior portion of the scar (where double potentials fuse) to the IVC will disrupt the circuit and eliminate the tachycardia (Figure 32.5).

Typical AFL can be associated with RA atriotomy tachycardia sequentially or simultaneously (dual loop re-entry). A small series[25] reported only postatrial septal defect surgical closure patients. Ablation of one circuit will unmask the other. Ablation of both circuits is necessary for clinical control of recurrent atrial arrhythmias.

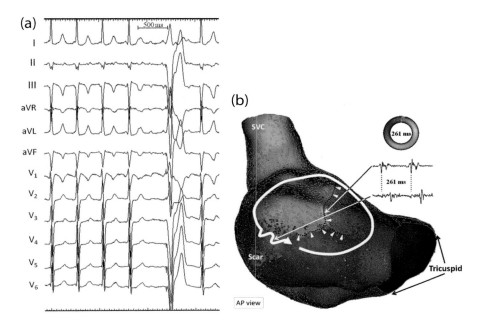

Figure 32.5 (a) Atypical (incisional) RA free wall AFL in a patient with previous mitral valve repair and RA incision (negative flutter wave in V₁). (b) Ultra-high density mapping (Rhythmia) of RA showing the CCW macro-re-entry in the RA free wall around a central obstacle represented by the surgical incision (line of double potentials and block—black dashed line). AP: anterior view.

SPONTANEOUS RA FREE WALL AFL

Kall and colleagues reported on a six-patient series of non CTI-dependent AFLs presenting with a typical AFL ECG pattern.[24] Most had structural heart disease with biatrial dilation, some had prior cardiac surgery but none had previous RA atriotomy (except one for whom the atriotomy scar was not involved in the circuit). The surface ECG was judged identical to that of typical CCW flutter (negative in the inferior leads in all). Nevertheless, in two patients, the authors described spontaneous polarity inversion in the inferior leads during ongoing flutter. An example is shown in Figure 32.6, where a large lateral RA circuit was observed and the participation of the crista terminalis was excluded. Ablation was successful after creation of a line between the inferior part of the circuit and the IVC.

UPPER LOOP RE-ENTRY

Upper loop re-entry (ULR) tachycardia is a non CTI-dependent re-entrant circuit involving the upper portion of the RA. Its circuit has been incompletely characterized. The superior vena cava and the upper crista terminalis serve as the zone of functional block.[26] The rotation can be CW or CCW but always crosses the upper portion of the crista terminalis where ablation is successful in eliminating the circuit.[27] This circuit will typically have a shorter cycle length, but frequently presents with flutter wave morphologies similar to CW typical AFL in the inferior leads (positive), as in the majority of cases, activation of the septum and LA occurs with inferiorly directed forces. An ECG algorithm for differentiating ULR from CW AFL was proposed[28]: negative, isoelectric (flat) or extremely low positive amplitude (<0.07 mV) wave in lead I was suggestive of ULR (regardless of the rotation), whereas CW flutter wave was constantly positive in lead I. However, definitive diagnosis of ULR requires detailed intra-cardiac mapping.

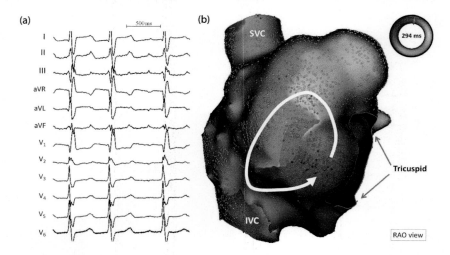

Figure 32.6 (a) RA free wall AFL in a patient with previous CTI ablation but with spontaneous free wall scar; note the negative p-wave in V1 suggesting the region of interest for detailed mapping. (b) Ultra-high density mapping (rhythmia) of RA showing the CCW macro-re-entry in the RA free wall around a scar area. RAO: right anterior oblique.

OTHER ATYPICAL RA AFL

Several other atypical right AFL circuits have been described. Although uncommon, septal flutters after prior surgery involving this area have been reported.[14] They are usually characterized by a biphasic or isoelectric flutter morphology in V_1, but no ECG pathognomonic pattern exists, and definitive diagnosis is solely based on intracardiac activation and entrainment mapping.

ATYPICAL LA AFL

A vast majority of these AFL occur in patients with previous AF radiofrequency catheter ablation. They are less frequent after surgery (incisional LA flutters[29]) or in native[30] (but diseased and "spontaneously" scarred) LA.

With the increasing number of AF ablation procedures, the incidence of atypical LA AFL is constantly increasing and it has become a frequent, yet difficult to treat, arrhythmia. Many various circuits[31-34] (with macro-re-entrant, micro-re-entrant, or focal propagation types) may occur in the LA, highly dependent of the previously created LA lesions[35]; the ECG of LA flutter is particularly difficult to characterize, as it may be similar for various circuit locations. Significant modification of intra and inter-atrial propagation after circumferential pulmonary vein (PV) isolation (and even more after more extensive lesions), is almost always accompanied by a flutter wave distortion and may also distort sinus P-wave, making ECG interpretation more difficult and occasionally inaccurate.[36]

In order to describe ECG characteristics of atypical LA AFL, when surface F waves are continuous without a clear isoelectric interval, it has been proposed[31] to determine the polarity in each lead of the 12-lead ECG by examining the F-wave polarity during the 80 ms before the tallest peak positive deflection in lead V_1 (see Figures 32.7–32.10). Most frequent postablation LA flutters are perimitral, roof-dependent (around ipsilateral PV), and PV-dependent AT (focal or micro-re-entry). Only three types have been relatively well characterized for their ECG aspect: perimitral/roof-dependent macro-re-entries and focal ATs from reconnected PVs.

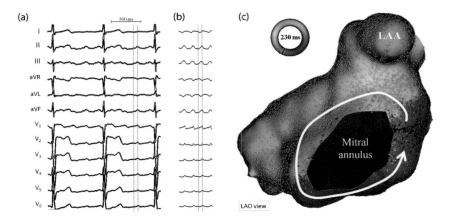

Figure 32.7 Counterclockwise mitral annular flutter. (a and b) Surface ECG examples of CCW PM AFL. The red-dotted lines encompass the 80 ms before the peak of the P-wave in V_1; note the inferiorly directed P-wave axis (see text). (c) Ultra-high density mapping (Rhythmia) of the LA showing the CCW macro-re-entry in the LA around the mitral annulus. LAO: left anterior oblique; LAA: left atrial appendage.

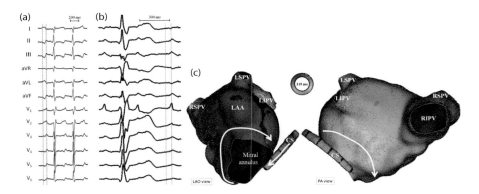

Figure 32.8 Clockwise mitral annular flutter. (a and b) Surface ECG examples of CW PM AFL; note the initial superiorly directed P-wave morphology (see text for details). The red dotted lines encompass the 80 ms before the peak of the F wave in V_1. (c) Ultra-high density mapping (Rhythmia) of the LA showing the CW macro-re-entry in the LA around the mitral annulus. LAO: left anterior oblique; PA: posterior view; LAA: left atrial appendage; CS: coronary sinus; LS: left superior, LI: left inferior; RS: right superior; RI: right inferior; PV: pulmonary vein.

PERIMITRAL FLUTTER

The perimitral flutter (PMF), probably the most frequent flutter post AF ablation[33,37] is a macro-re-entrant circuit rotating around the MA; sometimes, scars in the LA wall may alter the circuit, by partially deviating it from the MA (in case of scar/lines of block adjacent to the MA) or creating the substrate for a second circuit (double loop re-entries). In a similar way to typical (RA, CTI-dependent) flutter, PMF circuit may propagate in CCW or CW directions (both seem to be equally frequent[37]).

ECG characteristics of PMF have been described.[31] CCW MA flutter (Figure 32.7) is positive in the inferior and precordial leads (with a "pattern break"—negative component

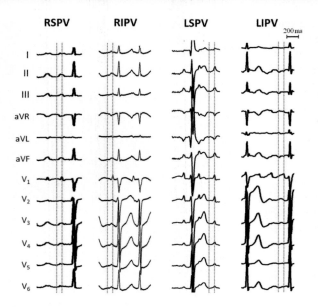

Figure 32.9 Twelve-lead ECGs from patients with focal ATs originating from the right superior pulmonary vein (RSPV), right inferior (RI) PV, left superior (LS) PV, and the left inferior (LI) PV. The red dotted lines encompass the 80 ms before the peak of the F wave in V_1.

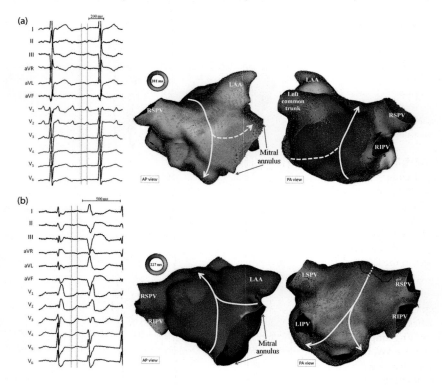

Figure 32.10 ECG and ultra-high density mapping (rhythmia) of the LA showing the roof-dependent macro-re-entry in the LA. (a) The circuit is descendent on the anterior wall (AW) and ascendant on the posterior wall (PW). (b) The circuit is ascendant on the AW and descendant on the PW.

in V_2) and had a significant negative component in leads I and aVL. The ECG characteristics are similar to those of left PV AT or left appendage AT (in case of CCW PMF) except for the unique pattern break in V_2 suggesting earliest activation of the P-wave being generated by activation medial to the left atrial appendage just under V_2). A negative component in lead I, when present, also helps in differentiating CCW PMF (negative in I) from left PV ATs (isoelectric). The CS activation sequence when coupled with the ECG information also helps to distinguish between these entities: a proximal to distal CS activation indicates CCW MA flutter whereas distal to proximal activation would be seen with left PV ATs.

CW MA flutter (Figure 32.8) demonstrated the converse limb lead morphology with a significant negative F-wave in the inferior leads and positive F-wave in leads I and aVL. Precordial leads are positive in V_1 and V_2 then have an initial negative component in V_3–V_6. The pattern is somewhat similar to typical CCW AFL. A positive F wave in lead I was best at differentiating CW PMF (positive) from CCW RA FL (isoelectric to slightly negative). CS activation sequence also helps to distinguish between these entities with a distal to proximal CS activation differentiates CW MA flutter from CCW typical (RA) flutter.[31,38]

FOCAL ATs FROM RECONNECTED PVs

ATs after AF ablation can be due to re-entry of variable size using gaps in the line surrounding the PV or to focal PV discharges. PV-related ATs can sometimes manifest with a flutter ECG aspect in case of associated slow intra-atrial propagation resulting from the previous atrial ablation.

Focal left ATs have similar features to those initially described for premature beats originating from the PV.[39] A small isoelectric baseline between P-waves is present in all 12 leads in a majority of cases (Figure 32.9). Other common ECG features are positivity throughout the precordium and inferior axis (although inferior PV ATs may have an initial negative component or could be completely negative when originating from the bottom of an inferior PV [Figure 32.9]). Left PV AT have wider p-waves, are usually flat or biphasic in lead I and negative in aVL; typically they are bifid in V_1 (but possibly in the other precordial leads) as well as in the inferior leads (the so-called "notch," "M shape," or "double hump").[40] Right PV ATs are characterized by a late peaking positive P-wave in V_1 (after an initial possibly negative component) and remain positive throughout the precordial leads; lead I has a significant positive component, and lead aVL is flat or biphasic.[31,34]

ROOF-DEPENDENT AFL

Most frequently, roof-dependent AFL occurs in patient with a previous "roof line."[41] Gaps across the roof represent isthmuses of slow conduction for flutters turning around the ipsilateral PV pairs.[32] These circuits (Figure 32.10) may travel across the roof in a postero-anterior direction (the wavefront being ascendant on the posterior wall [PW] and descendant on the anterior wall [AW]) or in an antero-posterior direction (in this case, the wavefront is ascendant on the AW and descendent on the PW). Lateralized gaps in the roof or conduction disturbances in the LA may direct the wavefront around one PV pair or another.

The surface ECG characteristics of roof-dependent AFL have been recently published.[42] Previously, the CS activation pattern and timing have been integrated into an algorithm of diagnosis of post-LA ablation AT.[38] In our experience,[42] both forms share common characteristics in the precordial leads: positive high amplitude waves in V_1 and V_2 with a rapidly decreasing amplitude afterward (often isoelectric in V_3–V_6). When the impulse is descending on the AW, the flutter pattern has an inferiorly directed axis (small positive waves in the inferior leads) with late negativity in lateral leads (I, aVL). The opposite is often seen in roof-dependent AFL when the wavefront is ascending on the AW: superior axis (negative waves in the inferior leads) with a possible late positivity in lateral leads (I, aVL). Nevertheless, LA scarring and dual loop re-entries (one roof-dependent and another LA loop, often perimitral) may alter ECG characteristics of these flutters.

LEFT SEPTAL AFL

Spontaneous[43] or postlesion septal LA AFL may occur. The authors defined CW and CCW left septal rotation as seen from inside the LA. The flutter wave is best seen in V_1 ($\pm V_2$) (positive in case of CCW rotation and negative in case of CW rotation), whereas the limb leads and the remaining precordial leads most of the time reveal very low voltage or flat F-wave morphology.

ANTERIOR WALL AFL

Atypical AFL circuits in the LA may be located in areas not concerned by a previous ablation.[29,44,45] A series of patients with circuits confined to the AW has been reported.[45] While a majority of these patients have sinus rhythm ECG characteristics suggestive of impaired anterior LA conduction, the proposed distinctive ECG flutter wave morphology included a discrete –/+ or +/–/+ aspect in inferior leads.

OTHER LA FLUTTERS

Other circuits in the LA have been described. A re-entrant circuit involving the musculature of the CS[46] was similar to typical flutter on the surface ECG. PW circuits due to electrically silent areas in patients with heart disease have also been described[29,44] but without a systematic report of the ECG aspect. Circuits involving both atria have also been reported.[47] The recent availability of rapid, ultra-high density mapping systems with multielectrode automated annotation allows detailed visualization of the propagation. This may be extremely valuable in the context of limited reliability of entrainment techniques. The information obtained with such detail will also give us more insight in terms of the ECG patterns associated with the different atrial flutter and the alteration in these patterns associated with specific scar characterization.

After transecting the initially defined "critical" isthmus of unique flutter circuits related to prior ablation, tributaries of this primary isthmus[48] (sometimes at distance) may be used by the continuing flutter circuit (with a longer cycle length). Eventually, all components of the isthmus will require ablation to abolish that particular flutter.

CONCLUSION

Atrial flutters have characteristic ECG morphologies which should be used for an accurate diagnosis. A systematic approach is key to successful ECG-based diagnostic of the origin of atrial flutters.

The flutter wave should be analyzed on all the 12 leads, and maneuvers slowing the AV conduction (like carotid sinus massage, Valsalva maneuver, and adenosine administration) should be used in order to avoid P-wave distortion by a superimposing T-wave. Analysis of the P-wave polarity may be difficult in case of a continuous undulation without isoelectric interval. In these cases, the use of the onset and peak of the flutter wave in V_1 is a helpful reference; the preceding 80 ms should be used for polarity diagnosis in the other leads.

Atrial flutter occurs in a significant number of cases in the context of previous atrial lesions (ablation or surgery); if these pre-existing lesions are extensive, the P-wave may be altered and interpretation more difficult. ECG recordings in sinus rhythm reflect the extent of atrial scar and conduction disturbances; if a sinus P-wave still has a familiar sinus P-wave morphology in a given patient then the 12 lead during flutter will typically be helpful for atrial flutter localization. ECG-based diagnosis and pre-procedural preparation should also include detailed knowledge of previous atrial lesions. Since "critical isthmuses" depend on local slowing of the conduction velocity, specific lesions "predispose" to certain AT. Limited scar after PV isolation alone may give rise to subsequent PV tachycardia

P/F wave morphology for AT/AFl after AF ablation

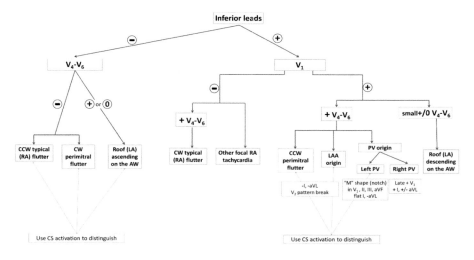

Figure 32.11 Algorithm based on P/F-wave morphology for distinguishing AT/AFL after AF ablation.

(but CTI-dependent flutter may also occur); on the contrary, a previous mitral line pre-disposes to PMF. Diagnostic accuracy of the 12-lead ECG during the atrial flutter may be enhanced by assessing CS activation.

The common ECG patterns may be integrated into an algorithm to diagnose the origin of atrial flutter on the surface ECG (Figure 32.11).

LIST OF ABBREVIATIONS

AF	atrial fibrillation
AFL	atrial flutter
AT	atrial tachycardia
AW	anterior wall
CCW	counterclockwise
CS	coronary sinus
CTI	cavo-tricuspid isthmus
CW	clockwise
ECG	electrocardiogram
IVC	inferior vena cava
LA	left atrium
LLR	lower loop re-entry
PMF	perimitral flutter
PV	pulmonary vein
PW	posterior wall
RA	right atrium
RF	radiofrequency
SVC	superior vena cava
ULR	upper loop re-entry

1. Saoudi N, Cosio F, Waldo A, et al. Classification of atrial flutter and regular atrial tachycardia according to electrophysiologic mechanism and anatomic bases: A statement from a joint expert group from the working group of arrhythmias of the European Society of Cardiology and the North American Society of Pacing and Electrophysiology. *J Cardiovasc Electrophysiol.* 2001;12:852–866.

2. Garcia-Cosio F, Pastor Fuentes A, Nunez Angulo A. Arrhythmias (iv). Clinical approach to atrial tachycardia and atrial flutter from an understanding of the mechanisms: Electrophysiology based on anatomy. *Rev Esp Cardiol (English ed.).* 2012;65:363–375.

3. Bun SS, Latcu DG, Marchlinski F, Saoudi N. Atrial flutter: More than just one of a kind. *Eur Heart J.* 2015;36:2356–2363.

4. Teh AW, Kistler PM, Kalman JM. Using the 12-lead ecg to localize the origin of ventricular and atrial tachycardias: Part 1. Focal atrial tachycardia. *J Cardiovasc Electrophysiol.* 2009;20:706–709; quiz 705.

5. Medi C, Kalman JM. Prediction of the atrial flutter circuit location from the surface electrocardiogram. *Europace.* 2008;10:786–796.

6. Puech P, Latour H, Grolleau R. Le flutter et ses limites. *Arch Mal Coeur Vaiss.* 1970;63(1):116–144.

7. Saoudi N, Nair M, Abdelazziz A, et al. Electrocardiographic patterns and results of radiofrequency catheter ablation of clockwise type I atrial flutter. *J Cardiovasc Electrophysiol.* 1996;7:931–942.

8. Ndrepepa G, Zrenner B, Deisenhofer I, et al. Relationship between surface electrocardiogram characteristics and endocardial activation sequence in patients with typical atrial flutter. *Zeitschrift fur Kardiologie.* 2000;89:527–537.

9. Latcu DG, Bun SS, Arnoult M, et al. New insights into typical atrial flutter ablation: Extra-isthmus activation time on the flutter wave is predictive of extra-isthmus conduction time after isthmus block. *J Interv Card Electrophysiol.* 2013;36:19–25; discussion 25.

10. Bernstein NE, Sandler DA, Goh M, et al. Why a sawtooth? Inferences on the generation of the flutter wave during typical atrial flutter drawn from radiofrequency ablation. *Ann Noninvasive Electrocardiol.* 2004;9:358–361.

11. Milliez P, Richardson AW, Obioha-Ngwu O, et al. Variable electrocardiographic characteristics of isthmus-dependent atrial flutter. *J Am Coll Cardiol.* 2002;40:1125–1132.

12. Chugh A, Latchamsetty R, Oral H, et al. Characteristics of cavotricuspid isthmus-dependent atrial flutter after left atrial ablation of atrial fibrillation. *Circulation.* 2006;113:609–615.

13. Cheng J, Cabeen WR, Jr., Scheinman MM. Right atrial flutter due to lower loop reentry: Mechanism and anatomic substrates. *Circulation.* 1999;99:1700–1705.

14. Yang Y, Cheng J, Bochoeyer A, et al. Atypical right atrial flutter patterns. *Circulation.* 2001;103:3092–3098.

15. Maury P, Duparc A, Hebrard A, et al. Prevalence of typical atrial flutter with reentry circuit posterior to the superior vena cava: Use of entrainment at the atrial roof. *Europace.* 2008;10:190–196.

16. Cheng J, Scheinman MM. Acceleration of typical atrial flutter due to double-wave reentry induced by programmed electrical stimulation. *Circulation.* 1998;97:1589–1596.

17. Nakagawa H, Lazzara R, Khastgir T, et al. Role of the tricuspid annulus and the eustachian valve/ridge on atrial flutter: Relevance to catheter ablation of the septal isthmus and a new technique for rapid identification of ablation success. *Circulation.* 1996;94:407–424.

18. Iesaka Y, Yamane T, Goya M, et al. A jump in cycle length of orthodromic common atrial flutter during catheter ablation at the isthmus between the inferior vena cava and tricuspid annulus; evidence of dual isthmus conduction directed to dual septal exits. *Europace.* 2000;2:163–171.

19. Yang Y, Varma N, Badhwar N, et al. Prospective observations in the clinical and electrophysiological characteristics of intra-isthmus reentry. *J Cardiovasc Electrophysiol.* 2010;21:1099–1106.

20. Saoudi N, Latcu DG. Intra-isthmus reentry: Another form of typical atrial flutter? *J Cardiovasc Electrophysiol.* 2010;21:1107–1108.

21. Latcu DG, Bun SS, Saoudi N. Intra-isthmus reentry: Diagnosis at-a-glance. *Europace.* 2013;15:414–419.

22. Bun SS, Latcu DG, Prevot S, et al. Characteristics of recurrent clockwise atrial flutter after previous radiofrequency catheter ablation for counterclockwise isthmus-dependent atrial flutter. *Europace.* 2012;14:1340–1343.

23. Zhang S, Younis G, Hariharan R, et al. Lower loop reentry as a mechanism of clockwise right atrial flutter. *Circulation.* 2004;109:1630–1635.

24. Kall JG, Rubenstein DS, Kopp DE, et al. Atypical atrial flutter originating in the right atrial free wall. *Circulation.* 2000;101:270–279.

25. Shah D, Jais P, Takahashi A, et al. Dual-loop intra-atrial reentry in humans. *Circulation.* 2000;101:631–639.

26. Tai CT, Liu TY, Lee PC, et al. Non-contact mapping to guide radiofrequency ablation of atypical right atrial flutter. *J Am Coll Cardiol.* 2004;44:1080–1086.

27. Tai CT, Huang JL, Lin YK, et al. Noncontact three-dimensional mapping and ablation of upper loop re-entry originating in the right atrium. *J Am Coll Cardiol.* 2002;40:746–753.

28. Yuniadi Y, Tai CT, Lee KT, et al. A new electrocardiographic algorithm to differentiate upper loop re-entry from reverse typical atrial flutter. *J Am Coll Cardiol.* 2005;46:524–528.

29. Ouyang F, Ernst S, Vogtmann T, et al. Characterization of reentrant circuits in left atrial macroreentrant tachycardia: Critical isthmus block can prevent atrial tachycardia recurrence. *Circulation.* 2002;105:1934–1942.

30. Fukamizu S, Sakurada H, Hayashi T, et al. Macroreentrant atrial tachycardia in patients without previous atrial surgery or catheter ablation: Clinical and electrophysiological characteristics of scar-related left atrial anterior wall reentry. *J Cardiovasc Electrophysiol.* 2013;24:404–412.

31. Gerstenfeld EP, Dixit S, Bala R, et al. Surface electrocardiogram characteristics of atrial tachycardias occurring after pulmonary vein isolation. *Heart Rhythm.* 2007;4:1136–1143.

32. Chae S, Oral H, Good E, et al. Atrial tachycardia after circumferential pulmonary vein ablation of atrial fibrillation: Mechanistic insights, results of catheter ablation, and risk factors for recurrence. *J Am Coll Cardiol.* 2007;50:1781–1787.

33. Jais P, Matsuo S, Knecht S, et al. A deductive mapping strategy for atrial tachycardia following atrial fibrillation ablation: Importance of localized reentry. *J Cardiovasc Electrophysiol.* 2009;20:480–491.

34. Wasmer K, Monnig G, Bittner A, et al. Incidence, characteristics, and outcome of left atrial tachycardias after circumferential antral ablation of atrial fibrillation. *Heart Rhythm*. 2012;9:1660–1666.

35. Chugh A, Oral H, Lemola K, et al. Prevalence, mechanisms, and clinical significance of macroreentrant atrial tachycardia during and following left atrial ablation for atrial fibrillation. *Heart Rhythm*. 2005;2:464–471.

36. Bun SS, Ricard P, Hugues T, et al. P-wave modifications after wide area circumferential ablation of atrial fibrillation. *Eur Heart J*. 2009;30 (Abstract Supplement):121.

37. Latcu DG, Squara F, Massaad Y, et al. Electroanatomic characteristics of the mitral isthmus associated with successful mitral isthmus ablation. *Europace*. 2015;18(2):274–280.

38. Pascale P, Shah AJ, Roten L, et al. Pattern and timing of the coronary sinus activation to guide rapid diagnosis of atrial tachycardia after atrial fibrillation ablation. *Circ Arrhythm Electrophysiol*. 2013;6:481–490.

39. Yamane T, Shah DC, Peng JT, et al. Morphological characteristics of p waves during selective pulmonary vein pacing. *J Am Coll Cardiol*. 2001;38:1505–1510.

40. Kistler PM, Sanders P, Fynn SP, et al. Electrophysiological and electrocardiographic characteristics of focal atrial tachycardia originating from the pulmonary veins: Acute and long-term outcomes of radiofrequency ablation. *Circulation*. 2003;108:1968–1975.

41. Hocini M, Jais P, Sanders P, et al. Techniques, evaluation, and consequences of linear block at the left atrial roof in paroxysmal atrial fibrillation: A prospective randomized study. *Circulation*. 2005;112:3688–3696.

42. Casado Arroyo R, Laţcu DG, Maeda S, et al. Coronary sinus activation and ECG characteristics of roof-dependent left atrial flutter after pulmonary vein isolation. *Circ Arrhythm Electrophysiol*. 2018;11(6):e005948. doi:10.1161/CIRCEP.117.005948.

43. Marrouche NF, Natale A, Wazni OM, et al. Left septal atrial flutter: Electrophysiology, anatomy, and results of ablation. *Circulation*. 2004;109:2440–2447.

44. Jais P, Shah DC, Haissaguerre M, et al. Mapping and ablation of left atrial flutters. *Circulation*. 2000;101:2928–2934.

45. Jais P, Sanders P, Hsu LF, et al. Flutter localized to the anterior left atrium after catheter ablation of atrial fibrillation. *J Cardiovasc Electrophysiol*. 2006;17:279–285.

46. Olgin JE, Jayachandran JV, Engesstein E et al. Atrial macroreentry involving the myocardium of the coronary sinus: A unique mechanism for atypical flutter. *J Cardiovasc Electrophysiol*. 1998;9:1094–1099.

47. Namdar M, Gentil-Baron P, Sunthorn H et al. Postmitral valve replacement biatrial, septal macroreentrant atrial tachycardia developing after perimitral flutter ablation. *Circ Arrhythm Electrophysiol*. 2014;7:171–174.

48. Asirvatham SJ, Stevenson WG. Editor's perspective: The isthmus of uncertainty. *Circ Arrhythm Electrophysiol*. 2014;7:175–177.

INDEX

Note: Page numbers in italic and bold refer to figures and tables, respectively.